Atlas of Adult
Electroencephalography

Second Edition

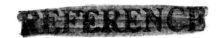

Atlas of Adult Electroencephalography

Second Edition

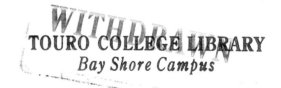

Warren T. Blume, M.D., F.R.C.P.C.
Masako Kaibara, R.E.T.
G. Bryan Young, M.D., F.R.C.P.C.
London Health Sciences Centre
University Hospital, EEG Department
The University of Western Ontario
London, Ontario, Canada

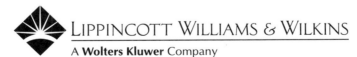
LIPPINCOTT WILLIAMS & WILKINS
A **Wolters Kluwer** Company
Philadelphia · Baltimore · New York · London
Buenos Aires · Hong Kong · Sydney · Tokyo

Acquisitions Editor: Anne M. Sydor
Developmental Editor: Pamela Sutton
Production Editor: Robin E. Cook
Manufacturing Manager: Colin Warnock
Cover Designer: Mark Lerner
Compositor: Maryland Composition
Printer: Edwards Brothers

MT

Library of Congress Cataloging-in-Publication Data

Blume, Warren T. (Warren Thomas)
   Atlas of adult electroencephalography/Warren T. Blume, Masako Kaibara, G. Bryan Young.—2nd ed.
       p.; cm.
   Companion v. to: Current practice of clinical EEG/edited by J. Ebersole and T.A. Pedley and Atlas of paediatric electroencephalography.
   Includes bibliographical references and index.
   ISBN 0-7817-2996-3
   1. Electroencephalography—Atlases. I. Kaibara, Masako. II. Young, G. Bryan (Gordon Bryan) III. Current practice of clinical EEG. IV. Atlas of paediatric electroencephalography. V. Title.
   [DNLM: 1. Electroencephalography—Atlases. WL 17 B658a 2001]
   RC386.6.E43 C87 2001
   616.8′047547—dc21   2001029914

   Care has been taken to confirm the accuracy of the information presented and to describe generally accepted practices. However, the authors, editors, and publisher are not responsible for errors or omissions or for any consequences from application of the information in this book and make no warranty, expressed or implied, with respect to the currency, completeness, or accuracy of the contents of the publication. Application of this information in a particular situation remains the professional responsibility of the practitioner.
   The authors, editors, and publisher have exerted every effort to ensure that drug selection and dosage set forth in this text are in accordance with current recommendations and practice at the time of publication. However, in view of ongoing research, changes in government regulations, and the constant flow of information relating to drug therapy and drug reactions, the reader is urged to check the package insert for each drug for any change in indications and dosage and for added warnings and precautions. This is particularly important when the recommended agent is a new or infrequently employed drug.
   Some drugs and medical devices presented in this publication have Food and Drug Administration (FDA) clearance for limited use in restricted research settings. It is the responsibility of the health care provider to ascertain the FDA status of each drug or device planned for use in their clinical practice.

10 9 8 7 6 5 4 3 2 1

5-20-03

To our spouses, Lydia, Imao, and Christie, and to our children, Christine, Sonia, Valerie, Kaede, Naomi, Taro, Stewart, Andrew, and Megan.

Contents

Foreword to the First Edition .... *ix*

Foreword to the Second Edition .... *xi*

Preface to First Edition .... *xiii*

Preface to the Second Edition .... *xv*

Acknowledgements .... *xvii*

1. Introduction *1*

2. Artifacts *7*

3. Normal Phenomena *41*

4. Focal Epileptiform Phenomena *173*

5. Generalized Epileptiform Phenomena *233*

6. Epileptiform Abnormalities: Seizures *283*

7. Nonepileptiform Abnormalities *353*

8. EEG in the Intensive Care Unit (ICU) *469*

9. Digital Electroencephalography *501*

References *533*

Subject Index *535*

Foreword to the First Edition

Atlas of Adult Electroencephalography, which complements *Current Practice of Clinical Electroencephalography* (D.D. Daly and T.A. Pedley, eds.), contains selected sample EEGs of normal adult subjects compared with typical records from patients with forms of epilepsy and various non-epileptiform abnormalities, including coma.

Both David Daly and Warren Blume received postdoctoral training in the Department of Electroencephalography at the Montreal Neurological Institute. Blume then studied electroencephalography with Donald Klass at the Mayo Clinic. He has developed, with the aid of one of his assistants, Masako Kaibara, an outstanding department of electroencephalography at the University of Western Ontario in London, where he is professor of neurology in the Department of Clinical Neurological Sciences. He specializes in epilepsy and clinical neurophysiology.

The present atlas contains many selected EEG tracings on a 16-channel apparatus, representing a wide spectrum of normal and abnormal electroencephalograms in adult subjects and neurological patients.

Blume and Kaibara also provide succinct descriptive interpretations of each record in light of clinical problems presented by the patients in question. Their atlas will be most useful in training electroencephalographers and gives highly experienced and thoughtful interpretations of the significance of EEG records for the diagnosis of many neuropathological conditions encountered in the clinical practice of neurology and neurosurgery.

Herbert H. Jasper, O.C. F.R.S.C.
Department of Physiology
Université de Montréal
Montreal, Quebec, Canada

Foreword to the Second Edition

It gives me great pleasure to introduce the second edition of the *Atlas of Adult Electroencephalography*.

The first edition of this book was highly acclaimed. For example, in a review for the *American Journal of EEG Technology*, Dr. Charles E. Henry, the eminent pioneer of EEG, wrote that he had been collecting EEG atlases for more than 50 years and that this atlas was "clearly the best of the lot." The second edition is a condign successor.

Developing skill in the visual analysis and interpretation of EEGs requires extensive exposure to the myriad of normal patterns, abnormal patterns, and artifacts that can occur and then judging their significance under the tutelage of an expert electroencephalographer. Outstanding features of this atlas are the excellent illustrations of the many diverse variations in EEG patterns together with detailed comments and explanations for each of them. Looking at any page of this atlas gives one the feeling that one is in a live teaching session and looking over the shoulder of a master electroencephalographer. The result is an important contribution to EEG education not only for the beginner but also for the continuing education of the practitioner.

In keeping with the changes in EEG practice and the expanding range of EEG applications, this second edition of the atlas contains welcome additional chapters on digital electroencephalography and on the EEG in the intensive care unit.

In the foreword and preface to the first edition of this book, Dr. Herbert H. Jasper and the authors mentioned that it was intended to complement another book. Clearly, however, this second edition is a monument that can very well stand on its own.

Donald W. Klass, M.D.

Preface to First Edition

Confident interpretation of electroencephalograms requires full appreciation of their many patterns. As the morphology of EEG phenomena may be affected by age, state of alertness, and other simultaneously occurring wave forms, their appearance may vary within and among EEGs. This atlas presents EEG phenomena not only in their "classical" forms, but, whenever possible, in their variants as well. To solidify the image of such patterns, several examples of most phenomena are presented. By simulating EEG reading sessions, this atlas attempts to bridge the gap between textbook presentation of EEG phenomena and their appearance in clinical practise.

This work complements its companion volume, *Current Practice of Electroencephalography*, edited by D.D. Daly and T.A. Pedley, which comprehensively presents EEG theory, the usual appearance of patterns, and their clinical significance. Legends under the figures in this atlas indicate their principal instructive features and provide concise data about the phenomena illustrated. These legends link the illustrations to the text of the companion volume and other works. In some instances, where a gradation exists between normal and abnormal wave forms, examples are presented in which the identity of the wave form shares characteristics of each to illustrate that a strict demarcation line is not present in all cases. For clarity, many illustrations include only 8 or 12 channels of a 16 or 18 channel recording.

The sequence of presentation follows that of *Current Practice*. Following a brief introduction, examples of common artifacts are presented; normal phenomena follow. This sequence follows that which we advise every electroencephalographer to use when assessing an EEG: Is the wave form artifactual? Is it normal? Is it abnormal?

A conservative approach to EEG interpretation has been adopted, reflecting our belief that errors are more likely to result from an overly narrow concept of normality than the converse.

Brief descriptions of principal artifactual, normal, and abnormal phenomena precede each major chapter.

Apiculate is a term commonly used to describe any sharply contoured feature. As expected, this word appears frequently throughout this atlas.

Warren T. Blume
Masako Kaibara

Preface to the Second Edition

The *Atlas of Adult Electroencephalography,* 2nd ed. forms part of a trio of companion volumes on electroencephalography by Lippincott Williams & Wilkins: *Current Practice of Clinical EEG,* edited by J. Ebersole and T.A. Pedley and *Atlas of Pediatric Electroencephalography* by ourselves.

Warren Blume and Masako Kaibara welcome Dr. G. Bryan Young as co-author. In addition to his counsel on several aspects of the *Atlas,* he authored a new section on EEG in the intensive care unit, a burgeoning aspect of clinical electroencephalography.

We have also added a chapter illustrating advantages and pitfalls of digital EEG. This chapter will likely grow considerably in the future as this capability augments.

As before, this volume emphasizes waveform identification through location, frequency, morphology, purity of rhythmicity (from sinusoidal to arrhythmic), relationship to state, and augmenting and attenuating factors. The atlas presents several examples of the same phenomena to sharpen the reader's concept of their essential characteristics and their variability. Gradations from normal and abnormal appear. Examples distorted by competing cerebrally originating waveforms or artifacts are included to reflect clinical practice. Although all illustrations are derived from 16 or 18 channel recordings, many figures contain only relevant channels for clarity of display.

The figure legends have received considerable attention to complement each figure and to maximize the learning experience.

Warren T. Blume
Masako Kaibara
G. Bryan Young

Acknowledgements

Our laboratory has long benefitted from the fruitful interaction of many colleagues—neurologists and technologists—who share our fascination for the infinite complexity of EEG phenomena. These individuals include: Dr. Richard S. McLachlan, Dr. Samuel Wiebe, D. Kent McNeill, Daniel C. Jones, Neda Lubus, Lisa Tapsell, Giannina Holloway, Dorota Ociepa, and Martin Kelly. Paula De Monte, Cathy Johnson, and Bonnie Jamieson performed some of the earlier EEGs. John Lemieux, computer systems analyst, provided the wave form simulations and some illustrations. Karen Bailey gave secretarial expertise.

Our photographers, Steve Mesjarik, Jim Moyer, and Kathy Stuart are to be congratulated for their great competence and meticulous attention to detail.

George Moogk contributed his considerable artistic expertise.

Maria Raffa played a major role in bringing this atlas together through her diligence and high quality editorial performance.

Finally, the professionalism of Lippincott Williams & Wilkins has been appreciated.

Chapter 1

Introduction

ELECTRODE PLACEMENT

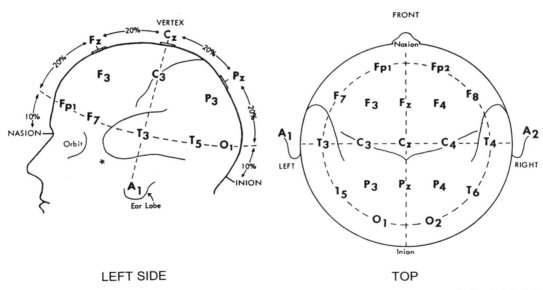

LEFT SIDE   TOP

FIG. 1–1. International 10–20 electrode placement system (1). Electrode placements indicated in this atlas conform to this system. *Mandibular notch electrode (2).

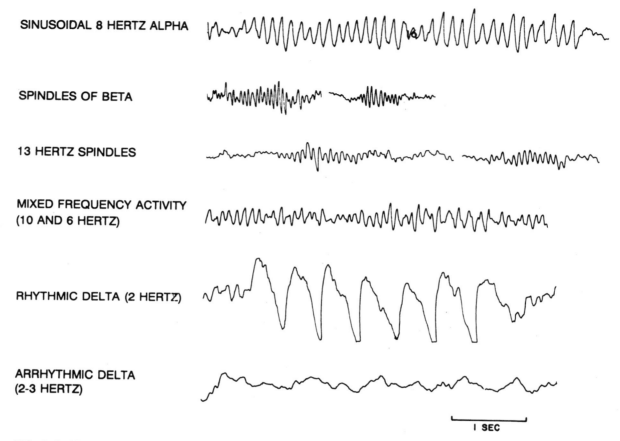

SINUSOIDAL 8 HERTZ ALPHA

SPINDLES OF BETA

13 HERTZ SPINDLES

MIXED FREQUENCY ACTIVITY
(10 AND 6 HERTZ)

RHYTHMIC DELTA (2 HERTZ)

ARRHYTHMIC DELTA
(2-3 HERTZ)

I SEC

FIG. 1–2. Various wave forms. "Classical" appearance of several types of wave forms which appear in this atlas.

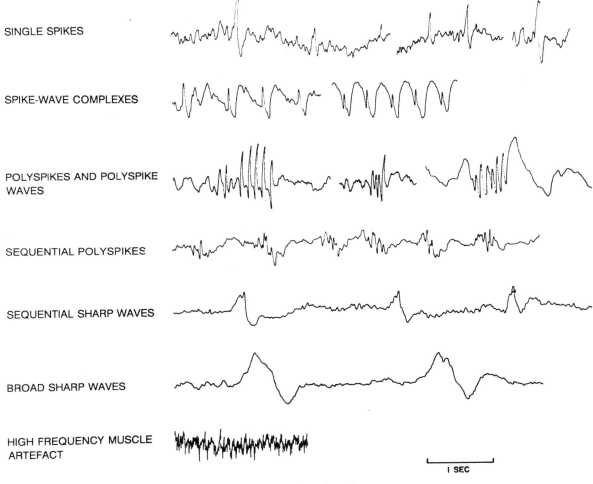

SINGLE SPIKES

SPIKE-WAVE COMPLEXES

POLYSPIKES AND POLYSPIKE
WAVES

SEQUENTIAL POLYSPIKES

SEQUENTIAL SHARP WAVES

BROAD SHARP WAVES

HIGH FREQUENCY MUSCLE
ARTEFACT

I SEC

FIG. 1–2. *(continued)*

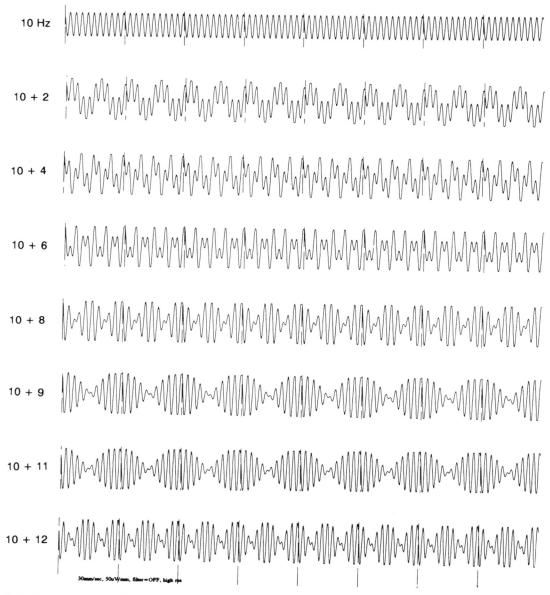

FIG. 1–3. Morphologies of superimposed sine waves of several frequencies. Sine waves of several frequencies usually appear together in clinical EEG to produce complex wave forms. This feature should be recognized in assessing such phenomena. This collage illustrates a simple 10 Hz sine wave which is then combined with those of other frequencies. The (*10 + 2*) resembles alpha activity with an underlying pulse artifact. The (*10 + 4, 10 + 6, 10 + 8*) are reminiscent of some posterior phenomena such as posterior slow of youth. The (*10 + 9, 10 + 11, 10 + 12*) mimic "alpha beating" resulting from narrowly separate alpha rhythms.

Montages: Advantages and Disadvantages

The following text lists the benefits and limitations of principal montages appearing in this atlas. While bipolar runs better localize focal or regional features, the morphology of widespread phenomena appear best on referential montages.

Longitudinal bipolar, "double banana"

- Best overall survey montage.
- Adequately lateralizes and localizes most EEG phenomena.
- If expanded to 18 channels, depicts sagittal events.
- Omits anterior-inferior temporal leads.
- Potentials with longitudinal fields may cancel.
- May not establish supra–Sylvian—infra–Sylvian relationships.

Fp1-F3	Fp1-F7
F3-C3	F7-T3
C3-P3	T3-T5
P3-O1	T5-O1
Fp2-F4	Fp2-F8
F4-C4	F8-T4
C4-P4	T4-T6
P4-O2	T6-O2

Coronal bipolar montage with sagittal leads

- Effective when laterality is established by longitudinal bipolar montage.
- Establishes supra–Sylvian—infra–Sylvian relationships.
- Confirms anterior-posterior topology.
- Records anterior-inferior temporal potentials.
- Predicts involvement of ear references (A1,2) in subsequent referential recordings.
- Appropriate initial sleep montage as it depicts V-waves, spindles.
- Detects sagittal events.
- Unless expanded beyond 16 channels, omits frontopolar, occipital leads.
- Unreliable for potentials of uncertain laterality.

F7-F3	T5-P3
F3-Fz	P3-Pz
Fz-F4	Pz-P4
F4-F8	P4-T6
T3-C3	F7-F8
C3-Cz	T3-T4
Cz-C4	M1-M2
C4-T4	T5-T6

Coronal-bipolar without sagittal leads

- Same general advantages/disadvantages as coronal montage described earlier.
- Provides better anterior-inferior temporal coverage.
- M2-M1 linkage in this manner and position for ease in visual assessment.

M1-F7	M2-M1
F7-F3	M1-T5
F3-F4	T5-P3
F4-F8	P3-P4
F8-M2	P4-T6
M1-T3	T6-M2
T3-C3	
C3-C4	
C4-T4	
T4-M2	

Coronal-bitemporal bipolar
- Use only when significant extratemporal phenomena have been excluded.
- Mandibular notch electrodes (M1,2) record anterior-mesial temporal spikes as effectively as sphenoidal leads (2).
- Coronal component better detects temporal spikes with longitudinal fields.

Cz-C3	Fp1-F7
C3-T3	F7-T3
T3-M1	T3-T5
M1-M2	T5-O1
M2-T4	Fp2-F8
T4-C4	F8-T4
C4-Cz	T4-T6
F7-F8	T6-O2

Anterior coronal bipolar
- May distinguish among frontal polar (Fp1,2), inferior frontal (F7,8), and anterior-temporal (A1,2; M1,2) involvement.
- Useful for frontal sagittal versus parasagittal field assessments.

M1-F7	M2-M1
F7-Fp1	M1-T3
Fp1-Fp2	T3-C3
Fp2-F8	C3-CZ
F8-M2	CZ-C4
F7-F3	C4-T4
F3-Fz	T4-M2
Fz-F4	
F4-F8	

Ear (A1,2) or mandibular notch (M1,2) referential
- Depicts morphologies of widespread wave forms.
- Reliably lateralizes most phenomena.
- Assesses symmetry of normally bilateral phenomena such as alpha, beta, mu, spindles.
- Moderate A1,2/M1,2 involvement distorts depiction of parasagittal potentials.
- Smaller fields difficult to visually appreciate.
- ECG potentials may be prominent.

Fp1-A1	F7-A1
Fp2-A2	F8-A2
F3-A1	T3-A1
F4-A2	T4-A2
C3-A1	T5-A1
C4-A2	T6-A2
P3-A1	
P4-A2	
O1-A1	
O2-A2	

Average reference (a.k.a. common average reference)
- Clearly depicts events with a restricted field.
- Localizes spikes with multiple phases producing ambiguous fields on bipolar montages.
- Events with widespread fields may "contaminate" a reference, either obscuring a localizing component or falsely localizing more diffuse ones.

Inputs 1-avg

Central sagittal (Cz) reference
- Useful for temporal events as reference external to field.
- Heavily involved in V-waves and other sleep potentials.

Inputs 1-Cz

Chapter 2

Artifacts

Electrode (Figs. 1, 2, 4–8)
- Abrupt, bizarre-appearing potentials.
- Differ markedly from cerebrally originating background activity.
- Superimposed upon background activity.
- Usually confined to single electrode.

Faulty Ground (Fig. 9)
- 60 Hz.
- Other potentials which do not blend with ongoing cerebral originating activity.
- In many or all channels.

Instrumental (Fig. 10)
- Affects single channel.

Eye Movement (Figs. 11–17)
- Cornea 100 mV positive compared to retina.
- Upward rotation of ocular globe on eye blinking or closure. Fp1, Fp2 become more positive, create downward deflections when connected to other standard scalp leads.
- Lateral eye movements create opposite polarities at F7, F8; that is, leftward movement increases positivity at F7 and decreases positivity (increases negativity) at F8.

Muscle (Figs. 18, 19)
- Very brief potentials.
- Single or multiple.
- May obscure EEG.
- Principally temporal, frontal, and occipital areas; may be diffuse.
- High-frequency filtering produces spike-like or beta-like appearance.
- Frontal spikes rarely resemble muscle artifact.

Glossokinetic (Figs. 20–23)
- Bursts of diffuse delta.
- Field varies according to tongue position.
- Usually accompanied by bursts of muscle artifact.
- Tip of tongue has negative DC potential with respect to its base.

Regularly Repetitive Muscle Potentials (Figs. 24, 25)
- Tremor.
- Focal motor seizures.
- Segmental myoclonus, i.e., palatal.

Cardiac (Figs. 26, 27)
- R-wave most prominent.
- A1 usually positive.
- A2 usually negative.
- Appears at O1,2 if neck is short.

Pulse (Figs. 28, 29)
- Periodic waves.
- Smooth or sharply contoured.
- Time-locked to electrocardiogram (ECG).
- 200 msec delay to wave peak.

Metals (Fig. 30)
- Abrupt spike-like brief single or multiphasic potentials.
- From dental fillings moving against each other.

Subgaleal Fluid (Figs. 31–33)
- Attenuates potentials by "salt bridge" or increased distance of EEG generators from electrodes.
- More apparent on bipolar montages.

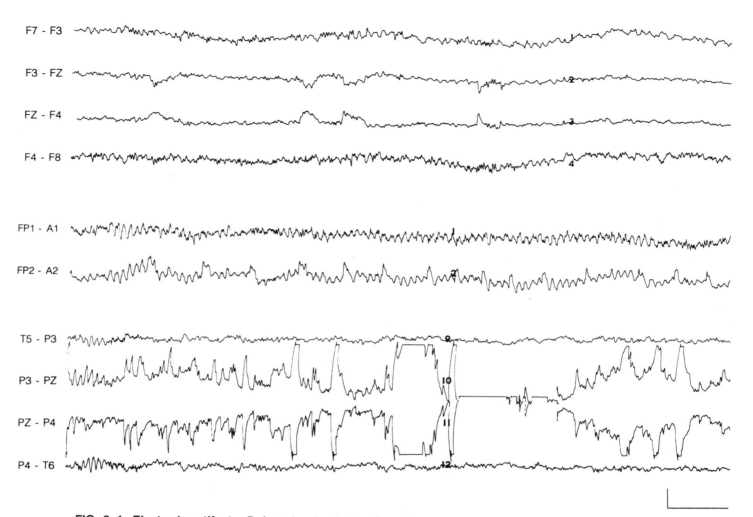

FIG. 2–1. Electrode artifacts. Defects in electrical and mechanical continuity of one electrode can produce bizarre, often sudden electrode potentials which differ markedly from ongoing background activity, do not blend with other simultaneously recorded activity, and appear only in derivations involving one electrode. In the top segment, such activity appears uniquely at Fz and has various bizarre shapes. Such intermittent activity can reflect high impedance or even popping of bubbles within the electrode jelly. On occasion, such activity can be repetitive and share morphology of periodic lateralized epileptiform discharges (PLEDs) or a focally originating seizure as in the center tracing. These repetitive potentials represent Fp2 artifact because they did not spread at all to adjacent channels (not shown) and are superimposed upon normal background activity. They bore no relationship to ECG (not shown). The high voltage and persistent nature of the Pz artifact in the bottom segment is the type produced by a faulty connection between the electrode and its wire or by its receptacle in the jackbox. Defects in conductive paste or jelly usually do not create such high voltage and sustained potentials. Calibration signal 1 sec, 50μV.

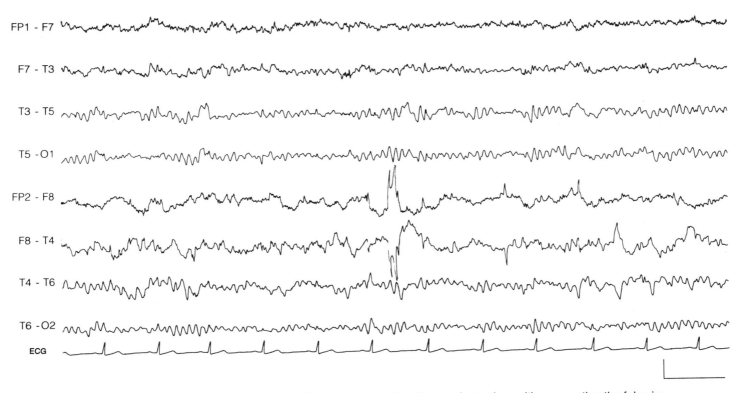

FIG. 2–2. Adjacent artifacts. Electrode artifacts may occur in adjacent electrode positions, creating the false impression that arrhythmic delta activity and/or spikes are present. Thus, the delta activity at F8 and T4 here is entirely artifactual as suggested by (a) the electropositive nature of the apiculate waves; spike-like artifacts are commonly electropositive, and (b) confinement of each artifactual waveform to a single electrode position. Note the normal background activity underlying the F8-T4 artifact. Calibration signal 1 sec, 50μV.

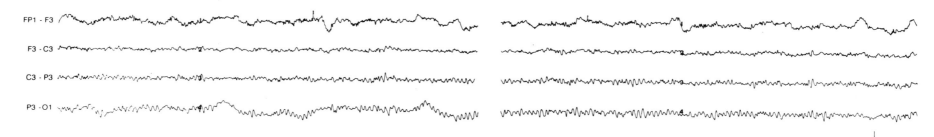

FP1 - F3

F3 - C3

C3 - P3

P3 - O1

FIG. 2–3. Head movement artifact during hyperventilation. Not all single electrode position artifacts represent technical faults. The low-frequency arrhythmic delta activity recorded at O1 during hyperventilation is not cerebrally originating because of the lack of associated "background" abnormality such as focal theta or attenuation and the lack of any spread to P3 as noted at the C3-P3 derivation (*left*). Stopping the head movement abolishes the artifact (*right*). Calibration signal 1 sec, 50μV.

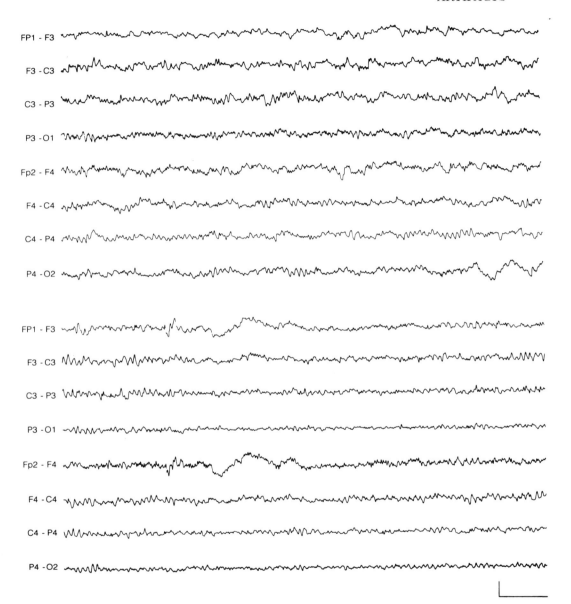

FIG. 2–4. Artifactual delta activity from multiple high-impedance electrodes. Suspicion that this apparently diffuse delta activity may be artifactual stems from the virtually normal background activity and from 60 Hz artifact in the P3-O1 derivation (*top*). Diminishing the impedance to acceptable levels eliminated the artifact (*bottom*). Calibration signal 1 sec, 100µV.

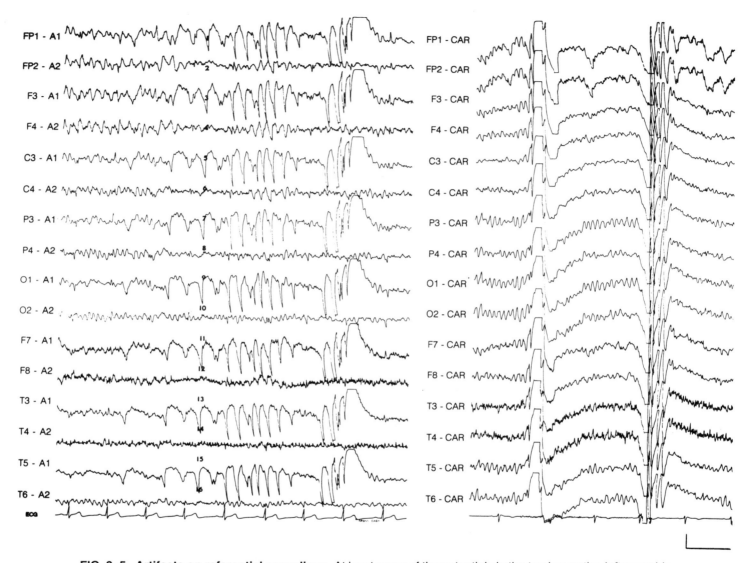

FIG. 2–5. Artifacts on referential recordings. At least some of the potentials in the tracing on the *left* resemble temporal spikes because the apiculate phase is electronegative. However, the similar voltage and wave form in all left-sided derivations indicate confinement of these potentials to A1; this would not occur with temporal spikes, where the involvement of F7, T3 and even Fp1 is usual. The common average reference (*right*) is vulnerable to head movement and to electrical charges in the environment, producing the widespread stereotyped potentials seen here. Although the first potential resembles a spike-wave, its identical appearance in all derivations identifies it as artifact; "generalised" spike-waves are always accentuated either anteriorly or posteriorly. Calibration signal 1 sec, 70μV.

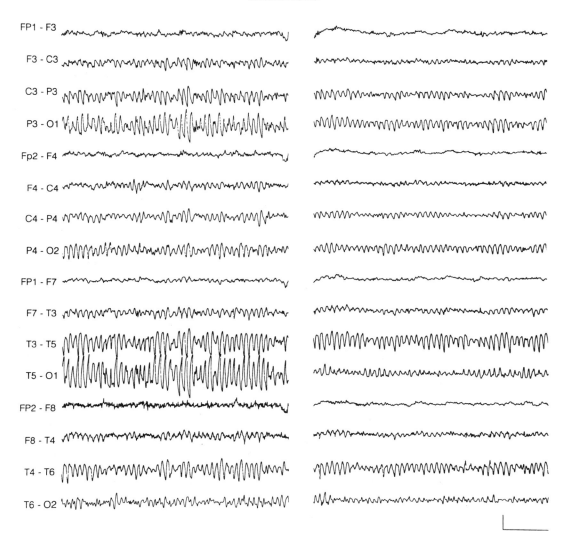

FIG. 2–6. Effect of interchange of electrodes on background activity. Erroneous substitution of Fz for O1 (*left*). Note the higher amplitude, out-of-phase alpha activity in the 4th and 12th channels (P3-Fz, T5-Fz). Tracing (*right*) after correction of erroneous substitution; alpha activity is only slightly higher in the left hemisphere, and the complete phase reversal of alpha activity is no longer present in the parasagittal leads. Normal phase reversals of alpha activity are present in the T5,6-O1,2 derivations. Montage labeling indicates *intended* linkages. Calibration signal 1 sec, 50μV.

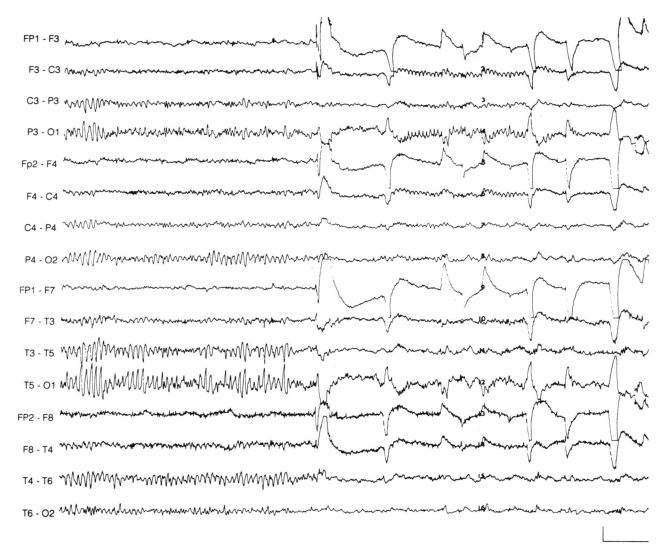

FIG. 2–7. Spurious amplitude asymmetry and other oddities from interchange of electrode positions. The several bizarre features of this recording can be explained by the erroneous interchange of Fz with O1. This produces an out-of-phase alpha activity of considerably higher voltage in the 4th and 12th channels (P3-Fz, T5-Fz), out-of-phase eye blinks because of the greater electropositivity at Fz than at either P3 or T5, and a mu rhythm from Fz in the 4th and 12th channels. Note the low-amplitude lambda activity in the technically correct derivations of P4-O2 and T6-O2. Montage labeling indicates *intended*, not actual linkages. Calibration signal 1 sec, 50μV.

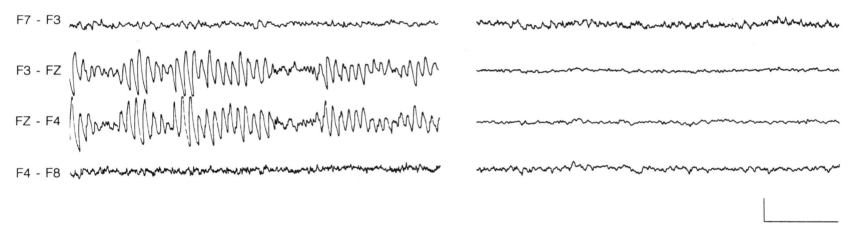

FIG. 2–8. Effect of interchange of electrodes on frontal activity. The tracing on the *left* illustrates erroneous interchange of Fz with O1, producing alpha activity in "F3-Fz" and "Fz-F4" derivations. Correction (*right*) reveals the normal low-voltage frontal activity. Suspect erroneous electrode interchange when high-amplitude activity is recorded on a coronal montage in derivations involving Fz, Cz, or Pz. Montage labeling indicates *intended* linkages. Calibration signal 1 sec, 70μV.

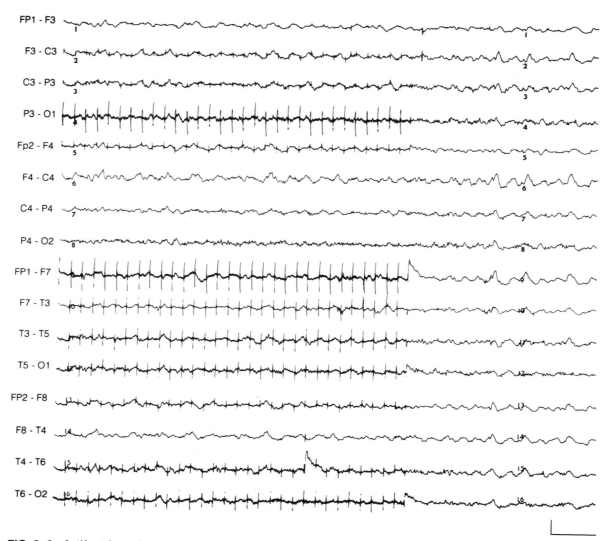

FIG. 2–9. Artifact from faulty ground electrode. A 4 Hz and 60 Hz artifact from the operating room transformer appears in most channels of this bipolar montage. Changing to a new ground lead (*last few seconds*) eliminated this artifact. Artifact from a faulty ground electrode does not always appear in all derivations. Calibration signal 1 sec, 70μV.

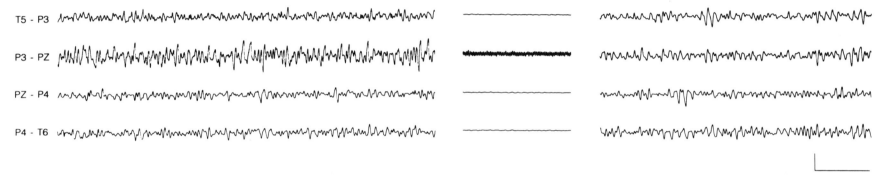

FIG. 2–10. Analog instrumental artifact. Instrumental artifact produces potentials in one channel which differ radically from electrical activity in adjacent channels. As it affects only one channel within this bipolar chain, it cannot reflect electrode malfunction. The higher (2 mm) alternating current test signal in this channel only (*middle segment*) confirmed this and suggested that the artifact resulted from incomplete connection of the master electrode selector when switching montages. Resetting the montage revealed normal cerebral activity (*right*). Calibration signal 1 sec, 50μV.

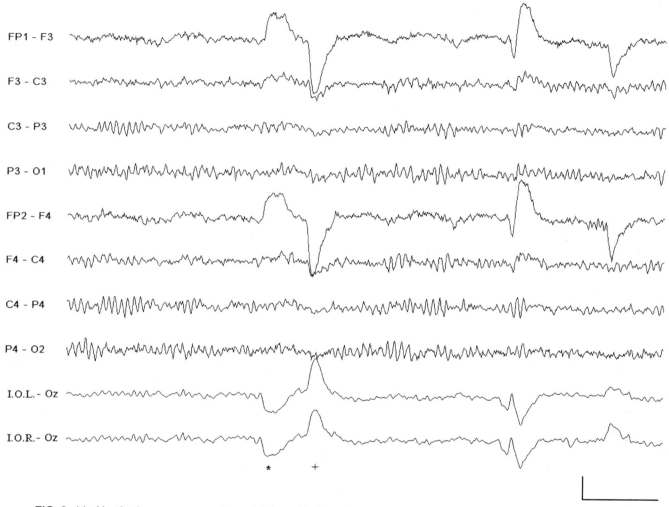

FIG. 2–11. Vertical eye movements and infraorbital leads. Electropositivity at the corneae produces a sudden negativity at Fp1,2 and positivity infraorbitally upon opening the eyes (*asterisk in 4th second*) and the opposite polarity upon their closure (+). Similar phenomena occur in the 8th second. IOL, IOR, infraorbital left, right. Calibration signal 1 sec, 50μV.

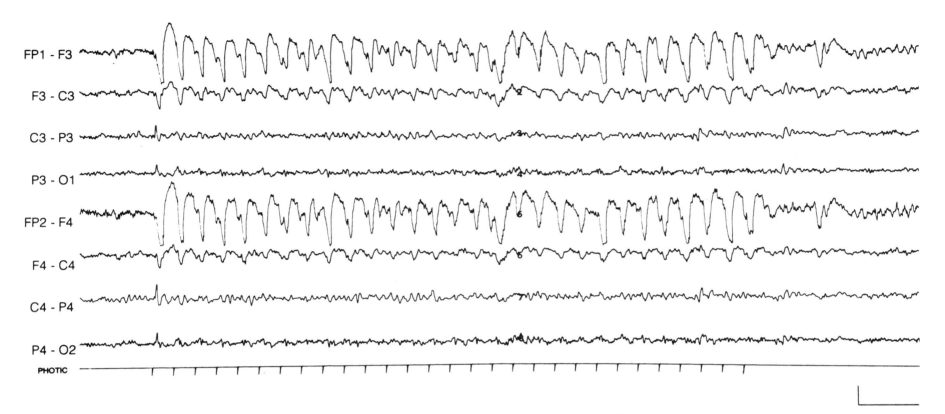

FP1 - F3

F3 - C3

C3 - P3

P3 - O1

FP2 - F4

F4 - C4

C4 - P4

P4 - O2

PHOTIC

FIG. 2–12. Eye flutter with photic stimulation. Three-Hz photic stimulation with the eyes open produces synchronous eye blinks followed by eye openings; each resulting positive-negative "complex" is preceded by a synchronous apiculate wave which presumably represents periocular muscle contraction. The resulting sequential complexes resemble spike-waves, but their primarily frontal polar location and the lockstep unison with the flash distinguishes them from the photoparoxysmal response. This sequence of spike-wave-like eye flutter is punctuated by a more obvious eye blink in the middle third of photic stimulation. Note the bisynchronous "on" response at the beginning of photic stimulation as an apiculate phenomenon. Calibration signal 1 sec, 50μV.

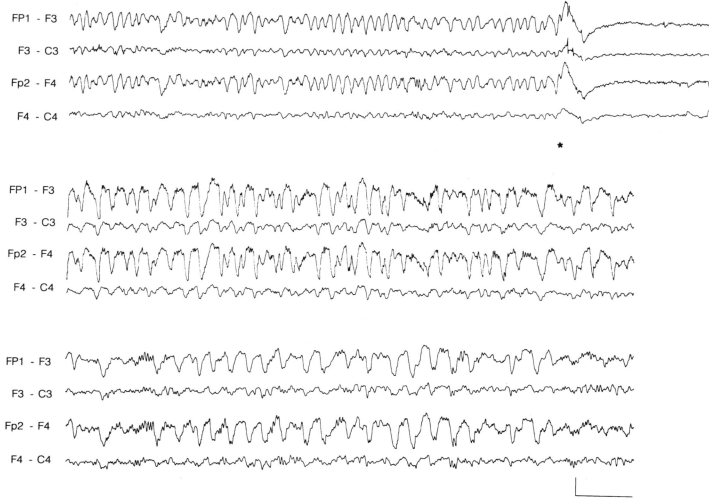

FP1 - F3

F3 - C3

Fp2 - F4

F4 - C4

FP1 - F3

F3 - C3

Fp2 - F4

F4 - C4

FP1 - F3

F3 - C3

Fp2 - F4

F4 - C4

FIG. 2–13. Eye blinks. Sequential eye blink artifacts are identifiable by their location at Fp1 and Fp2, their considerably lower amplitude at F3 and F4, and their response to eye opening (*left asterisk*). Note the bisynchronous downward potential in the frontal leads with an eye blink (*right asterisk*), the potential due to movement of the positive end of the ocular dipole towards the frontal polar electrodes suddenly creating a positive field centered near the frontal polar electrodes which extends somewhat posteriorly (3). Movement of the eyelids across the eyeball may contribute to this potential (4). At times, eye blink artifact may combine with higher-frequency background activity to resemble spike-waves (*center*) but the virtual confinement to the Fp1,2 electrodes would make this interpretation most unlikely. Calibration signal 1 sec, 50μV.

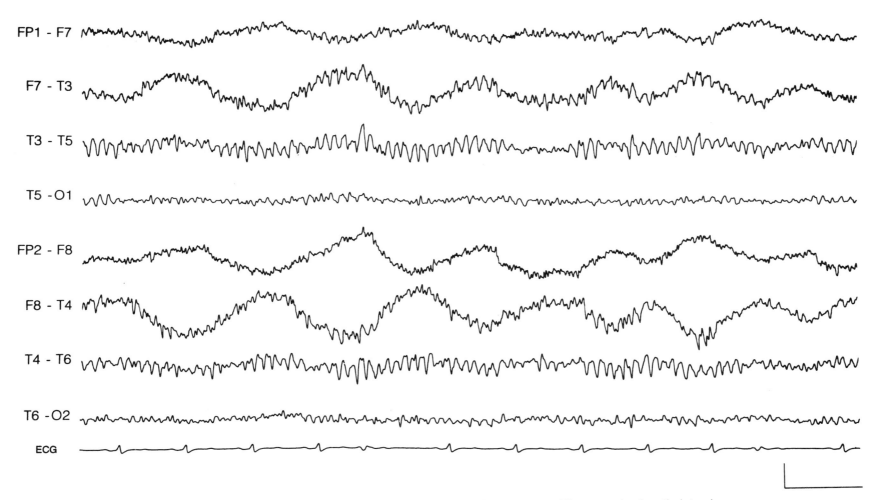

FIG. 2–14. Predominantly lateral eye movements on bipolar montage. These predominantly lateral eye movements are out-of-phase in derivations involving F7 and F8 electrodes, as an increase in positivity at one is associated with a decrease in positivity (more negative) in the other as recorded by these differential amplifiers. Calibration signal 1 sec, 50μV.

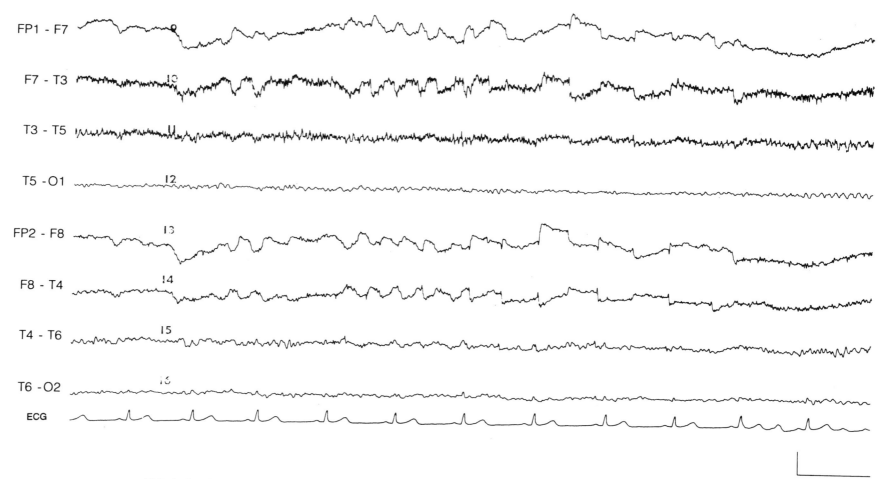

FIG. 2–15. Rapid lateral eye movements. Rapid lateral eye movements demonstrate the strict out-of-phase potentials between F7 and F8. Calibration signal 1 sec, 50 μV.

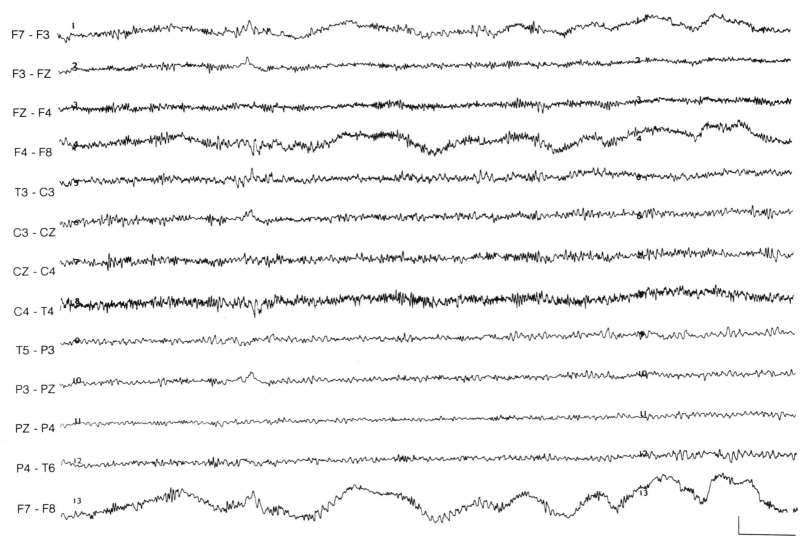

FIG. 2–16. Slow lateral eye movements on a coronal montage. Lateral eye movements produce opposite potentials at F7 and F8. Thus, a rightward eye movement would give increasing positivity at F8 and decreasing positivity at F7. As F7 and F8 are connected to input 1 and input 2 of their respective derivations on this coronal montage, the opposite changes of polarity produce pen deflections in the same direction, but summate in the F7–F8 derivation. These similar wave forms and the lack of associated disturbances in background activity, such as excess theta, distinguish this phenomenon from temporal delta activity. Calibration signal 1 sec, 100μV.

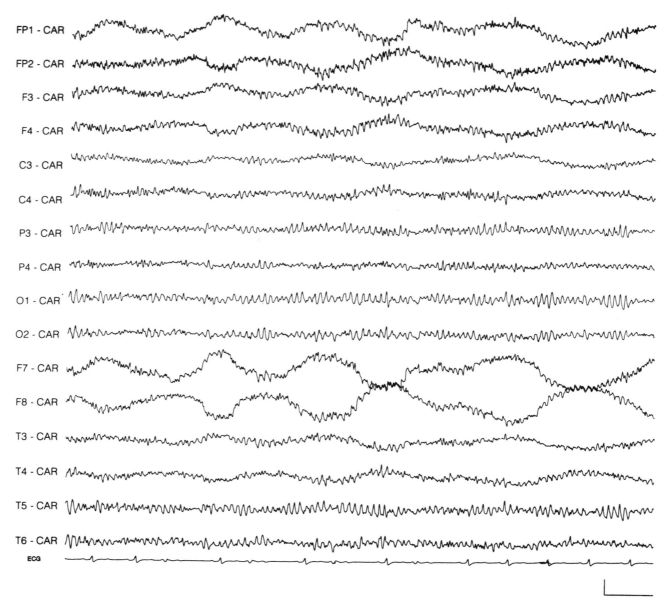

FIG. 2–17. Slow lateral eye movements on a common average reference montage. The slow lateral eye movements are out-of-phase between hemispheres, including the frontal and central derivations. Again, the lack of regional background abnormalities distinguishes such waves from frontal delta activity. Calibration signal 1 sec, 50μV.

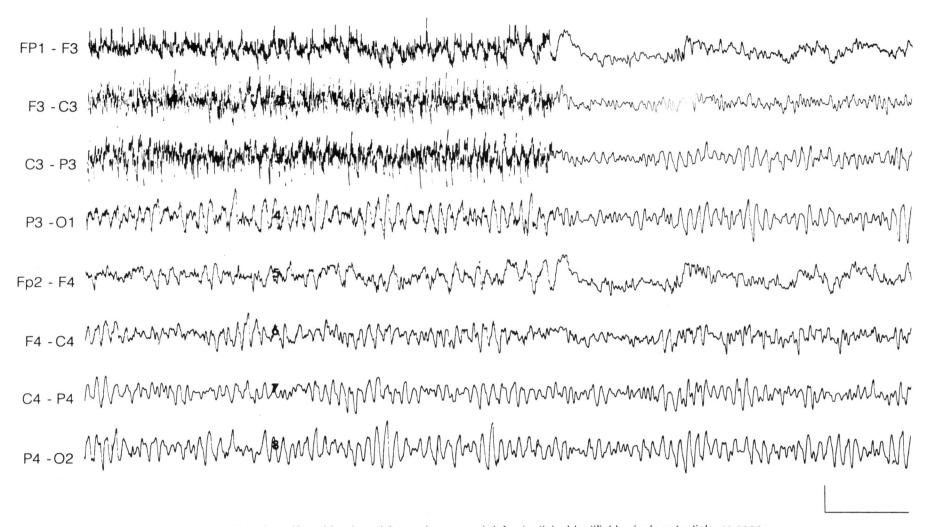

FIG. 2–18. Muscle artifact. Muscle activity produces very brief potentials. Identifiable single potentials, as seen at Fp1 and other positions here, may render background activity apiculate. Bursts of muscle potentials may obscure cerebral activity. This muscle activity was abolished in the last 4 seconds when the patient opened his mouth. Calibration signal 1 sec, 50μV.

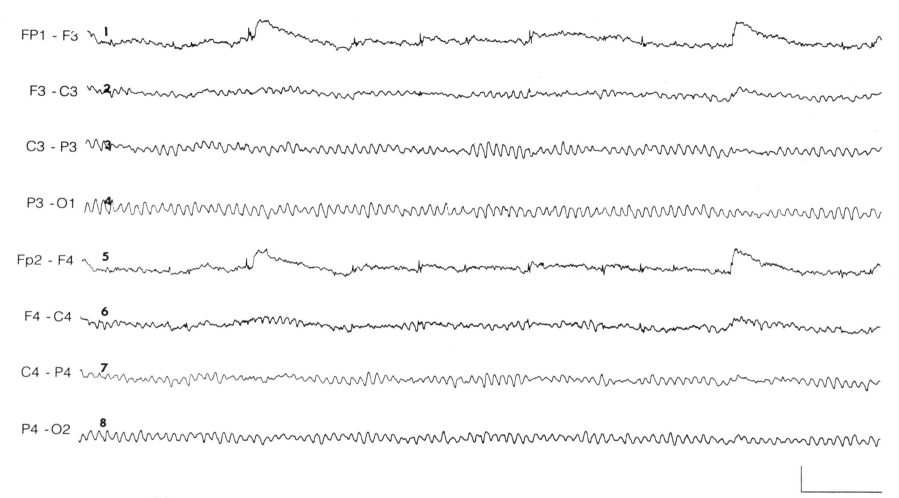

FP1 - F3   1

F3 - C3   2

C3 - P3   3

P3 - O1   4

Fp2 - F4   5

F4 - C4   6

C4 - P4   7

P4 - O2   8

FIG. 2–19. Periocular muscle artifact. The very brief potentials in the frontal polar regions (*Fp1, Fp2*) are produced by minimal contraction of periocular muscles. Downward ocular movements create negativity at Fp1 and Fp2, producing the upward pen deflections. Calibration signal 1 sec, 50μV.

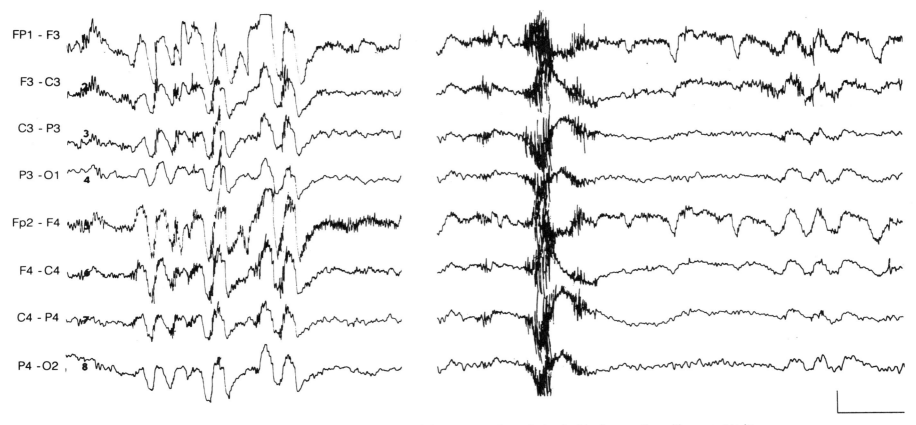

FIG. 2–20. Glossokinetic artifact. Movement of the tongue, whose tip is electrically negative with respect to its base, may produce widely distributed, low-frequency intermittent potentials that may resemble "projected rhythms." A burst of muscle potentials *may* precede such low-frequency waves, serving to differentiate glossokinetic potentials from "projected" activity. In the *left segment*, bursts of muscle potentials are accompanied by an equally long burst of diffuse rhythmic waves, both of which are characteristic of glossokinetic artifact. The first burst glossokinetic artifact in the second segment is dominated by muscle artifact, whereas the second burst of glossokinetic artifacts is dominated by rhythmic waves. Calibration signal 1 sec, 50μV.

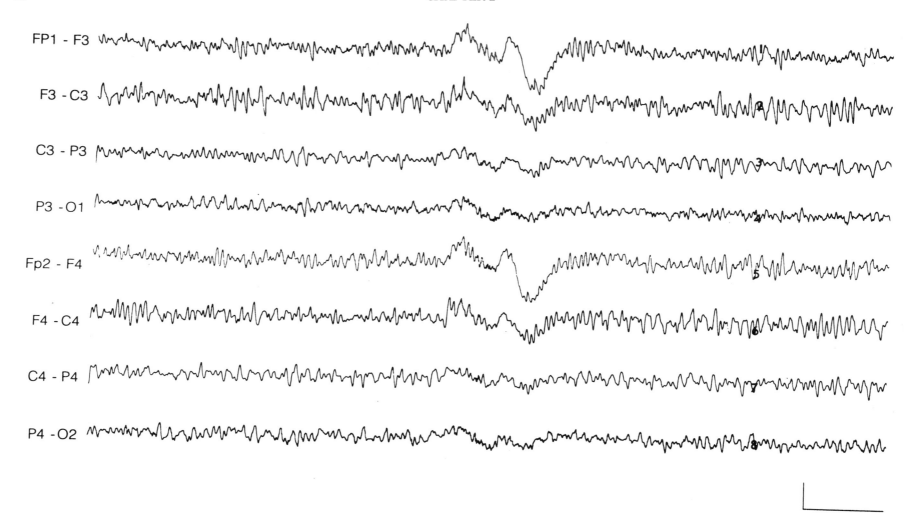

FIG. 2–21. Glossokinetic artifact. In this and the following two illustrations, glossokinetic artifact resembles "projected" rhythms; this is particularly prominent in the latter two tracings while the patient is talking. Such artifact may be produced by asking the patient to say "lilt" or "Tom thumb." True "projected" activity is often associated with a diffuse theta burst, which is not present in these samples. Calibration signal 1 sec., 50μV.

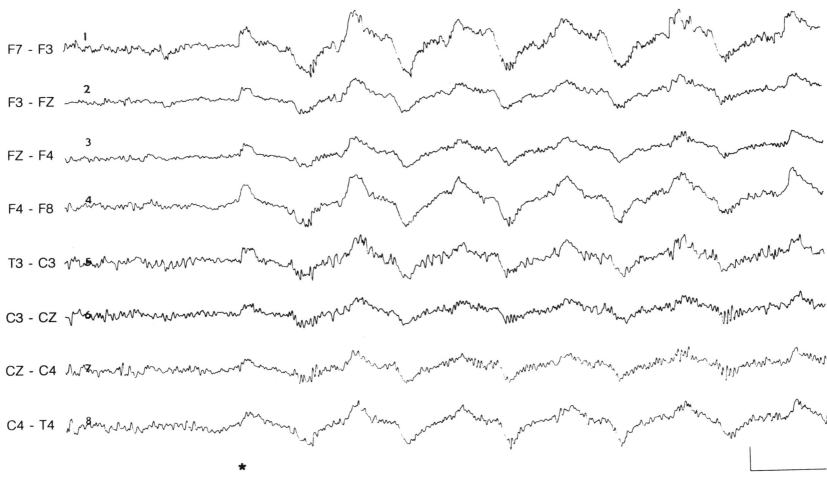

F7 - F3

F3 - FZ

FZ - F4

F4 - F8

T3 - C3

C3 - CZ

CZ - C4

C4 - T4

*

FIG. 2–22. Lateral glossokinetic artifact on coronal montage. The delta-free recording in the first seconds of this segment is subsequently marred by the subject wagging his tongue laterally (*asterisk*). Again, the artifactual nature of this delta activity is indicated by the normal background activity and its stereotyped appearance in many derivations. Calibration signal 1 sec, 50μV.

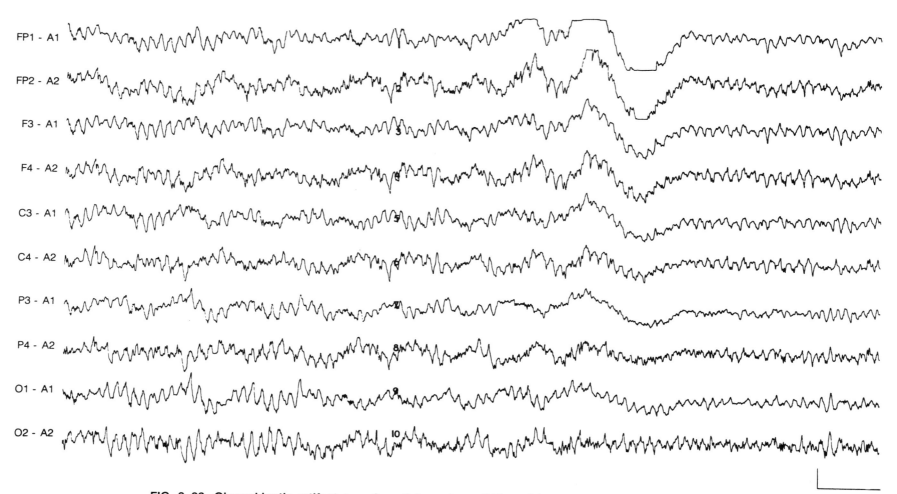

FIG. 2–23. Glossokinetic artifact on referential montage. Diffuse delta activity unaccompanied by excess theta should raise suspicion of artifact. A clue here is the out-of-phase delta in each hemisphere produced by the subject wagging his tongue laterally. Cessation of that activity during the last 3 seconds eliminated the delta. Calibration signal 1 sec, 50μV.

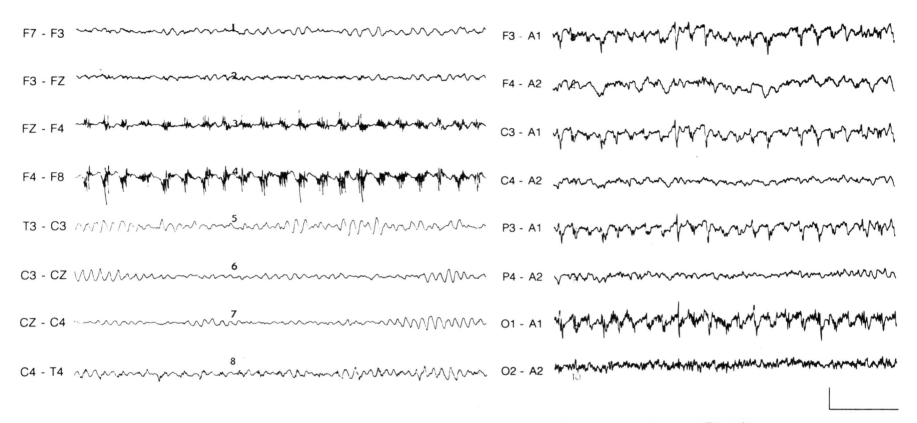

FIG. 2–24. Tremor. The 4 Hz rhythmic waves with accompanying bursts of muscle potentials seen at F4 on the bipolar montage are even more evident in the left-sided derivations on the ear referential montage. The rhythmic 4 Hz activity in synchrony with the tremor could be mistaken for cerebrally originating activity. Calibration signal 1 sec, 100μV.

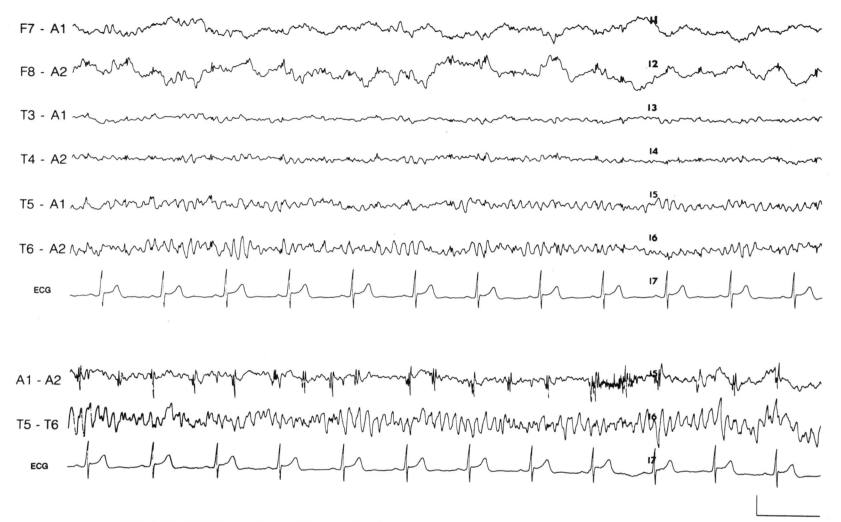

FIG. 2–25. Palatal myoclonus. 60 years. Muscle artifact at 100–200/min from palatal myoclonus produces potentials of metronomic regularity. Its rate (about 110/min) and morphology differ from those of the ECG. The lower section fully displays the myoclonus in the A1-A2 derivation, whereas it appears minimally in the ear reference montage (*upper*) at another point in recording. Calibration signal 1 sec, 70μV.

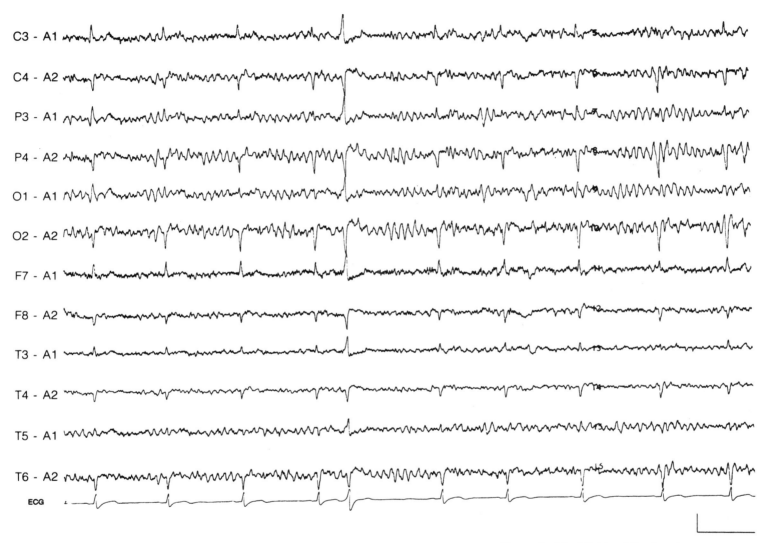

FIG. 2–26. Electrocardiogram (ECG) and referential montage. 71 years. Since electrical fields of the heart extend to the base of the skull, they may be detected by ear electrodes and therefore may be prominent on ear referential montages. The usual cardiac electrical axis produces an R-wave which is positive at A1 and negative at A2, accounting for the out-of-phase deflections in alternate hemisphere channels. An ECG monitor helps identify the large-amplitude premature contraction as cardiac and will more readily identify unusual-appearing cardiac artifacts due to arrhythmias or aberrant electrical conduction pathways. Calibration signal 1 sec, 50μV.

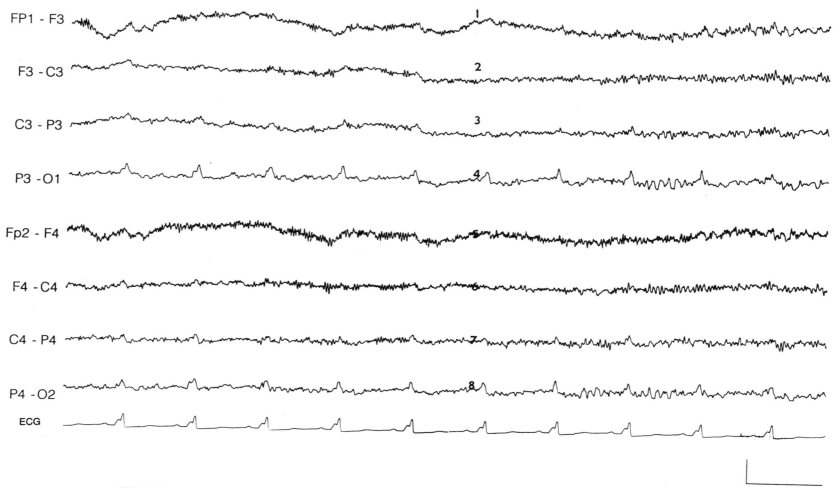

FP1 - F3

F3 - C3

C3 - P3

P3 - O1

Fp2 - F4

F4 - C4

C4 - P4

P4 - O2

ECG

FIG. 2–27. Electrocardiogram (ECG) artifact and bipolar montage. 74 years. Electropositive apiculate lambda-like potentials from occipital leads (O1,2) may be produced by the R-wave of the ECG in patients with short necks. An ECG monitor is most helpful. Calibration signal 1 sec, 50μV.

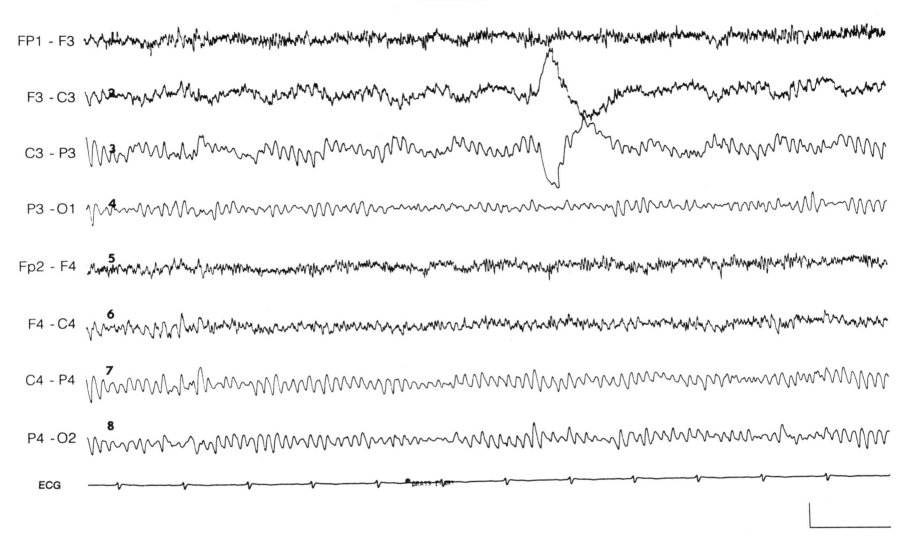

FIG. 2–28. Pulse artifact, smooth type. Rhythmic delta activity confined to a single electrode position (C3 here) likely represents pulse artifact. Although the position of an electrode on or near a scalp artery may produce this artifact, the latter may also represent high electrode impedance as reflected in the sudden high-amplitude electropositive artifactual deflection at C3 in the middle of the tracing. Calibration signal 1 sec, 50μV.

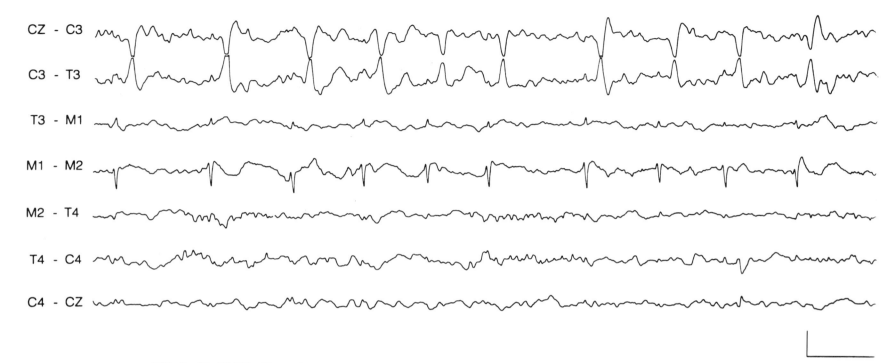

FIG. 2—29. PLEDs-like pulse artifact. Pulse artifact may appear as periodic sharply contoured potentials which are time-locked to ECG as depicted by the M1–M2 derivation. Note the invariable 200 msec delay between the R-wave and the pulse artifact peaks. Calibration signal 1 sec, 50μV.

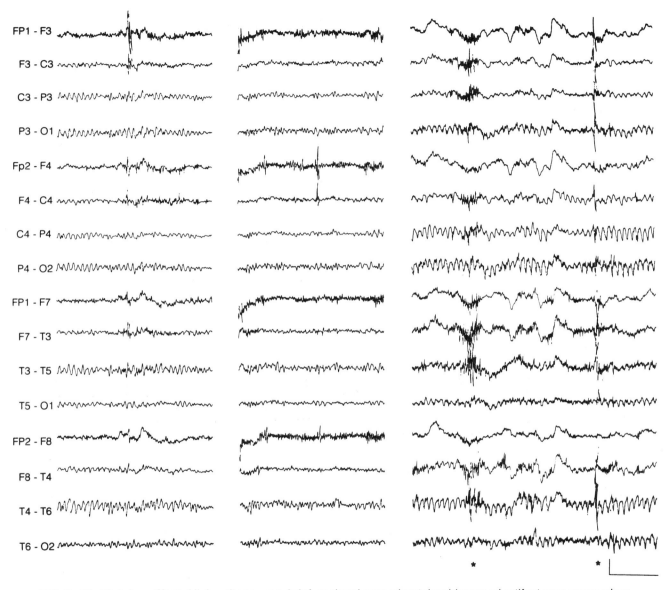

FIG. 2–30. Metals artifact. High-voltage, very brief, regional or moderately widespread artifact may occur when metals such as dental fillings rub against each other during mouth movements, as illustrated here. Such activity is usually more abrupt, higher in voltage, and briefer than muscle artifact. Thus, in the example on the *right*, the first burst of potentials (*left asterisk*) is muscular with glossokinetic artifact, whereas the last burst (*right asterisk*) is a metal artifact. A similar artifact occurs during electrocorticograms from "snaps" rubbing together. Calibration signal 1 sec, 50μV.

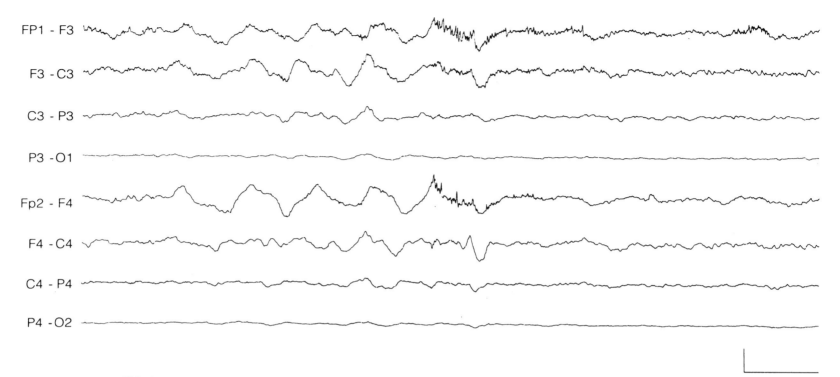

FIG. 2–31. Attenuation from subgaleal fluid. 59 years. Subgaleal edema or blood reduces amplitudes of background rhythms, particularly in bipolar recordings. Since comatose patients are usually nursed supine, such edema collects posteriorly. Possible mechanisms include a "salt bridge" or increased distance of electrodes from generators of cerebral potentials. It is quite possible that the arrhythmic delta activity, expressed principally anteriorly, is diffuse. Calibration signal 1 sec, 50μV.

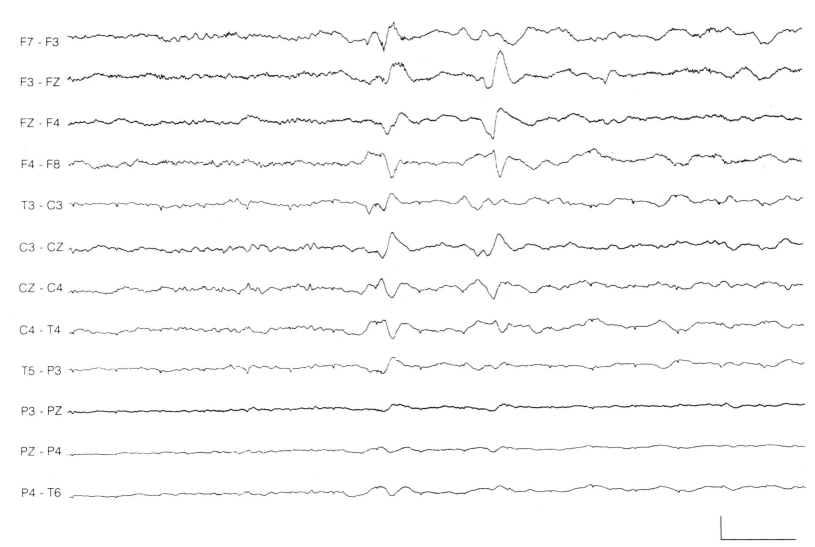

FIG. 2–32. Subgaleal fluid and coronal montage. Same patient as in Fig. 2–31 with posteriorly situated sub-galeal fluid. This fluid likely caused the attenuated potentials posteriorly. Note the persistent diffuse delta activity elsewhere and the blunted vertex waves. Calibration signal 1 sec, 50μV.

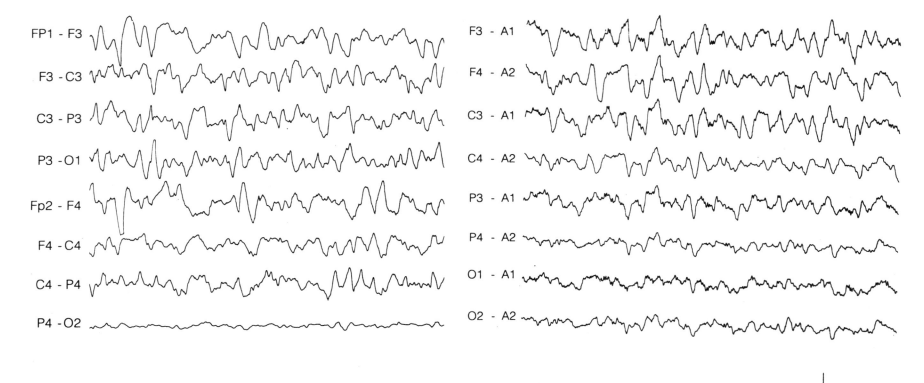

FIG. 2–33. Regional attenuation from subgaleal edema. 69 years. Scalp edema will attenuate EEG amplitude as occurs here in the parietal-occipital (P4, O2) regions on this bipolar montage. The referential recording shows that this attenuation also includes the left occipital (O1) region as indicated by the considerably lower voltage potentials at P4, O1 and O2 compared to more anterior positions. The attenuation at O1, displayed on the referential montage, is not apparent on the bipolar montage since P3 likely contributes most of the potentials to the P3-O1 derivation. Both members of the derivation pair must be attenuated or in complete synchrony for attenuation to occur as seen at the P4-O2 derivation. A1 and A2 record background potentials less than parasagittal leads. Calibration signal 1 sec, 70μV.

Chapter 3

Normal Phenomena

Alpha Rhythm (Figs. 1–24, 29, 30)
- 9–13 Hz; slows to 7–8 Hz in drowsiness.
- Sinusoidal or sharply contoured if beta present.
- Waxing and waning, that is, "beating," if composed of two close frequencies, for example, 9 and 10 Hz.
- Same dominant frequency in each hemisphere.
- Highest amplitude O1,2; P3,4; T5,6.
- Commonly extends to C3,4; A1,2; T3,4.
- Bilaterally symmetrical or higher right most common. Higher left also normal.
- Persistent symmetry > 50% produced by artifact or abnormality.
- Symmetry is variable within recording.
- Ear referential recording is the best measure of symmetry.
- Partial or complete "blocking" by eye opening or alerting; attenuation normally symmetrical.
- Low voltage ($< 15\mu$V) in some normals.

Slow Alpha Variant (Figs. 25–28)
- Saw-toothed wave form at above one-half alpha frequency from partial fusion of two alpha waves.
- Same location and reactivity as alpha.

Mu Rhythm (Fig. 20, 21)
- Arciform–apiculate negative and rounded positive phase.
- 10 (9–11) Hz.
- Intermingled with 20 Hz beta.
- C3,4 and Cz location; occasionally involves P3,4.
- Long epochs of unilateral expression common.
   - Normal if other central rhythms symmetrical.
   - Side-to-side shifts in maximum amplitude occur.
- Movement of contralateral or ipsilateral extremities (or its contemplation) blocks rhythm.
- Eye opening has no effect.
- High voltage over skull defect–breach rhythm.
- Apiculate phase may resemble spikes.

Beta (Figs. 15, 17, 31–37)
- Any rhythmic activity > 13 Hz.
- Some beta in all normals; amount varies.
- 14–40 Hz, 15–25 Hz most common.
- Usually sinusoidal; apiculate or arciform if competing frequencies; "beating" if close frequencies.
- May occur in bursts.
- Locations
   - Frontal—common.
   - Central—common, mixed with mu.
   - Posterior—fast alpha variant.
   - Diffuse—when abundant—medication effect.
- Usually $< 20\mu$V; occasionally 20–30μV.
- Amplitude and distribution increased by:
   - Drowsiness, light sleep, rapid eye movement (REM).
   - Skull defect.
   - Medication; especially benzodiazepines, barbiturates.
- Diffuse theta may accompany medication-induced excess beta.

Theta (Figs. 33, 34)
- Low-voltage ($< 30\mu$V) 4–7 Hz diffuse theta is a common component of normal recordings.
- More common in children and young adults than in older adults.

- Temporal theta.
   ≤ 10% of awake records in normal subjects over 60 years.
   Equal distribution bilaterally or twice as abundant on left.
   Single wave or brief bursts, separated by normal background.

Hyperventilation (Figs. 39–42)

- Sequence:
   Increase in diffuse theta.
   Rhythmic delta in bursts.
   Continuous rhythmic delta.
- Effect maximum anteriorly in most adolescents and adults.
- Maximum amplitude of delta bursts may shift from side to side.
- Multiple frequencies may create apiculate wave forms.
- Effect greatest in youth, with maximum effort and low serum glucose.
- Effect subsides in 60–90 seconds after hyperventilation (HV).
- May abnormally elicit focal spikes, generalized spike-waves, and focal delta or theta.
- Posthyperventilation period may contain newly appearing focal delta or theta as abnormalities.

Lambda Waves (Figs. 44–46)

- O1,2 principally; involve P3,4 and T5,6.
- Bilaterally synchronous.
- Diphasic or triphasic.
- Largest wave electropositive, lasting 100–200 msec.
- Usually < 20μV; rarely > 50μV.
- Evoked by scanning well-illuminated, patterned visual field.
- Present in 50% of normal EEGs.

Photic Stimulation (Figs. 47–55)

- ≤ 3 flashes/second.
   Electropositive evoked response.
   100 msec delay.
   Maximum O1,2 and T5,6.
   Variable anterior extension.
   Resembles lambda.
- ≥ 6 flashes/second.
   More rhythmic response.
   Time-locked to flash with harmonic or subharmonic frequencies.
   Initial response may resemble:
   ≤ 3 flashes/second response or lambda.
   V-wave.

- Responses larger in children, elderly.
- Responses symmetrical or asymmetrical, usually higher right.
- Responses not visible in many normal subjects.

Positive Occipital Sharp Transients of Sleep (POSTS) (Figs. 56–58)

- Also known as lambdoid waves.
- Monophasic.
- Sharply contoured.
- Electropositive.
- Bioccipital.
- Singly or in 4–5 second sequences.
- Occur in most normal subjects.

Wicket Spikes (Figs. 59–64, Chapter 4: Figs. 4–18, 19)

- Arciform waves.
- Negative phase apiculate.
- Positive phase rounded.
- Single or clusters.
- T3,4 or T3,4-F7-8.
- Unilateral or independent bilateral.
- No distortion of background rhythms.

Psychomotor Variant (Figs. 65–67)

- 5–7 Hz.
- Sharply contoured, often notched.
- Mid-anterior temporal regions.
- Parasagittal spread.
- Bursts or runs.
- Gradual onset and offset.
- Monomorphic; that is, without evolution.

Subclinical Rhythmic EEG Discharge of Adults (SREDA) (Figs. 68, 69)

- Sequential monophasic or biphasic apiculate waves mixed with rhythmic theta or delta.
- No morphological evolution.
- Abrupt onset; abrupt or gradual offset.
- Usually in wakefulness, occasionally in sleep.
- May occur after hyperventilation.
- Principally parietal, posterior temporal.
- Bisynchronous or unilateral.
- Occurs principally in elderly or middle age.

Drowsiness (Figs. 70–80)
- Alpha augments in amplitude and distribution, then disappears.
- Theta augments in amplitude and distribution.
- Beta increases, occasionally in bursts, then may decrease.
- Slow lateral eye movements.
- Occasional bursts of theta.
- Occasional 2–4 Hz waves, in bursts, in elderly.
- Brief epochs of drowsiness common in senility.

Vertex (V-) Waves (Figs. 43, 81–102, 106, 109)
- Bilaterally synchronous.
- Maximum amplitude at vertex (Cz).
- Extend to Fz, Pz; F3,4; C3,4; P3,4.
- May appear in sequences.
- Shifting asymmetries occur.
- Principal component may be positive.
- Principal component is usually a sharply contoured electronegative wave.
- May be preceded and/or followed by smaller waves of opposite polarity.
- Highest amplitude and sharpest in youth; become more blunt with age.
- Appear principally in light sleep but also in wakefulness, drowsiness, and at on-set of high-frequency flash stimuli.
- Rarely suppressed by focal pathology.

Spindles (Figs. 93–106)
- Rhythmic or arciform waves.
- In 2–3 second bursts, waxing and waning, giving spindle shape.
- Bilaterally synchronous and symmetrical, or asynchronous with symmetry of total spindle quantity.
- 13–14 Hz, Cz,3,4 with frontal spread in light stage 2 sleep.
- 10–12 Hz, Fz,3,4 in deeper stage 2 and stage 3 sleep.

Mitten Pattern (Figs. 96, 99)
- High voltage 400–500 msec waves at Fz-Cz with parasagittal spread.
- Notched in ascending phase by 100–125 msec wave.

K-Complexes (Fig. 97)
- Diphasic wave.
    Initial brief wave.
    Subsequent slower wave.
- Spindles superimposed on slower wave.
- Stage 2 sleep.

Rapid Eye Movement (REM) Sleep (Figs. 107, 108)
- Low voltage.

- Mixed frequencies; theta, beta, delta.
- Clusters of rapid conjugate vertical and/or horizontal eye movements.

Arousal (Figs. 109–119)
- Number, complexity and duration of phenomena vary directly with depth of sleep.
- From drowsiness: no intermediate waves or frontocentral beta.
- From light sleep:
    V-waves.
    Frontocentral alpha-theta.
- From deep sleep:
    High-voltage delta.
    Frontocentral alpha-theta.
- Duration: 1–5 seconds.

Small Sharp Spikes (Figs. 120–124, Chapter 4: Figs. 7, 10–12)
- Abrupt ascending slope.
- Steeper descending slope.
- Low amplitude following slow wave, same polarity as spike; or low am-plitude following potential as "dip" in background, polarity opposite to spike.
- Brief: < 50 msec.
- No disruption of background activity.
- Widespread field; dipole between hemispheres or within hemisphere.
- Cancellation between ear (A1,2) and posterior temporal lead (T5,6) common.
- Often appear bilaterally with maximum amplitude on one hemisphere.
- Single events; rarely as doublets.
- Adults and adolescents.
- Light, non-REM sleep.

Fourteen and Six Per Second Positive Spikes (Figs. 125–127)
- Positive component apiculate or arciform.
- Negative component smooth.
- Singly or in bursts.
- 13–17 Hz or 6–7 Hz; principally 14 or 6 Hz.
- Posterior temporal and adjacent areas.
- Widespread field.
- Best recorded with coronal or referential montages.
- < 1–2 seconds long.
- Drowsiness and sleep.
- Adolescents, young adults.

Six Per Second Spike-Waves (Figs. 127, 128, Chapter 5: Fig. 15–17)

- 5–7 Hz.
- Brief, low amplitude spike.
- Awake, drowsiness, not sleep.
- Bisynchronous.
- < 1 second duration.
- Two forms:
  Low amplitude, posterior.
  High amplitude, anterior.

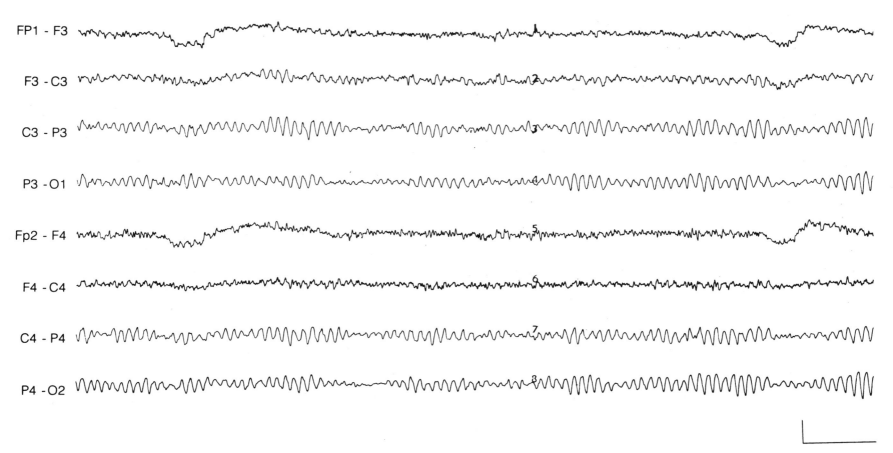

FIG. 3–1. Normal alpha activity. 62 years. Well regulated 9 Hz alpha activity. Its slight asymmetry, right higher, is well within normal limits. Beta activity is slightly lower in the left frontal region than right, but a greater quantity of EEG would have to be assessed before ascribing any significance to this asymmetry. Note the ocular movements in the 2nd and 10th seconds. Calibration signal 1 sec, 50μV.

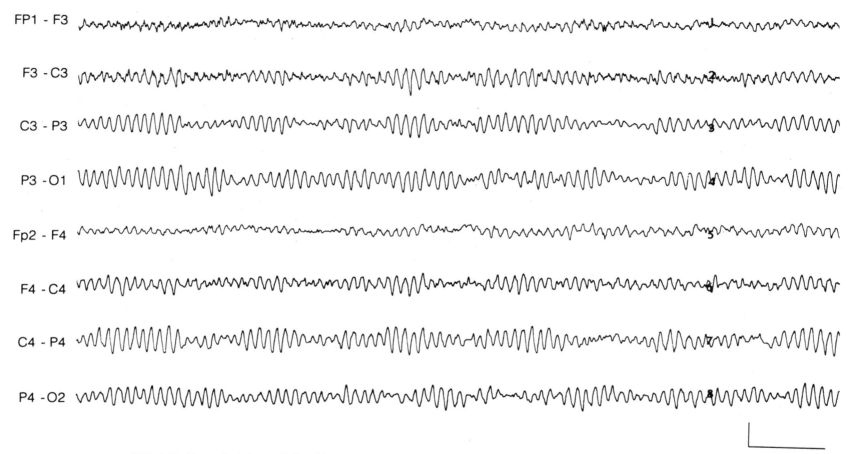

FIG. 3–2. Normal alpha activity. 83 years. 8–9 Hz alpha rhythm in an awake adult. Its waxing and waning amplitudes ("beating"), particularly in derivations C3-P3 and C4-P4, together with the incompletely sinusoidal nature of the rhythm suggest more than one frequency, in this case 8 and 9 Hz. The relative contributions of alpha and mu rhythm to the potentials in derivations F3-C3 and F4-C4 are not clear with the eyes closed. Alpha may extend to the central regions and rarely to the superior frontal areas. Calibration signal 1 sec, 70μV.

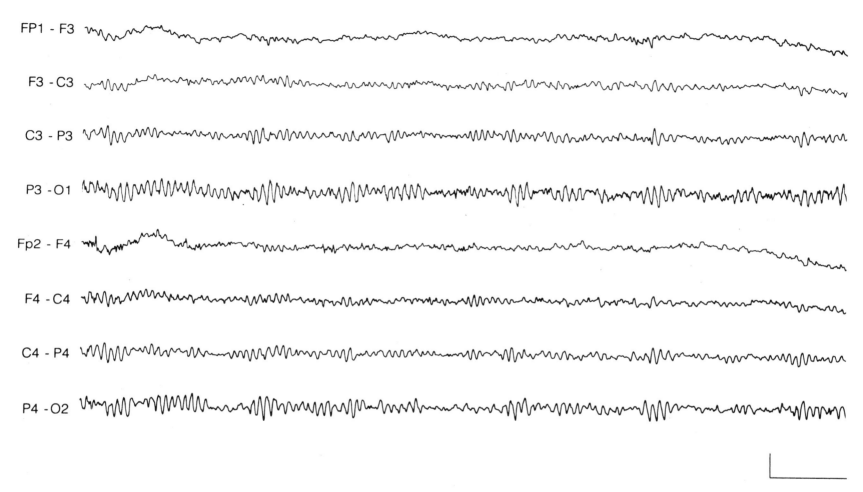

FP1 - F3

F3 - C3

C3 - P3

P3 - O1

Fp2 - F4

F4 - C4

C4 - P4

P4 - O2

FIG. 3–3. Normal alpha. 29 years. Well regulated minimally asymmetrical waxing and waning alpha activity with minimal competing wave forms. Calibration signal 1 sec, 70μV.

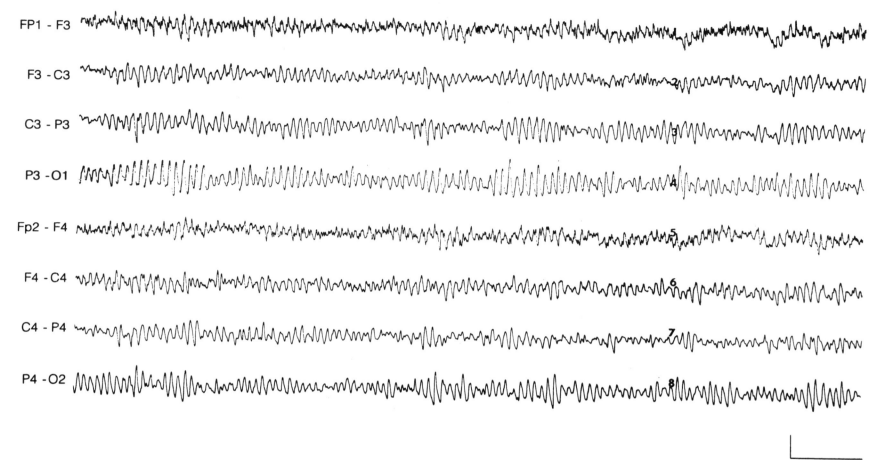

FIG. 3–4. Normal alpha activity. 80 years. 10–12 Hz alpha in this elderly patient. The lack of a pure sinusoidal wave form is due to the coexistence of other frequencies, in this instance principally beta. The slightly higher amplitude on the left may reflect not only a true voltage asymmetry but an asymmetry of field, as the alpha field may extend relatively more to P4 than to P3, causing some cancellation in the P4-O2 derivation. An ear referential montage would clarify this. Muscle potentials and beta activity contribute to the high-frequency wave forms at the Fp1-F3 and Fp2-F4 derivations. Note the very minimal theta activity of this age in this parasagittal bipolar montage, a normal feature. Calibration signal 1 sec, 50μV.

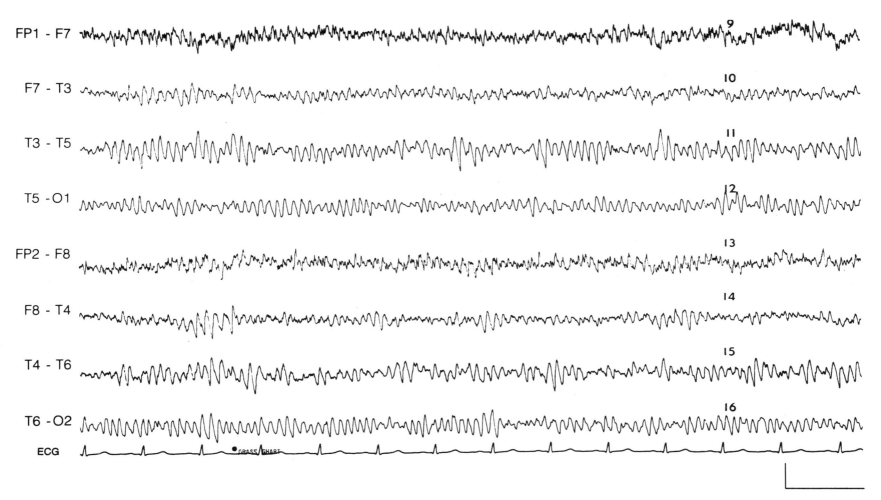

FIG. 3–5. Normal temporal activity for age. 80 years. Note the extension of alpha to the T3, T4 regions. Its occasional disruption at T3,4 is due to sporadic temporal theta activity, a normal finding at any age. The slow potentials in the Fp1-F7 and Fp2-F8 derivations are eye movements. Calibration signal 1 sec, 50μV.

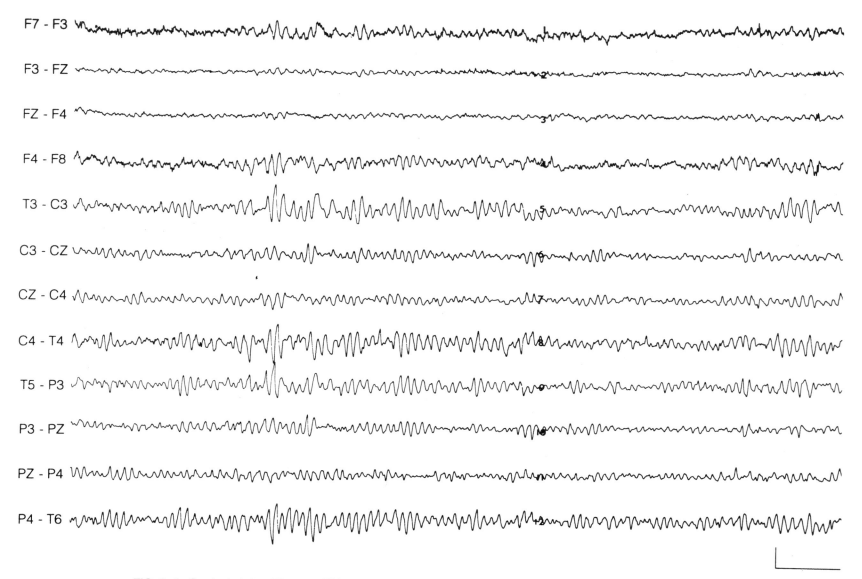

FIG. 3–6. Central alpha. 50 years. This coronal montage illustrates the extension of alpha activity to the central regions, although contribution by a mu rhythm cannot be excluded, since the eyes remain closed. The small amount of theta activity centrally (4th second) is not an abnormality. Note the relative paucity of frontal activity, which is usual in this montage. Calibration signal 1 sec, 50μV.

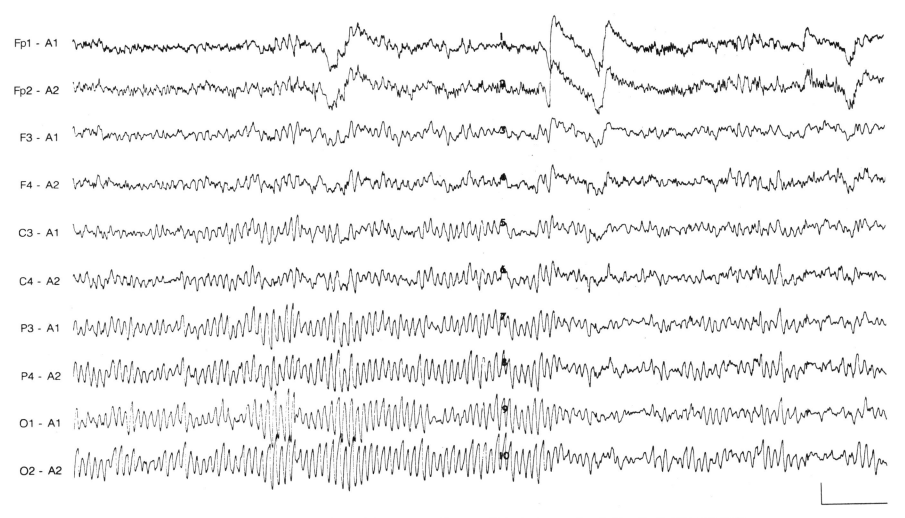

FIG. 3–7. Abundant alpha on referential montage. 18 years. Abundant, occasionally "beating" alpha activity is transiently and partially inhibited by eye blinking. Muscle potentials and beta activity contribute to the high-frequency waves of the frontal polar derivations, whose slight asymmetry has no significance. A normal amount of diffuse theta activity is revealed in the epoch of alpha attenuation. Such diffusely distributed activity is more evident on referential than bipolar montages. Calibration signal 1 sec, 50μV.

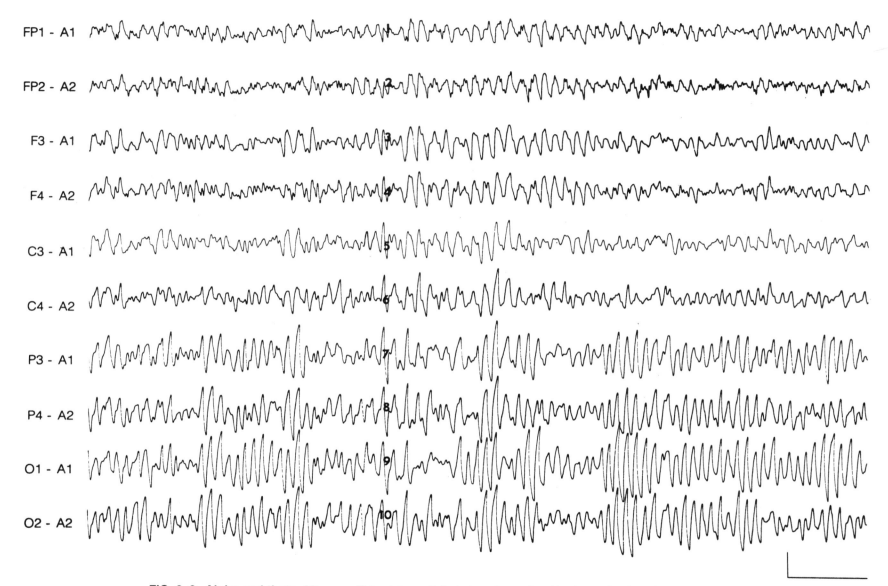

FIG. 3–8. Alpha and theta. 32 years. This alpha activity is largely confined to the parietal-occipital regions. Its combination with 6 Hz rhythms creates apiculate wave forms which are not spikes. The "beating" or waxing and waning of alpha activity likely represents the effect of two narrowly separate alpha frequencies. Note the 7 Hz theta anteriorly; this early sign of drowsiness occurs before the disappearance of alpha activity. Calibration signal 1 sec, 70μV.

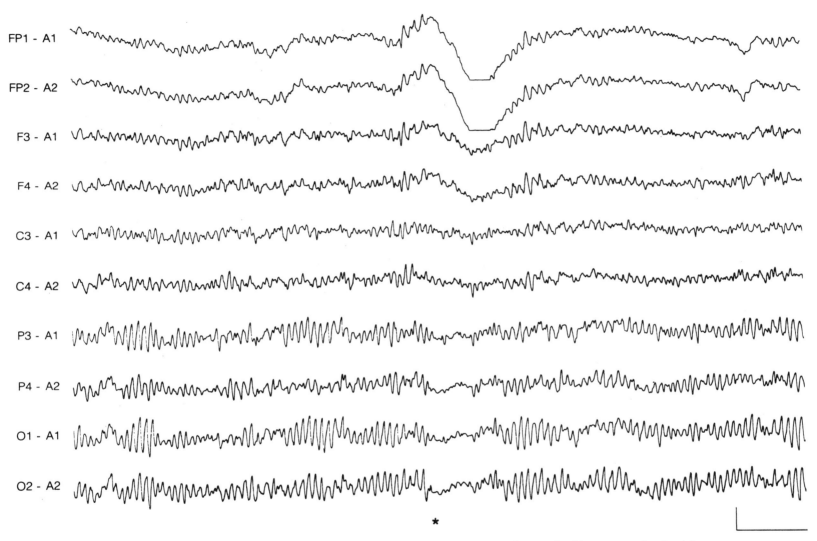

FP1 - A1

FP2 - A2

F3 - A1

F4 - A2

C3 - A1

C4 - A2

P3 - A1

P4 - A2

O1 - A1

O2 - A2

*

FIG. 3–9. Normal alpha asymmetry. 25 years. No clinical significance can be ascribed to even moderate alpha asymmetries if: (a) the alpha on each side is in itself normal, (b) there are no frequency differences exceeding 1 Hz, and (c) there are no other electrographic abnormalities. Note how the degree of asymmetry between P3 and P4 fluctuates with time. Slow eye movements create the delta activity of anterior derivations. The brief eye opening attenuates the alpha transiently (*asterisk*). Calibration signal 1 sec, 70μV.

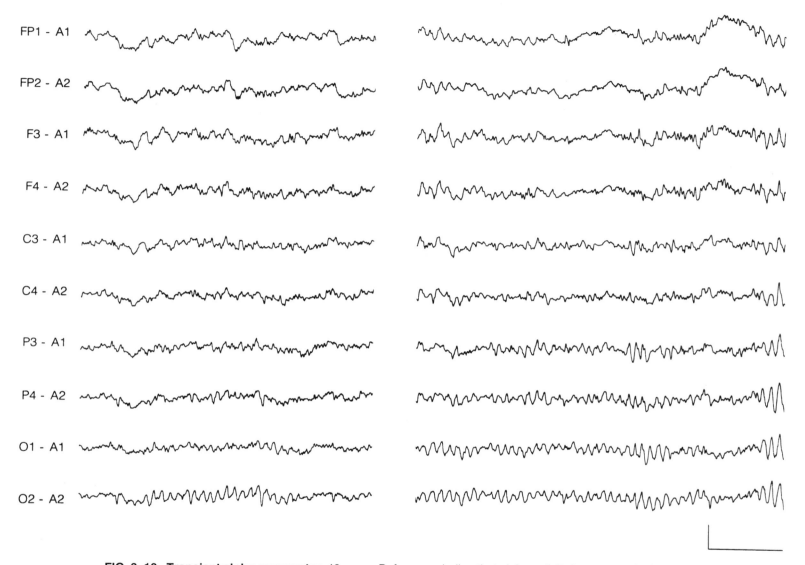

FIG. 3–10. Transient alpha asymmetry. 43 years. Before concluding that alpha activity is asymmetrical, assure that an adequate sample has been assessed. Note the symmetrical alpha activity in the second segment, whereas it is clearly less abundant in the left hemisphere in the first segment from the same recording. Such alpha activity is normal. This normal amount of diffuse theta and delta is more evident on ear reference than on bipolar montages. Eye movements contribute to the anterior delta activity. The normal "background" activity precludes such low-voltage delta activity from representing a cortical abnormality. Calibration signal 1 sec, 50μV.

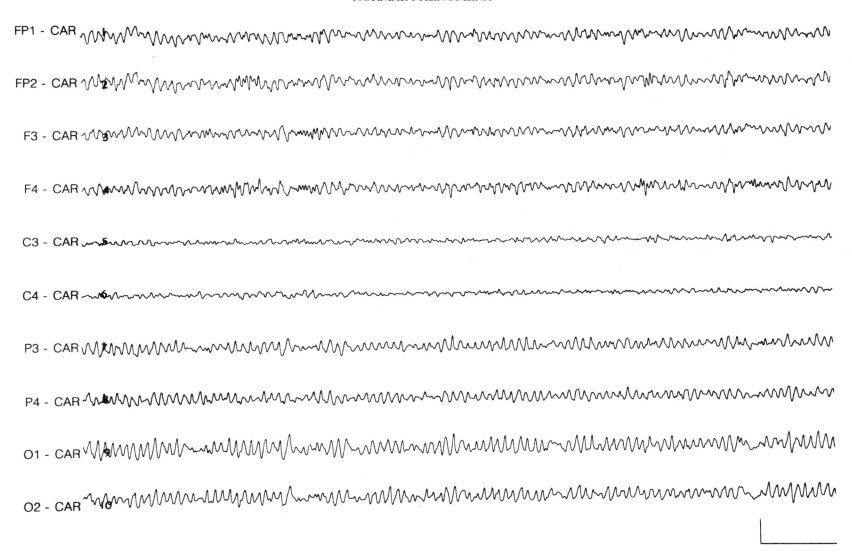

FIG. 3–11. Alpha and the common average reference (CAR). 23 years. The widespread field of alpha activity may enter the common average reference (CAR) and be expressed in derivations of frontal electrodes which are outside the alpha field. The alpha activity of "frontal" derivations is usually in the phase opposite to that seen in the occipital and parietal derivations which are within the alpha field. The minimal alpha seen in the 5th and 6th channels reflect a cancellation effect between the amount of alpha at C3,4 and that of the CAR. Calibration signal 1 sec, 50μV.

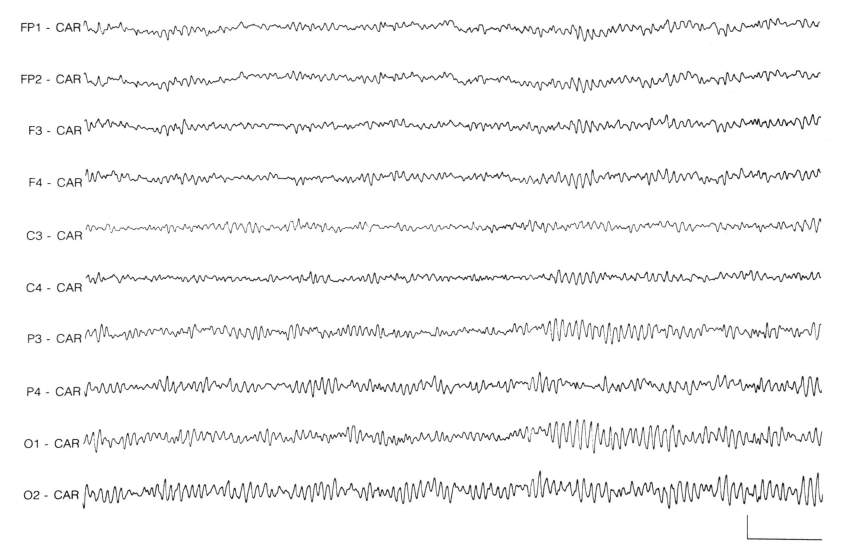

FIG. 3–12. Shifting alpha asymmetries. 25 years. The common average reference (CAR) also depicts alpha symmetry or shifts in asymmetry. Note the shifting alpha asymmetry from right dominant to left dominant in this tracing. This is clearly normal, because the alpha is normal on each side and there are no other electrographic abnormalities. Low-voltage delta activity underlying the alpha in the P3-CAR and O1-CAR derivations does not represent an abnormality as it is unassociated with any "background" disturbance. Calibration signal 1 sec, 70μV.

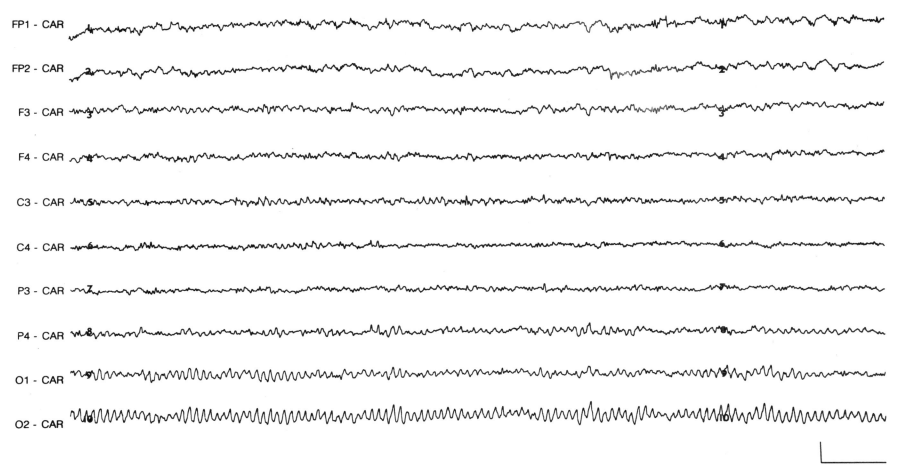

FIG. 3–13. Alpha asymmetry. 43 years. Even though the alpha is considerably more abundant in the right occipital (O2) as opposed to the left occipital (O1) region, adequate alpha appears in the latter, reducing somewhat the chance that this asymmetry has clinical significance. Calibration signal 1 sec, 50μV.

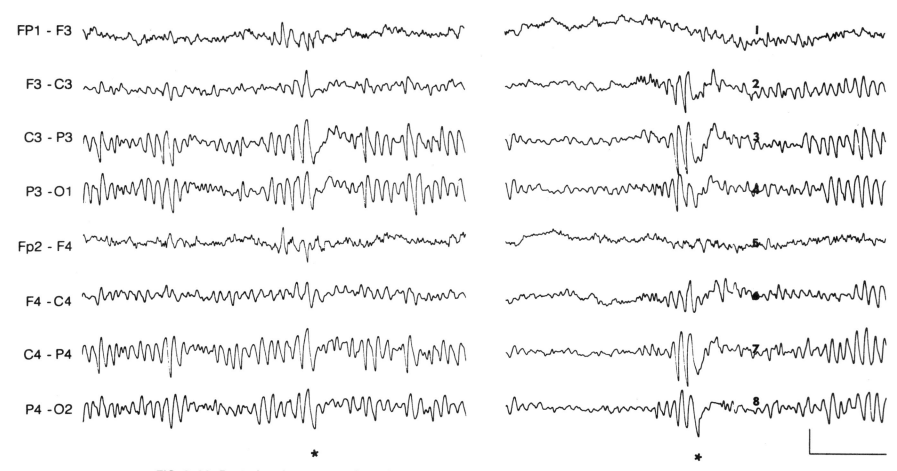

FIG. 3–14. Posterior slow waves of youth. 32 years. Posterior slow waves of youth as polyphasic potentials (5) may disrupt the alpha rhythm, creating a posteriorly situated spike wave-like phenomenon as seen here (*asterisks*). The 1 Hz activity underlying normal background rhythms in many derivations is not abnormal in youth. Youthful wave forms may normally persist into adulthood. Calibration signal 1 sec, 50μV.

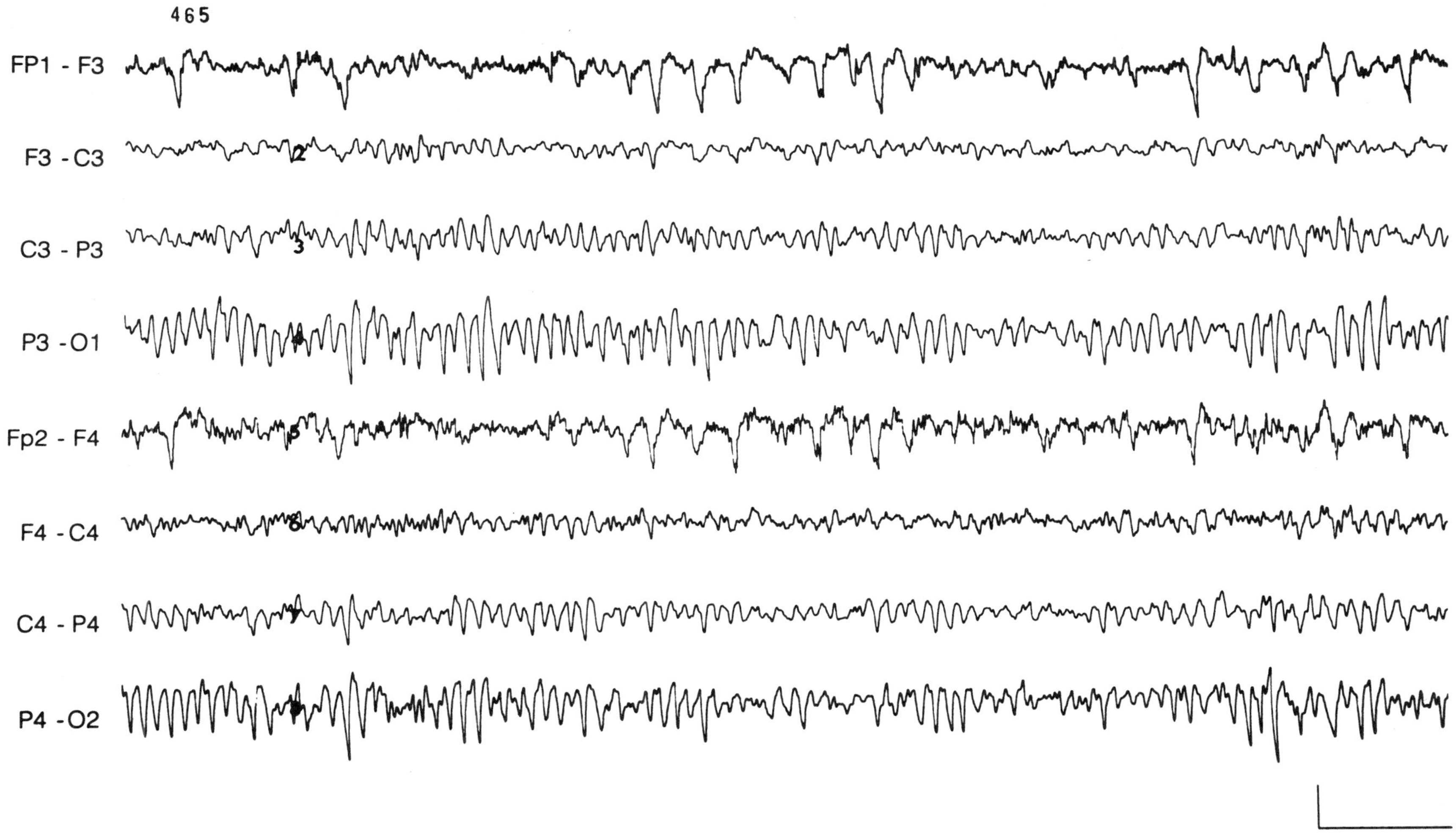

FIG. 3–15. **Alpha and beta.** 32 years. Posteriorly situated beta activity combines with 10 Hz alpha to create sharply contoured waves in the negative, in this case downward, phase of the wave forms. Eye blinks appear in the frontal polar derivations. Calibration signal 1 sec, 50μV.

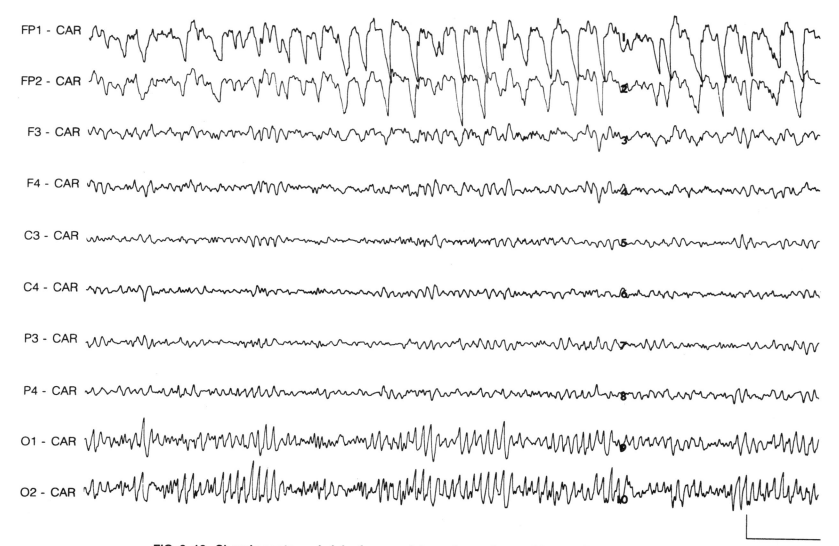

FIG. 3–16. Sharply contoured alpha from a mixture of wave forms. 32 years. Posterior beta activity, "fast alpha variant," may combine with the usual alpha activity to create sharply contoured arciform waves. Note the abundant eye blinks at Fp1, Fp2. Calibration signal 1 sec, 70μV.

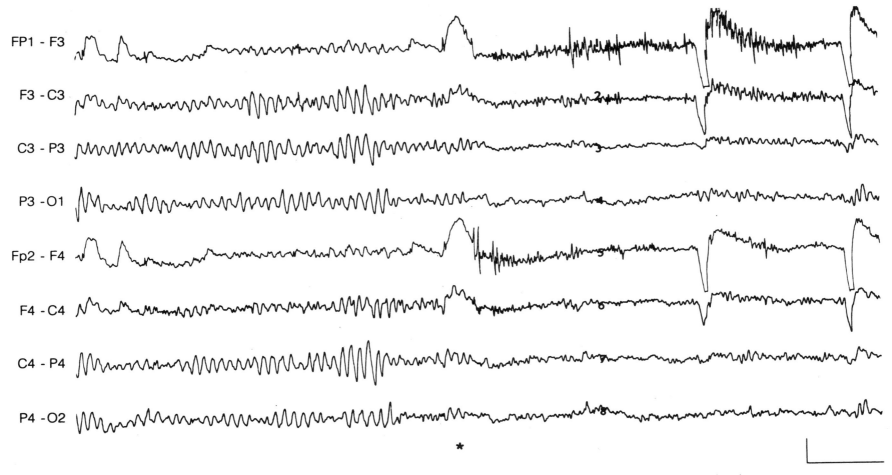

FIG. 3–17. Alpha attenuation with eye opening. 83 years. Eye opening (*asterisk*) completely abolishes the alpha activity in this example, leaving a central (C3, C4) beta rhythm and low-voltage lambda waves in the occipital derivations. Calibration signal 1 sec, 50µV.

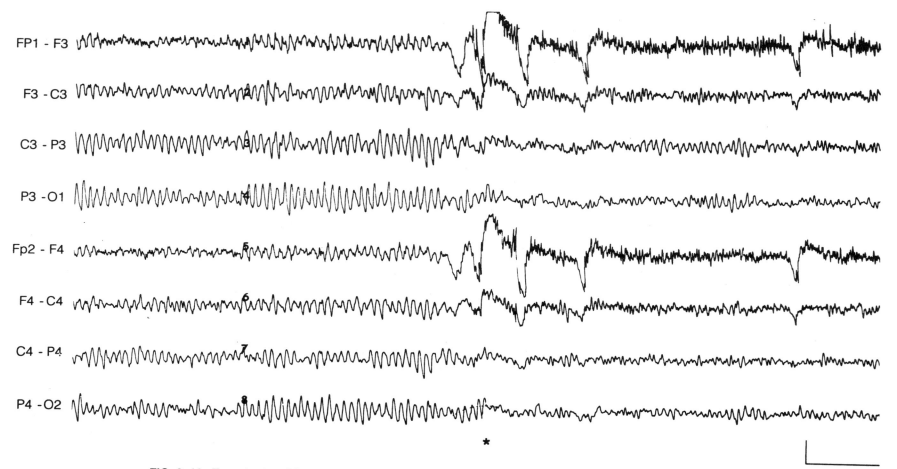

FIG. 3–18. Transient and incomplete alpha attenuation. 80 years. Eye opening (*asterisk*) only transiently attenuates the alpha activity, but such attenuation is sufficient to reveal beta activity (F3-C3, F4-C4) which was not evident while the eyes were closed because of the very considerable anterior extent of the alpha field. Beta activity combines with muscle activity in Fp1,2-F3,4 derivations. Note the minimal parasagittal theta activity in recordings of most normal elderly subjects. Calibration signal 1 sec, 50μV.

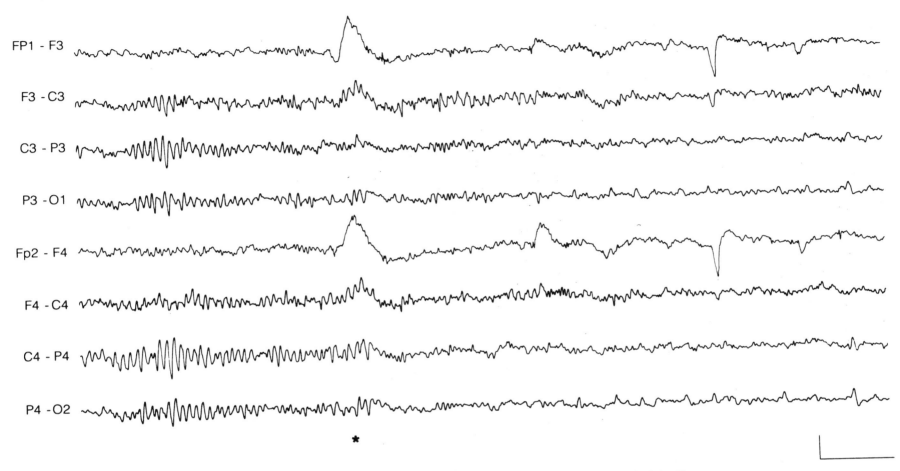

FIG. 3–19. Eye opening abolishes alpha activity. 25 years. Alpha activity is completely abolished by eye opening (*asterisk*), revealing 12 Hz and 25 Hz central rhythms which were partially hidden by the anterior extent of the alpha field when the eyes were closed. The principally electropositive monophasic or diphasic occipital potentials are lambda waves. Note the normal amount of 2–3 Hz very low-voltage delta activity, more evident with eyes open. Calibration signal 1 sec, 50μV.

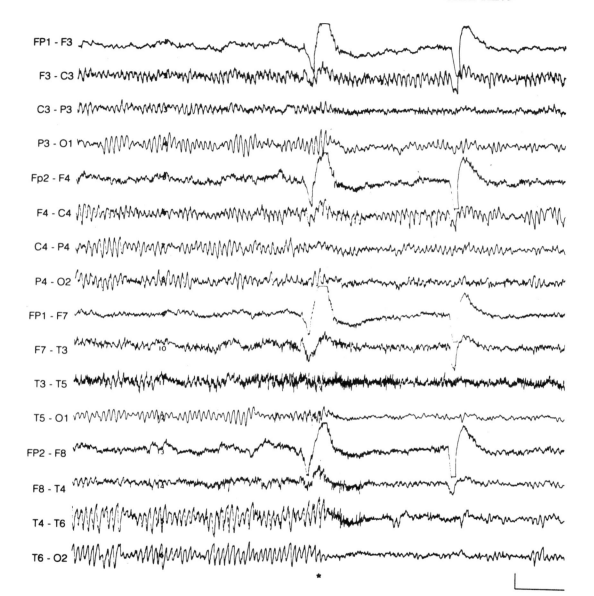

FIG. 3–20. **Eye opening reveals mu.** 18 years. Eye opening (*asterisk*) attenuates alpha activity, revealing a prominent mu rhythm at about the same frequency (10 Hz) as that of the alpha. Note that the left side mu rhythm appears principally at C3-P3 as evidenced by the downward deflection of the sharply contoured component at F3-C3, the electrical cancellation at C3-P3, and the corresponding upward deflection of the sharply contoured component at P3-O1. On the right, the mu field is more confined to C4 as there is no cancellation between C4 and P4. However, in each instance the field extends to the parietal regions (P3, P4), creating the false impression that the alpha has not fully attenuated. The lack of alpha at the T5-O1 derivation and its minimal presence at the T6-O2 derivation reveal the attenuation. Calibration signal 1 sec, 50μV.

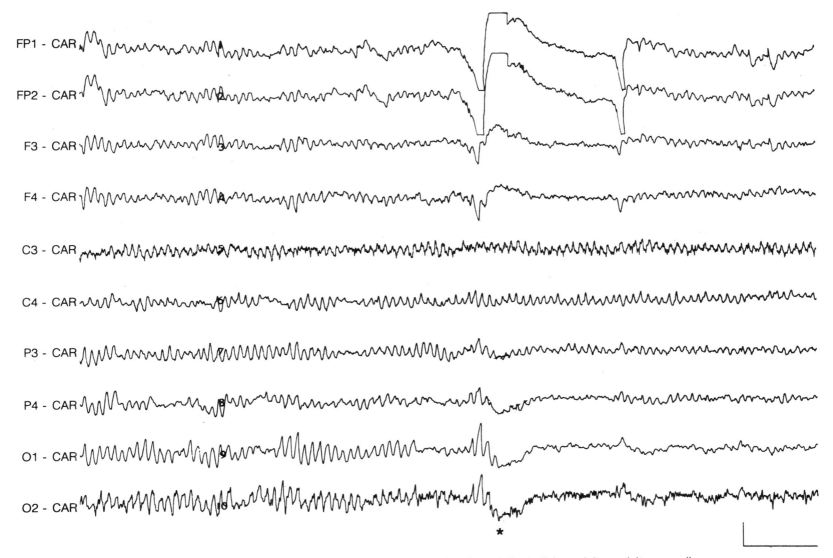

FIG. 3–21. Eye opening reveals mu. 18 years. Eye opening (*asterisk*) abolishes alpha activity, revealing a prominent mu rhythm bilaterally at the C3, C4 and P3, P4 regions. Although the alpha activity was completely abolished in the first 2 seconds after eye opening, the 10 Hz rhythm seen in the frontal derivations with the common average reference (CAR) suggests a minimal return of a diffuse 10 Hz rhythm which may partially cancel with the CAR in the occipital derivations but not in the frontal ones. Muscle potentials contaminate the mu rhythm at C3 and occipital potentials at O2. Calibration signal 1 sec, 70μV.

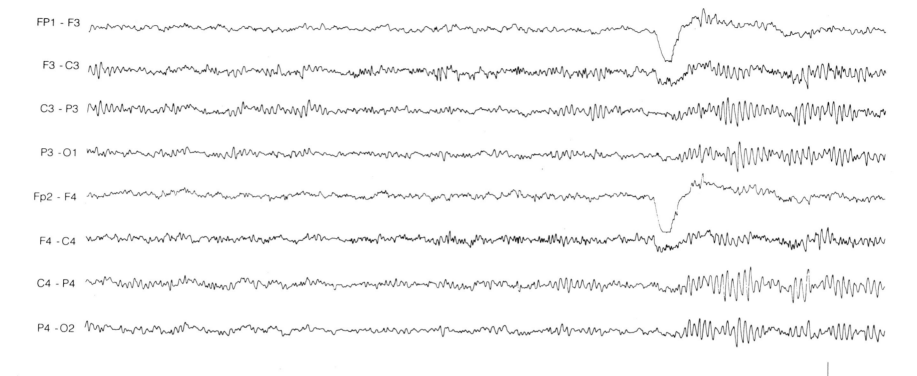

FIG. 3–22. Amorphous, then well organized normal EEG. 25 years. No abnormality appears in either the amorphous portion of this recording with the eyes open or in the more conventional-appearing portion with the eyes closed. Adequate central rhythms appear on either side with the eyes open; the slight left predominance has therefore no significance. At least part of the posterior delta activity may represent a pulse artifact; without any disturbance in posterior background activity, this delta activity should not be considered an abnormality. Calibration signal 1 sec, 50μV.

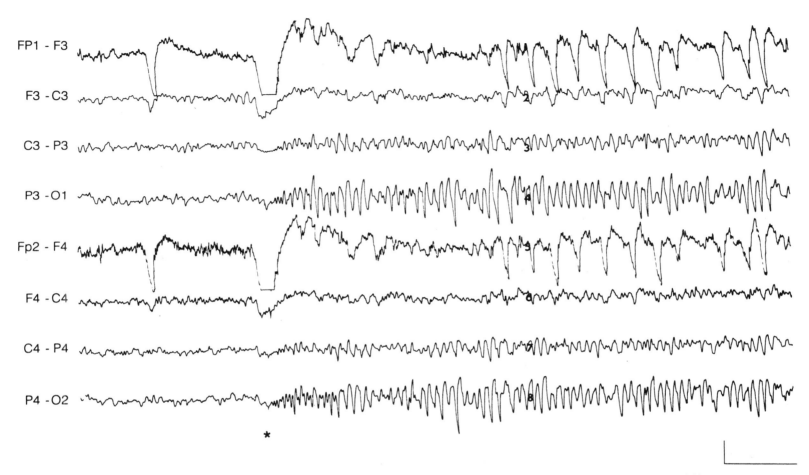

FIG. 3–23. Fast alpha variant. 32 years. Here, 20–25 Hz occipital waves appear upon eye closure (*asterisk*), largely replaced by alpha activity at the usual frequency within 1 second. Abundant eye blink artifacts appear at Fp1, Fp2. Calibration signal 1 sec, 50μV.

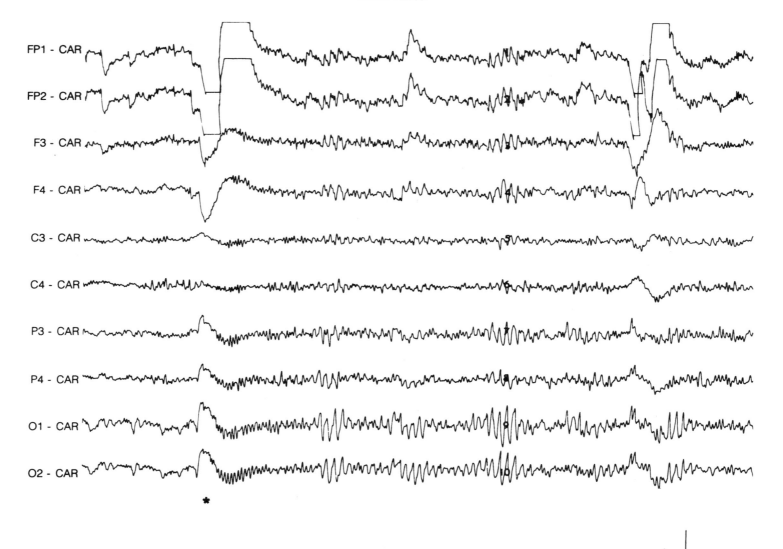

FIG. 3–24. Fast alpha variant on eye closure. 37 years. The fast alpha variant, a posteriorly situated beta rhythm that attenuates upon eye opening and which may be particularly prominent upon eye closure, combines with usual frequency alpha activity to create sharply contoured wave forms. Note the principally electropositive lambda waves in the occipital derivations in the first second prior to eye closure. The prominent upward deflecting potentials in the occipital and parietal derivations represent common average reference involvement of the eye blinks and are opposite in phase to those in the frontal derivations. The diffuse theta and minimal beta are well within acceptable normal limits. Calibration signal 1 sec, 50μV.

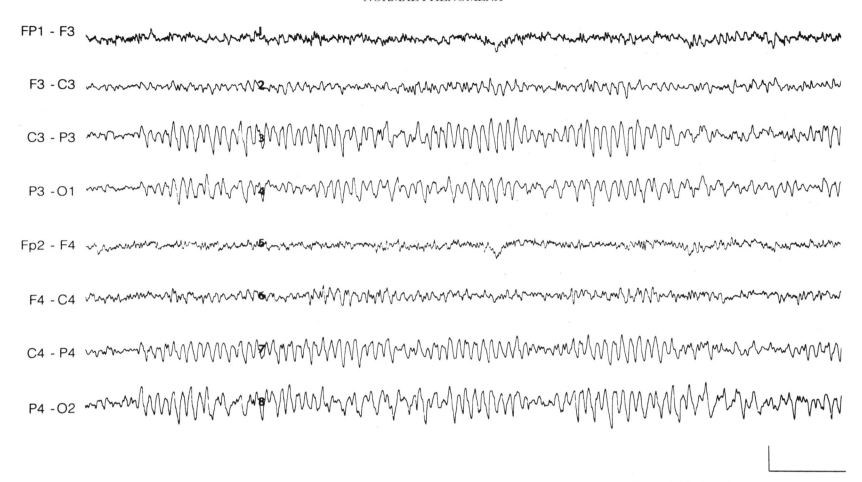

FIG. 3–25. Slow alpha variant. 67 years. This saw-toothed morphology may be created by the partial fusion of two alpha waves, creating a notched wave form at half the usual alpha frequency. This usually, but not always, appears with drowsiness. Note the usual alpha frequency in the C3-P3 and C4-P4 derivations, which is suddenly approximately halved in the P3,4-O1,2 derivations. The apiculate component of the alpha rhythm appears principally in the negative phase of the alpha waves, downgoing in this instance. Calibration signal 1 sec, 50μV.

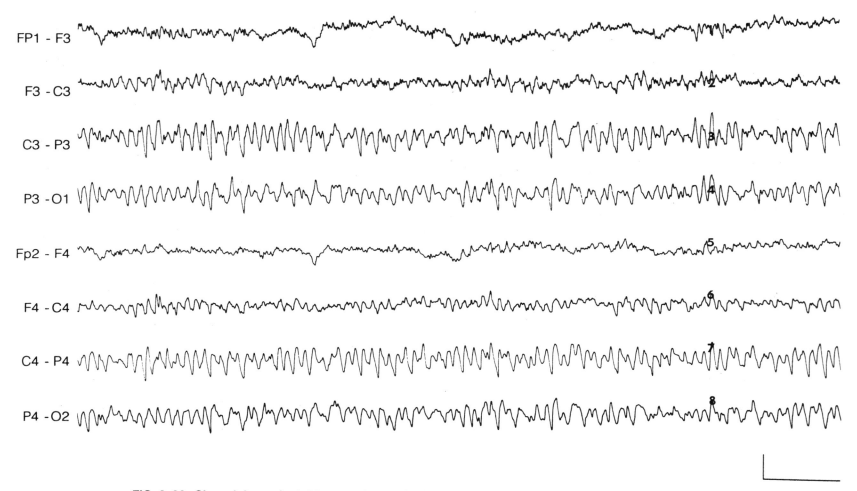

FIG. 3–26. Slow alpha variant. 60 years. An epoch where most of the alpha activity appears in the slow alpha variant form and is an entirely normal phenomenon. Delta activity in the frontal polar derivations represents slow eye movements. Calibration signal 1 sec, 50μV.

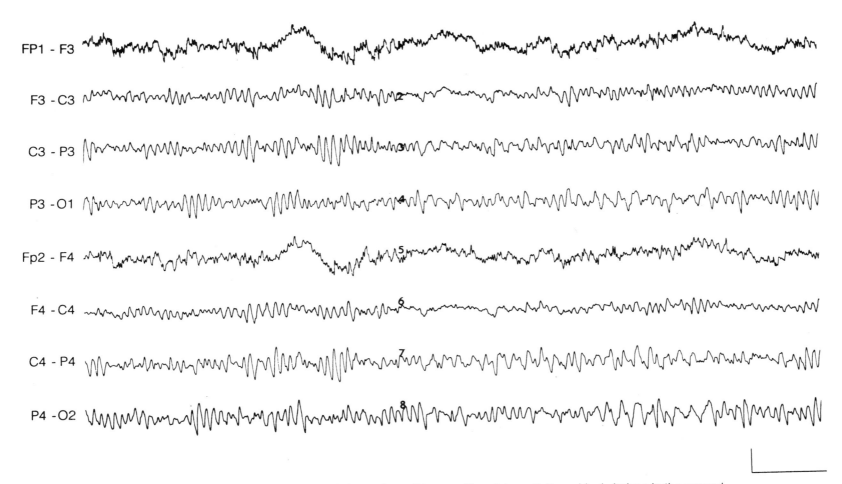

FIG. 3–27. Normal alpha and slow alpha variant. 27 years. The alpha activity suddenly halves in the second half of this segment, creating the slow alpha variant morphology which bears some resemblance to the "psychomotor variant" pattern. Slow eye movements and muscle artifact produce the wave forms in the frontal polar derivations. Calibration signal 1 sec, 50μV.

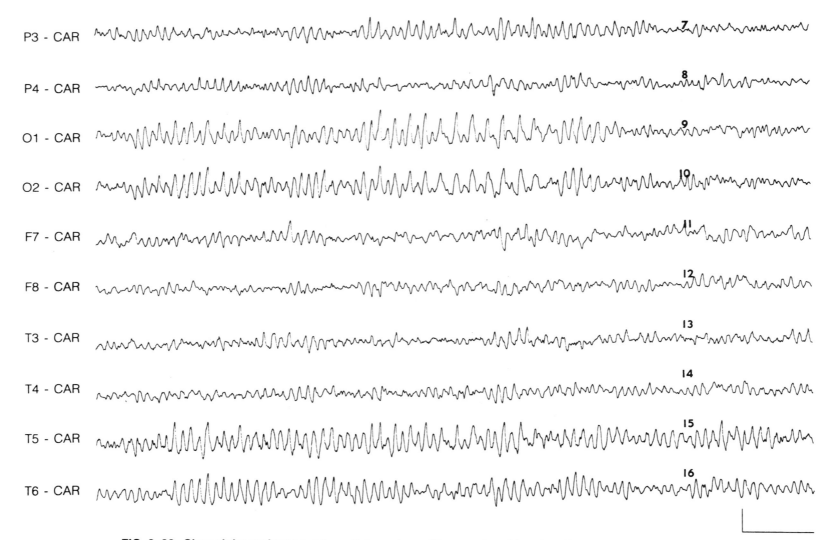

FIG. 3–28. Slow alpha variant on referential montage. 60 years. A sudden virtual halving of alpha frequency, creating the notched slow alpha variant form at occipital (O1, O2) and minimally at posterior temporal (T5, T6) regions. The apiculate component occupies the negative phase of the alpha rhythm, as was seen in the previous bipolar examples. Calibration signal 1 sec, 70µV.

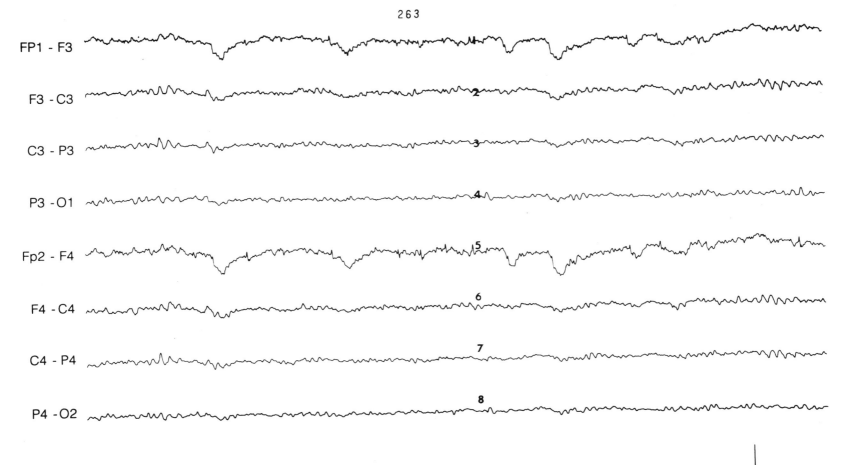

FIG. 3–29. Low-voltage alpha. 24 years. A minority of normal subjects may have minimal alpha activity. As seen in the first 2 seconds, the paucity of alpha allows the normal amount of theta to become more evident. The low-voltage "spikes" at Fp1 and Fp2 are orbicularis oculi muscle potentials. Calibration signal 1 sec, 50μV.

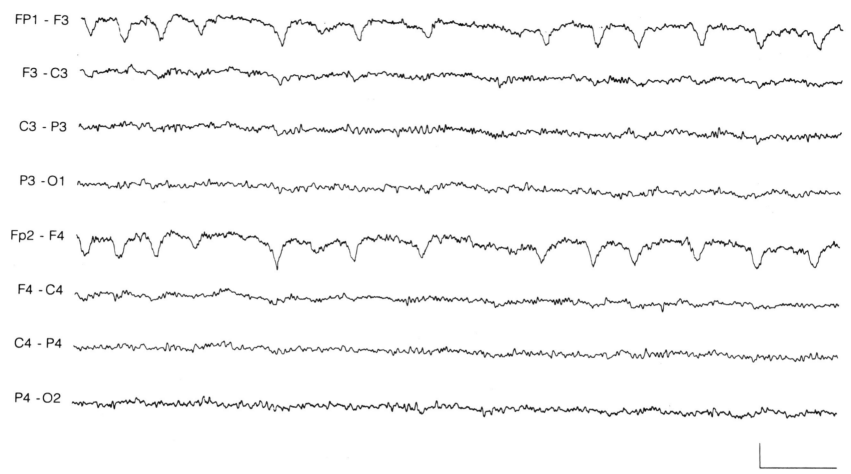

FIG. 3–30. Low-voltage alpha. 70 years. Minimal alpha activity allows other normal potentials to appear, such as diffuse beta and low-voltage delta. Calibration signal 1 sec, 50μV.

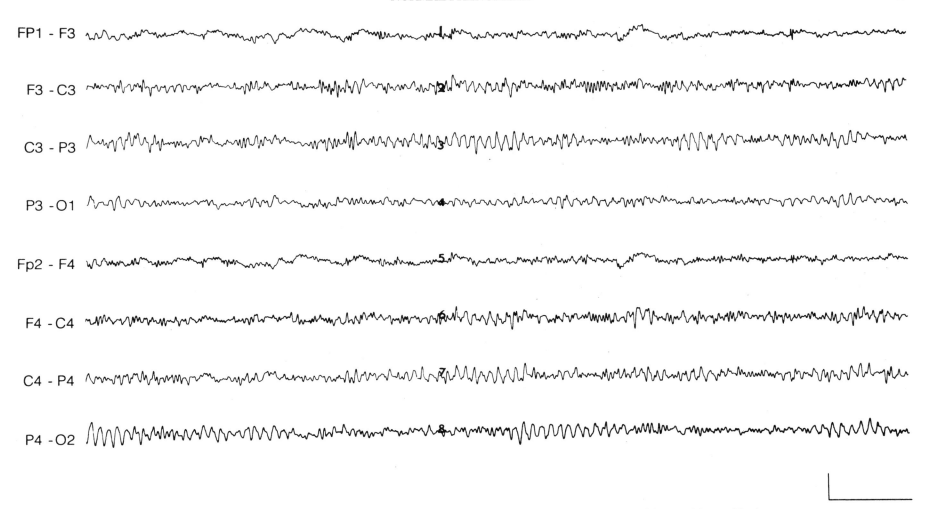

FIG. 3–31. Normal alpha and beta activity. 37 years. A small amount of diffuse beta activity combines with alpha activity to produce an arciform shape of the latter. Calibration signal 1 sec, 50μV.

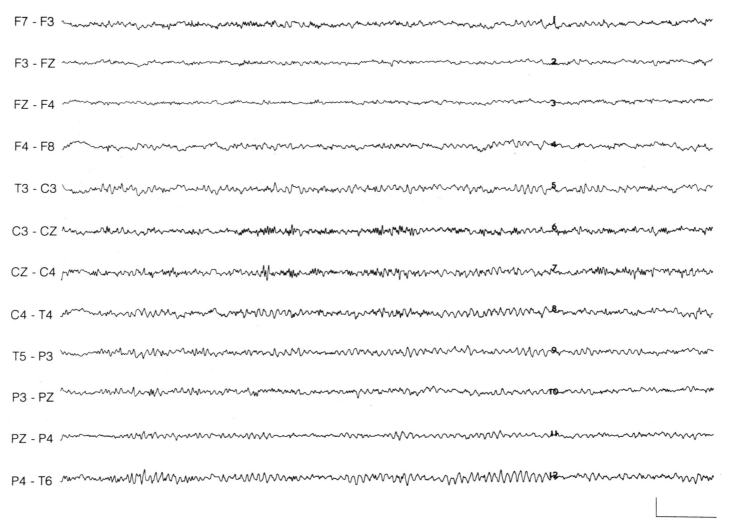

FIG. 3–32. Central beta. 39 years. Low-amplitude 20 Hz beta activity appears at the central vertex (Cz) and minimally diffusely in this coronal montage in an awake subject with the eyes closed. Its combination with a 9 Hz central rhythm produces occasional apiculate wave forms which are not spikes. Note the relative paucity of frontal activity as recorded on this montage. Note also the partial cancellation of alpha activity at the P3-Pz and Pz-P4 derivations, due to the widespread field of alpha activity. Calibration signal 1 sec, 50μV.

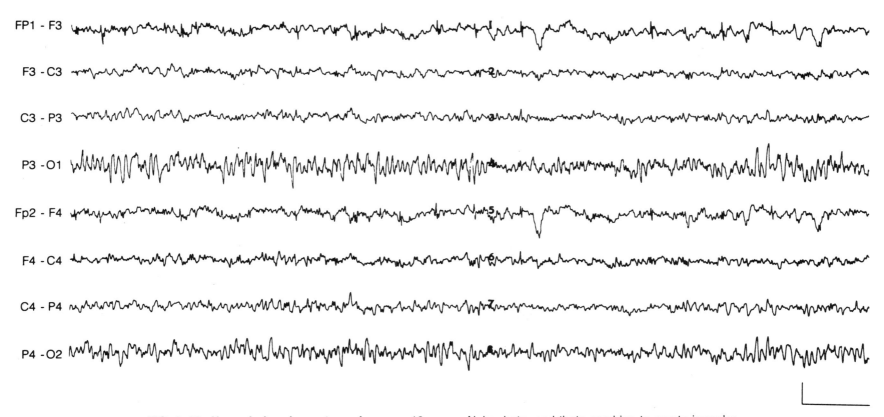

FIG. 3–33. Normal sharply contoured waves. 19 years. Alpha, beta, and theta combine to create irregular, sharply contoured wave forms, particularly in derivations containing occipital leads. The slightly higher alpha activity in the left hemisphere compared to the right is not abnormal because the alpha frequency is virtually the same in each hemisphere, the alpha abundance is adequate on each side, and there are no focal abnormalities. The very brief apiculate potentials in the frontal polar (Fp1,2) derivations (with occasional minimal spread to F3 and F4) represent orbicularis oculi muscle potentials. Calibration signal 1 sec, 70μV.

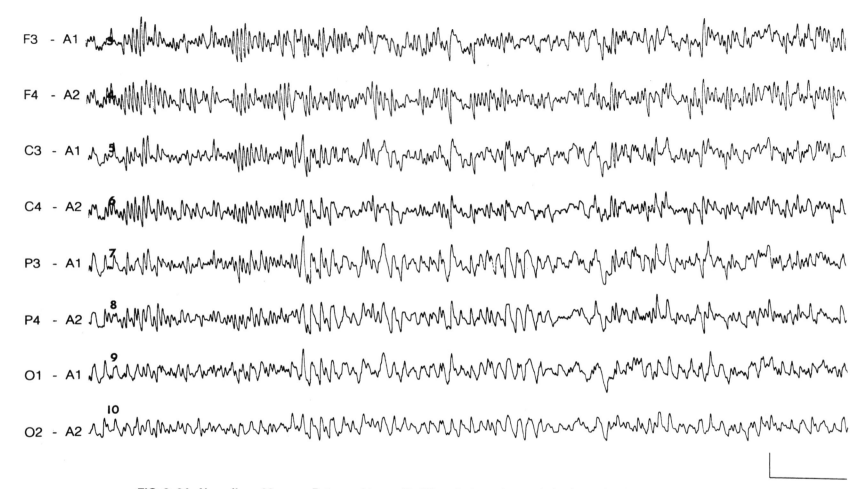

FIG. 3–34. No spikes. 23 years. Beta combines with diffuse theta and posteriorly situated alpha to produce many sharply contoured waves, none of which is a spike. These background components partially obscure the V-wave in the 5th second. Calibration signal 1 sec, 70μV.

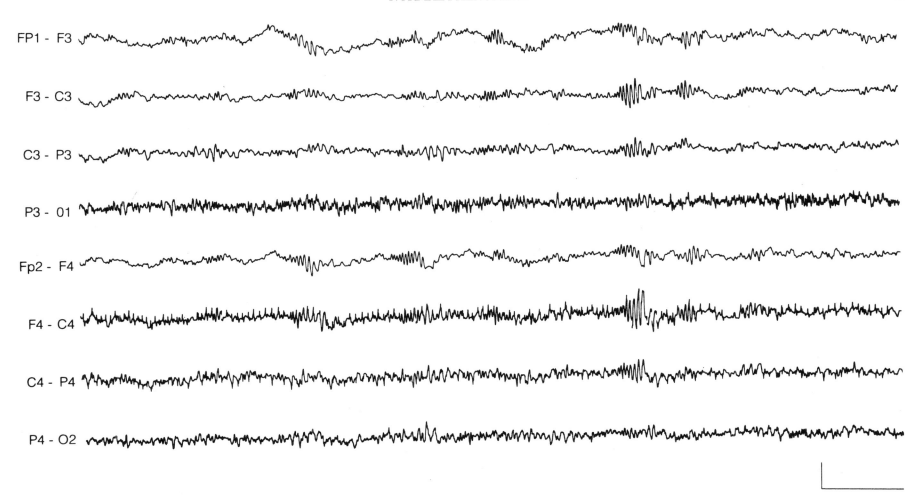

FIG. 3–35. Normal bursts of beta activity. 67 years. Amplitudes of beta activity can fluctuate suddenly, producing bursts superficially resembling polyspikes. The gradual crescendo of amplitude, the more sinusoidal wave form as opposed to spikes, and the lack of a prominent succeeding delta wave are clues that such phenomena are beta and not polyspikes. Muscle activity complicates the morphology in several channels. Calibration signal 1 sec, 50μV.

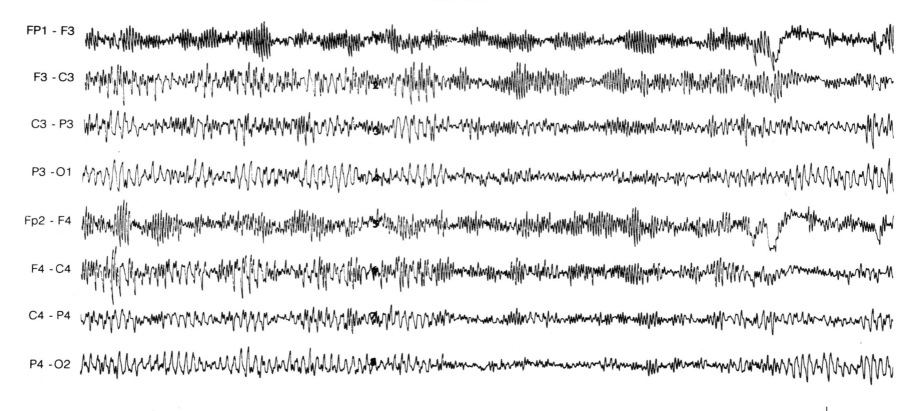

FP1 - F3

F3 - C3

C3 - P3

P3 - O1

Fp2 - F4

F4 - C4

C4 - P4

P4 - O2

FIG. 3–36. Beating of beta. 55 years. As does alpha, the amplitude of beta activity may wax and wane in a regular fashion, producing a "beating" appearance. Note that its combination with 10 Hz alpha (or mu) produces a particularly apiculate appearance in the first 5 seconds. Calibration signal 1 sec, 50μV.

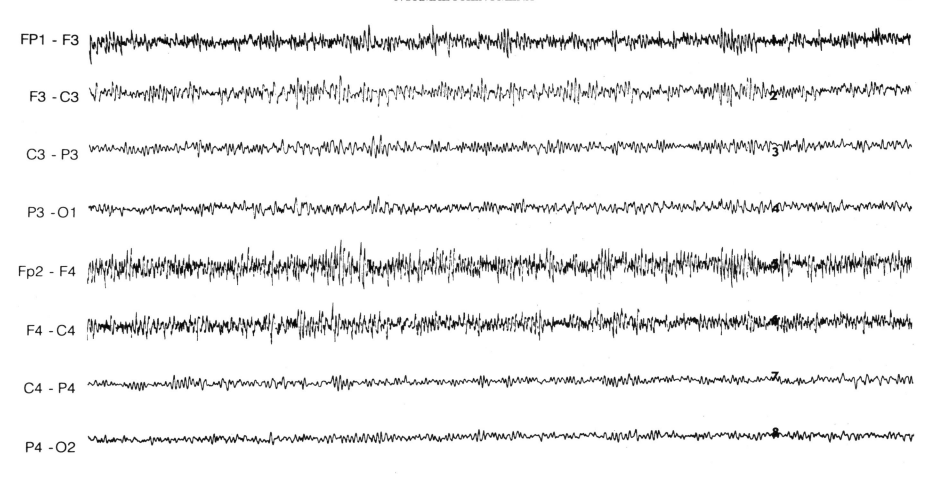

FIG. 3–37. Beta activity and muscle artifact. 55 years. Right frontal muscle artifact joins beta activity to produce a particularly dense appearance. This combination is only minimally present in the left frontal (Fp1-F3) derivation. Calibration signal 1 sec, 70μV.

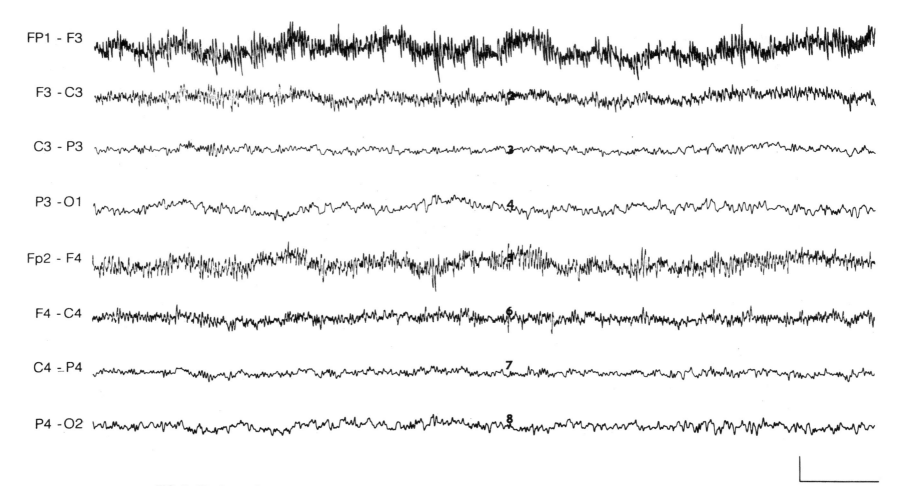

FIG. 3–38. Amorphous normal EEG. 18 years. When no rhythm, such as alpha activity, dominates a recording, the virtually equal competition of other waves for prominence creates a disorganized appearance. Artifacts such as head movement and frontalis muscle complicate the occipital and frontal rhythms, respectively. The lack of alpha activity reveals a normal amount of posteriorly situated beta and theta activity. Consider whether any abnormality is clearly evident; if not, the EEG should be interpreted as normal, as in this instance. Calibration signal 1 sec, 50μV.

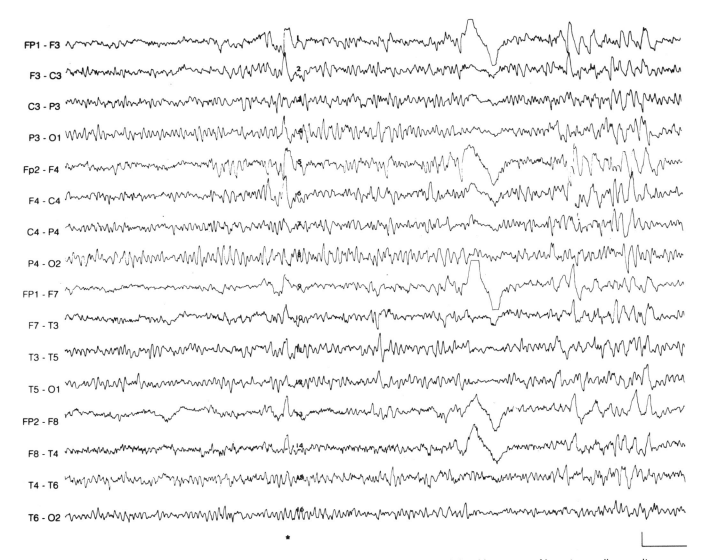

FIG. 3–39. Early hyperventilation response. 21 years. Initially, only a minimal increase of low- to medium-voltage theta activity appears joined (*asterisk*) by a single "projected" high-voltage theta wave. Then the quantity of theta augments for about 6 seconds before another, more sustained high-voltage theta burst occurs. The superimposition of hyperventilation (HV)-associated waves upon the resting background activity produces many sharply contoured waves, none of which is a spike. The single bifrontal delta wave between theta bursts is an eye opening-closing artifact. Calibration signal 1 sec, 50μV.

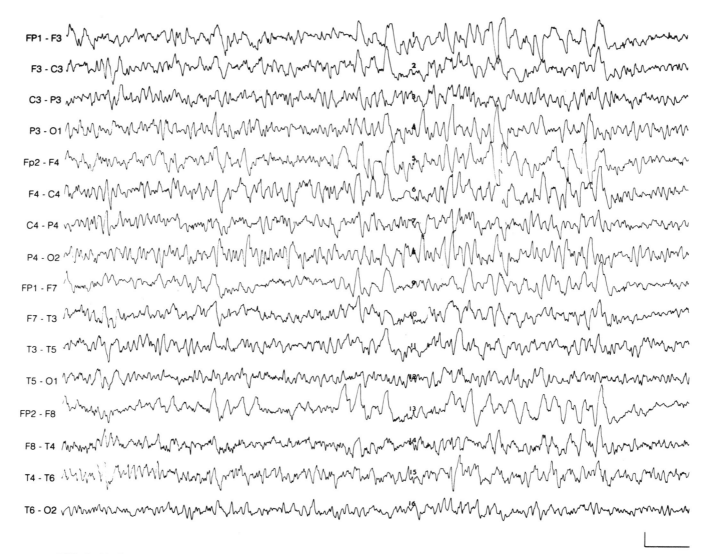

FIG. 3–40. Late hyperventilation. 21 years. More sustained high-voltage theta and delta whose amplitude shifts from side to side. Once again, the multiple sharply contoured waves are not spikes. Very slow delta activity at F7 and F8 are lateral eye movements, as they remain persistently out-of-phase. Calibration signal 1 sec, 50μV.

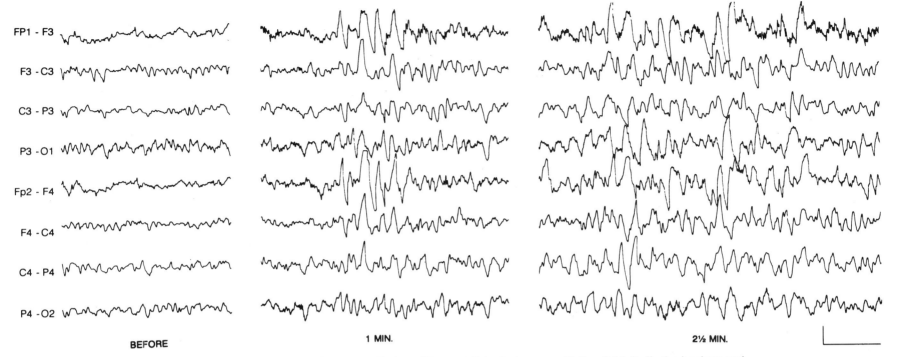

FP1 - F3

F3 - C3

C3 - P3

P3 - O1

Fp2 - F4

F4 - C4

C4 - P4

P4 - O2

BEFORE   **1 MIN.**   **2½ MIN.**

FIG. 3–41. Before, early, late hyperventilation. 17 years. Prior to hyperventilation (HV) (*left*), the background activity consists of alpha (*far left*), "slow alpha variant" (*far right*) and bilateral mu rhythm. Bursts of 200–300 msec high-voltage waves with intermingled sharply contoured waves characterize the early (1 minute) HV period (*center*); none of these sharply contoured waves could be considered a definite spike. Such high-voltage waves appear more persistent during late (2 1/2 minutes) hyperventilation (*right*). The magnitude of the HV response is not a criterion of its normality but is greater in youth, with hypoglycemia, and with HV effort. Calibration signal 1 sec, 50μV.

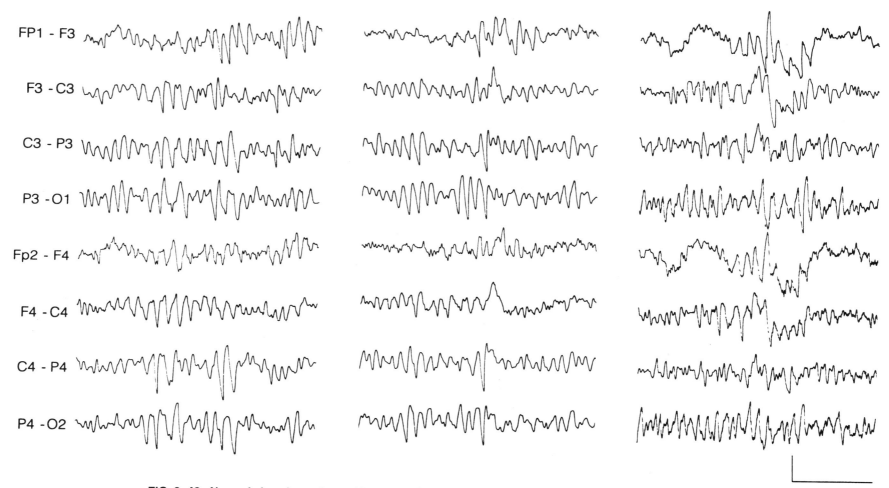

FIG. 3–42. Normal sharply contoured hyperventilation responses. 32 years. None of the bursts in these tracings contains a spike or spike-wave; instead, each is a result of the superimposition of hyperventilation-induced wave forms upon background activity. Calibration signal 1 sec, 50μV.

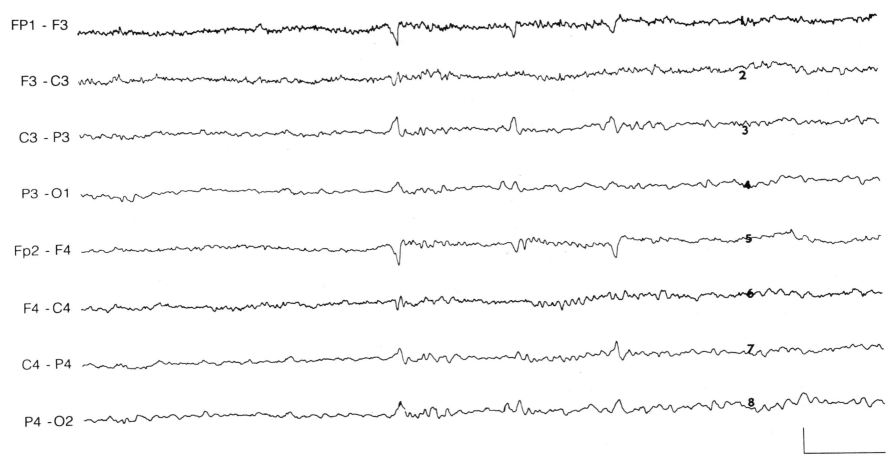

FP1 - F3

F3 - C3

C3 - P3

P3 - O1

Fp2 - F4

F4 - C4

C4 - P4

P4 - O2

FIG. 3–43. Light sleep after hyperventilation. 46 years. Hyperventilation and photic stimulation can occasionally be followed by non-REM sleep, as occurred here (6, 7). Note the symmetrical V-waves and low-amplitude 12 Hz spindles, the latter slightly more evident in the right hemisphere compared to the left. Calibration signal 1 sec, 70μV.

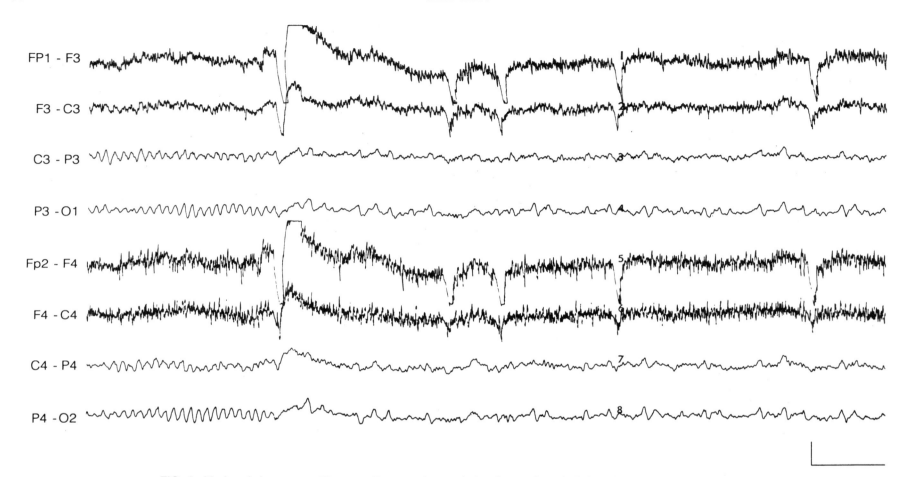

FIG. 3–44. Lambda waves. 62 years. Eye opening and visual scanning abolishes the alpha rhythm and produces bilaterally synchronous, primarily electropositive diphasic or triphasic waves whose positive phase lasts 100–200 msec. Although lambda waves spread to the parietal regions, their location is primarily occipital. Calibration signal 1 sec, 50μV.

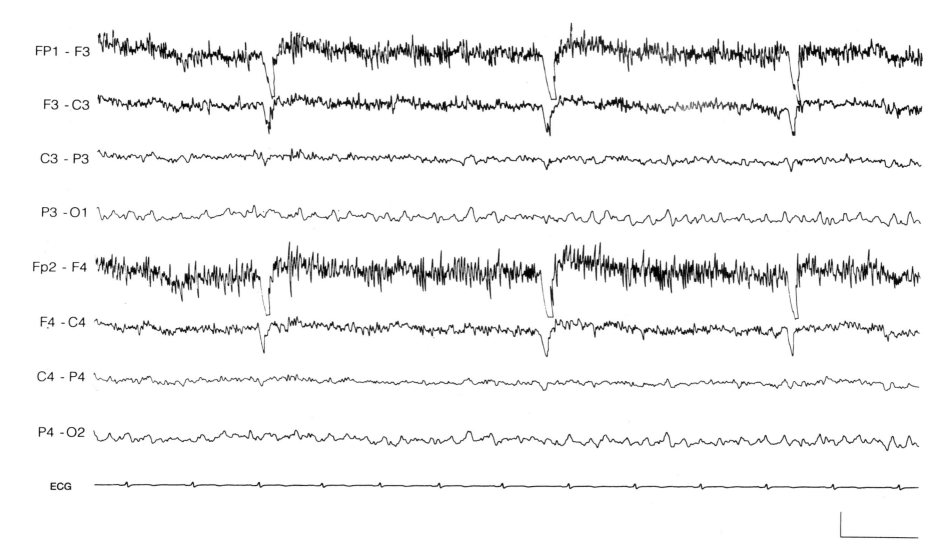

FIG. 3–45. Continuous lambda. 23 years. Virtually continuous lambda activity distinct from ECG potentials in an alert subject whose eyes are open and who is presumably scanning his visual field. Calibration signal 1 sec, 50μV.

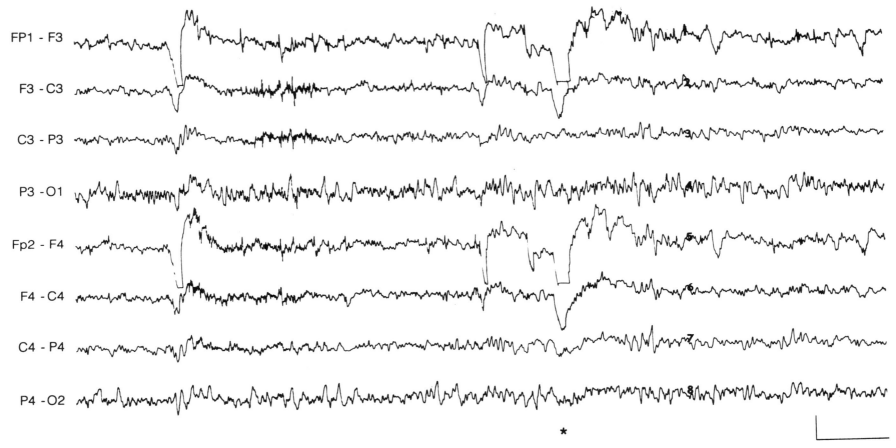

FIG. 3–46. Lack of abnormality equals normality. 19 years. Prominent lambda waves combine with beta activity in the occipital derivations to create a highly irregular but normal background activity. Eye closure (*asterisk*) has minimal effect because of the small amount of alpha activity present in this apparently anxious subject. Eye movements and frontal muscle potentials create irregular waves in the frontal polar derivations. A normal amount of theta activity, diffuse beta activity, and a burst of muscle potentials from swallowing add to the havoc. However, no abnormality can be identified. Calibration signal 1 sec, 70μV.

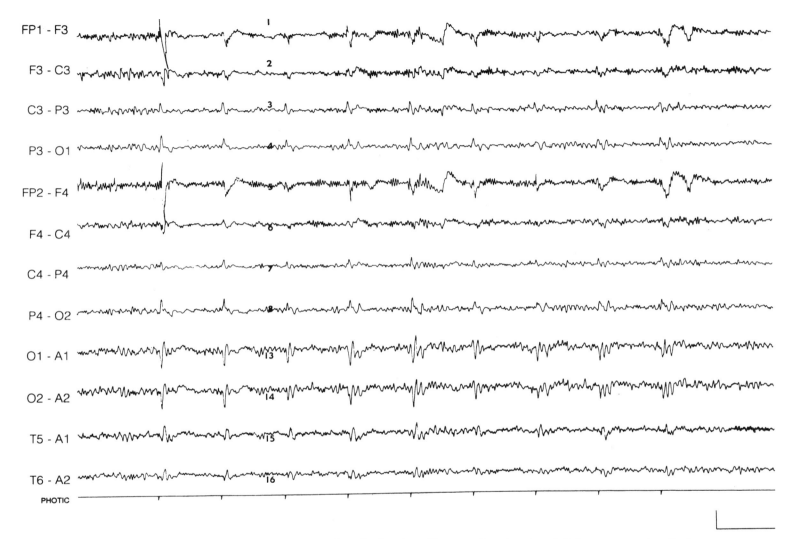

FIG. 3–47. Prominent photic response at low flash rates. 23 years. Prominent occipital response to low flash rates with the eyes open in an earlier-illustrated subject with prominent lambda waves suggesting a similar mechanism. Note the anterior extension of this response. Artifact at Fp1, Fp2 at 2 seconds. Calibration signal 1 sec, 70μV.

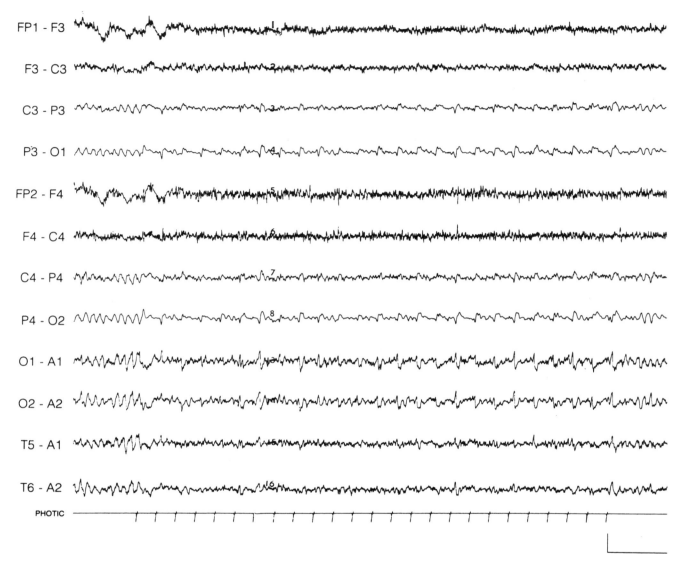

FIG. 3–48. Photic following response. 62 years. Prominent biphasic occipital response to low flash rate, which occurs in subjects with relatively prominent lambda, suggesting a similar mechanism. Muscle artifact obscures the frontal region activity bilaterally. Calibration signal 1 sec, 50μV.

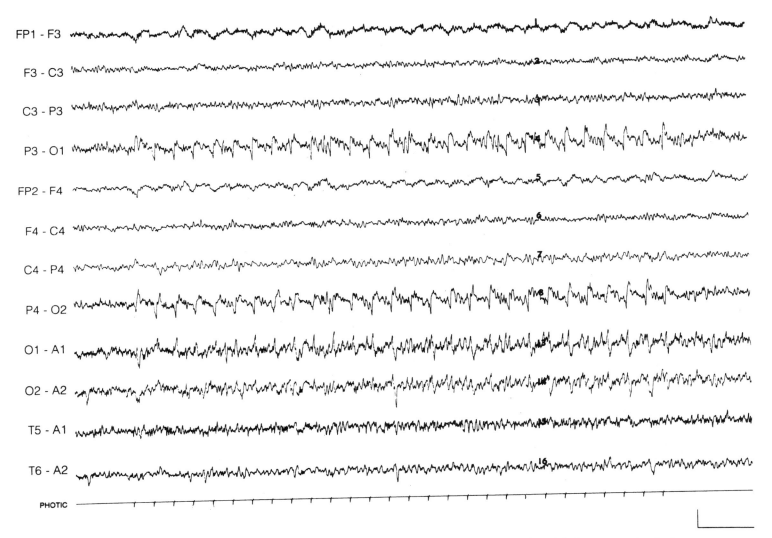

FIG. 3–49. Prominent photic response in the elderly. 77 years. The time-locked occipital response to photic driving may be larger in the elderly than in younger adults, as shown here at 3 flashes/sec. This amplitude increase has uncertain clinical significance. Note the prompt cessation of the response with the termination of the flash. Calibration signal 1 sec, 50μV.

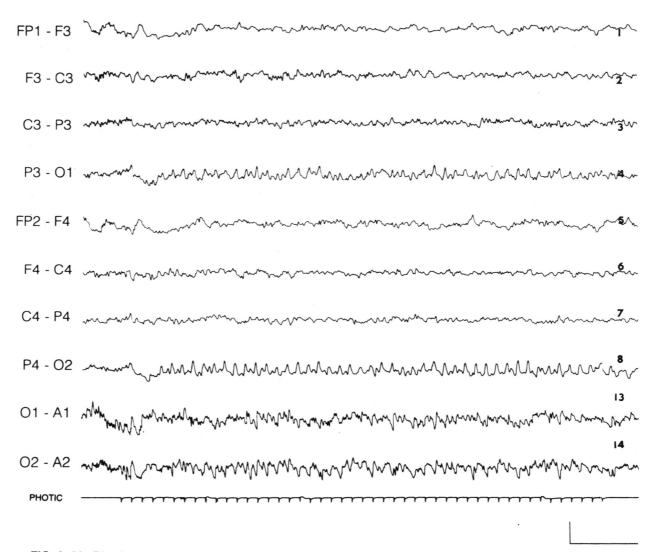

FIG. 3–50. Photic driving response. 40 years. Primarily electropositive diphasic bioccipital response to photic driving at 6 flashes/sec. Calibration signal 1 sec, 50μV.

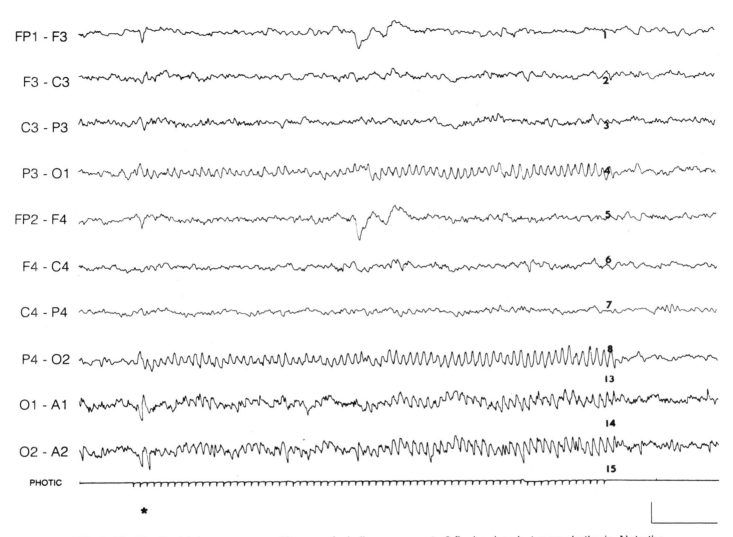

FIG. 3–51. Photic driving response. 40 years. A similar response to 9 flashes/sec but more rhythmic. Note the diffuse primarily electronegative potential at the onset of the flash rate (*asterisk*); this may be a vertex response representing alerting. Calibration signal 1 sec, 50μV.

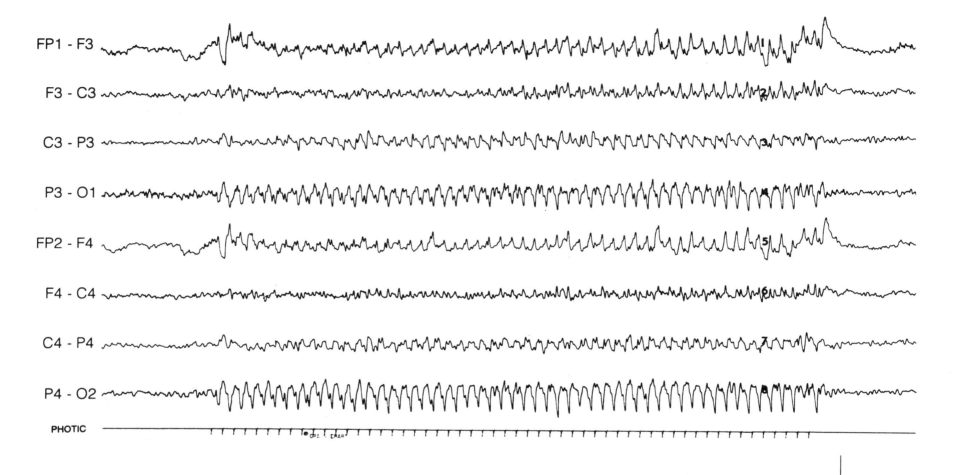

FIG. 3–52. Widespread field of photic driving. 76 years. In some subjects, the field of photic driving may extend far anteriorly, as illustrated here and in Fig. 3–53, without apparent clinical significance. The anteriorly recorded potentials probably do not represent an electroretinogram, because of the approximately 100 msec delay to the peak (8). The photic driving responses in these segments occasionally resemble spike-wave discharges, but these do not represent a photoparoxysmal response, because they are time-locked to the flash stimulus. A prominent bilaterally synchronous high-voltage potential initiates the photic response, termed an "on response." Calibration signal 1 sec, 50μV.

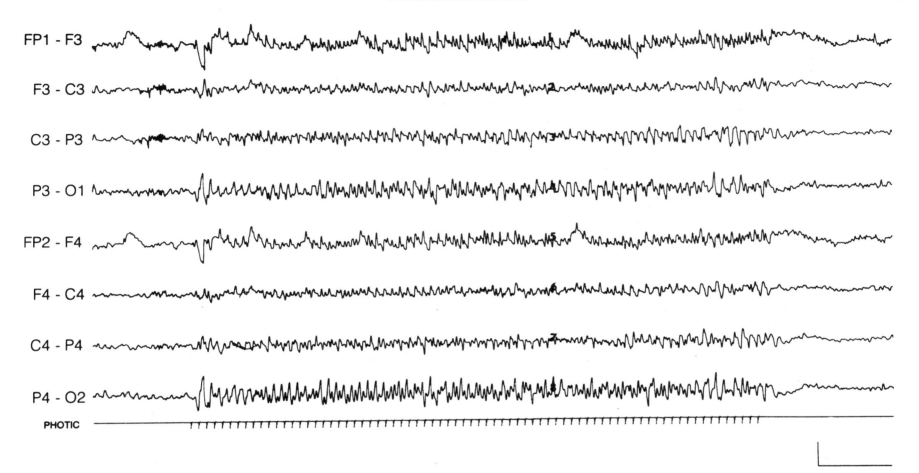

FIG. 3–53. Widespread field of photic driving. 76 years. Similar principles as in Fig. 3–52; including diffuse parasagittal involvement of the photic response, and the initial "on response." In addition, the response in this instance on occasion has double the frequency (20 Hz) as that of the flash rate (10 Hz). This is termed a "harmonic" of the fundamental flash rate and is a normal response. Calibration signal 1 sec, 50μV.

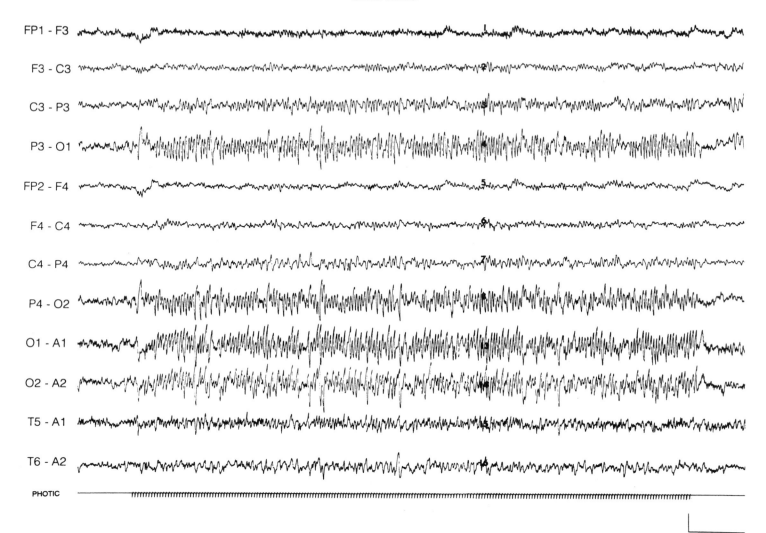

FIG. 3–54. Prominent photic response in the elderly. 77 years. The time-locked occipital response to photic driving may be larger in the elderly than in younger adults, as depicted in these two tracings of the response to 3 and 20 flashes/sec (Fig. 3–49). This amplitude increase has uncertain clinical significance. Note the prompt cessation of the response with the termination of the flash. Morphology of the initial "on" response differs from that of driving at 20/sec. Calibration signal 1 sec, 50 μV.

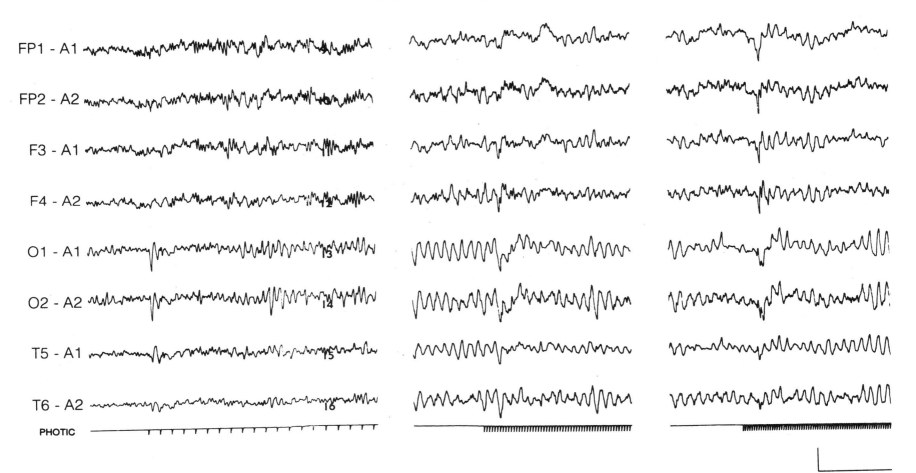

FIG. 3–55. Photic response at higher flash rates. 23 years. The single, immediate responses to higher-frequency (6, 25 and 30 Hz) photic stimulation resemble those to single flashes, whereas the subsequent photic driving at 6 flashes has a different morphology (*left*), and that at 25 and 30 flashes is not detectable (*center, right*). This suggests a different mechanism for photic driving at higher flash rates than that for single flashes and for photic onset, whose mechanism may be closer to that of positive occipital sharp transients of sleep (POSTS) and lambda waves (9). Calibration signal 1 sec, 70μV.

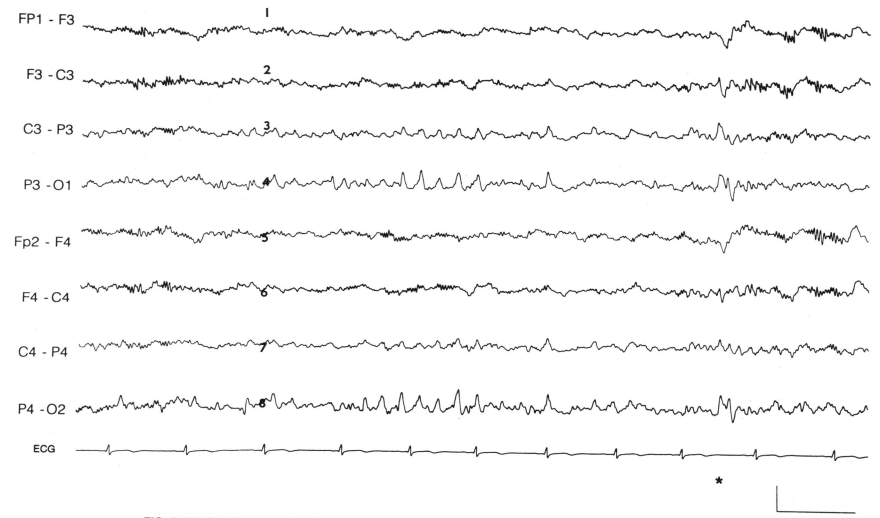

FIG. 3–56. Positive occipital sharp transients of sleep (POSTS) on bipolar montage. 23 years. Prominent single and sequential positive occipital sharp transients of sleep (POSTS) in very light sleep. Note the more widespread low-amplitude V-wave (*asterisk*). Calibration signal 1 sec, 70μV.

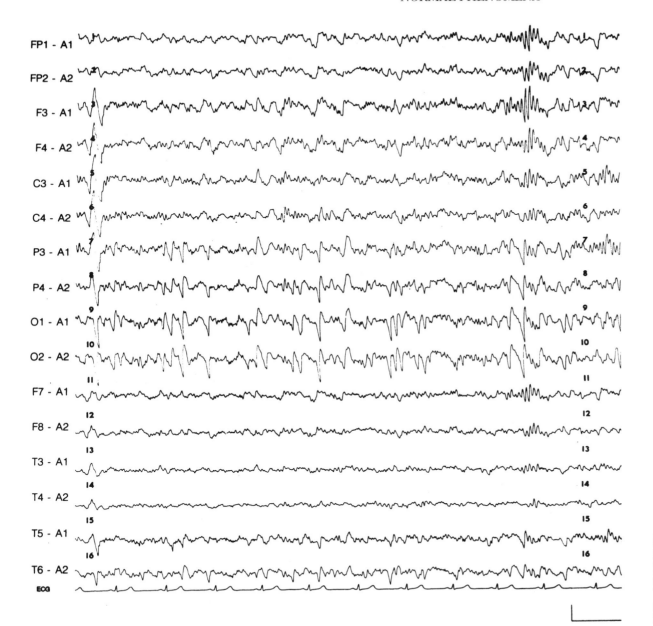

FIG. 3–57. Prominent POSTS. 23 years. Prominent bilaterally synchronous POSTS seen principally in the occipital (O1,O2) positions. The slight and shifting asymmetries have no significance. Their field contrasts with that of the spindle (tenth second) and that of the V-waves (first second). Calibration signal 1 sec, 70μV.

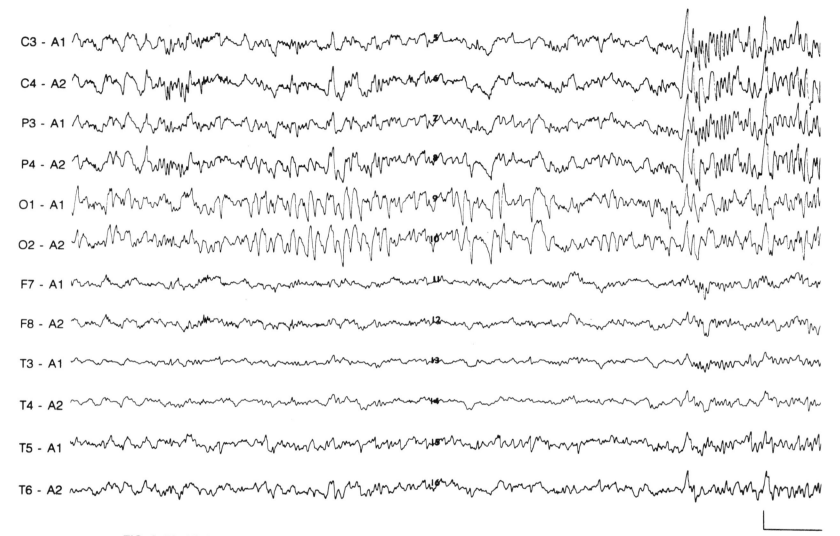

FIG. 3–58. High-frequency POSTS. 18 years. The sequential spike-like occipital waves are POSTS and not conventional spikes, because of the positive polarity of their spike-like potentials and the very minimal involvement of the posterior temporal regions (T5, T6). Note the V-waves and spindles in the last seconds. Calibration signal 1 sec, 50µV.

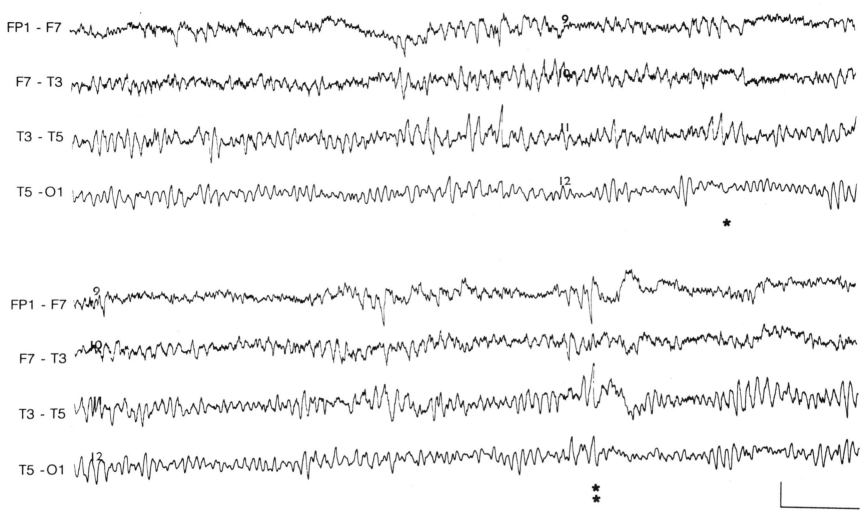

FIG. 3–59. Wicket spikes. 71 years. Described by Reiher and Lebel (10), these arciform temporal apiculate waves appear in clusters or singly in the temporal regions, in either the midtemporal or midanterior temporal area. As seen here, the morphology can present as innocent-appearing wave forms resembling mu (*asterisk*), or their amplitude may increase prominently so that they resemble abnormal anterior temporal spikes (*double asterisks*). The presence of intermediate-amplitude versions of the same phenomenon suggests the presence of a single phenomenon and not two. It can be difficult to make the distinction between the clinically innocent wicket spikes and anterior temporal spikes in some instances, particularly when a prominent aftercoming slow wave appears (*double asterisk*). In practice, we would consider all of these apiculate forms to be wicket spikes. This tracing depicts sequential samples of left temporal activity. Calibration signal 1 sec, 70μV.

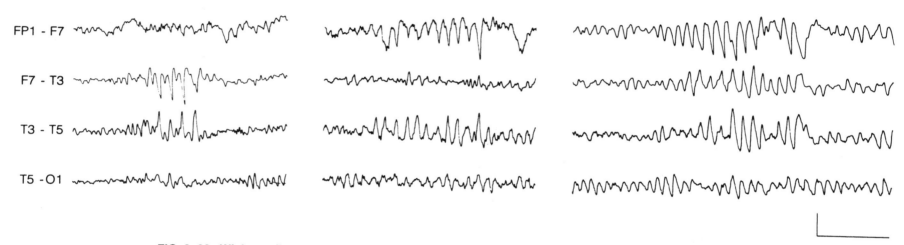

FP1 - F7

F7 - T3

T3 - T5

T5 - O1

FIG. 3–60. Wicket spikes. 21 years. Sequential electronegative wicket spikes at T3, T3-F7, and F7 with spread to T3. All of these wicket spikes appear as the sharply contoured negative components of 6–7 Hz rhythmic waves in the temporal region. Calibration signal 1 sec, 50μV.

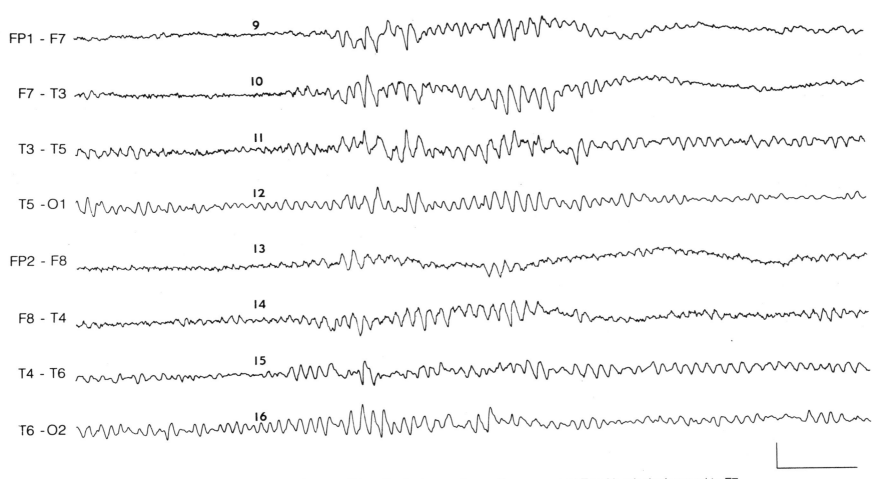

FIG. 3–61. Wicket spikes. 50 years. Primarily electronegative arciform waves at T3 with principal spread to F7 occurring as part of a burst of more sinusoidal 7 Hz bitemporal waves. The slow waves at F7 and F8 represent lateral eye movements. Calibration signal 1 sec, 70μV.

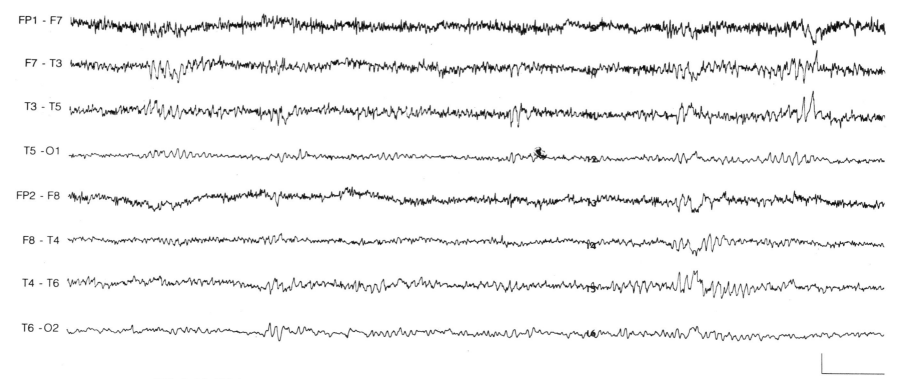

FIG. 3–62. Wicket spikes and theta. 76 years. Similar wicket spikes with theta seen over the left temporal (principally T3) and the right temporal (principally T4) regions, findings with no known clinical significance at this age. Muscle artifact, ever present in the temporal regions in many awake recordings, augments the sharply contoured nature of the wave forms over the left temporal area. Calibration signal 1 sec, 50μV.

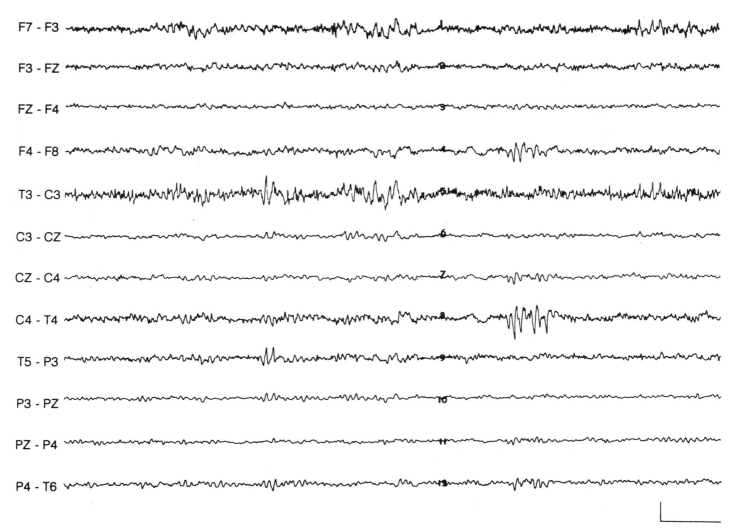

FIG. 3–63. Wicket spikes on coronal montage. 76 years. Wicket spikes, singly or in brief bursts with intermingled theta, appear at T3 and T4. Such discharges occasionally attain a moderately high voltage. Calibration signal 1 sec, 50μV.

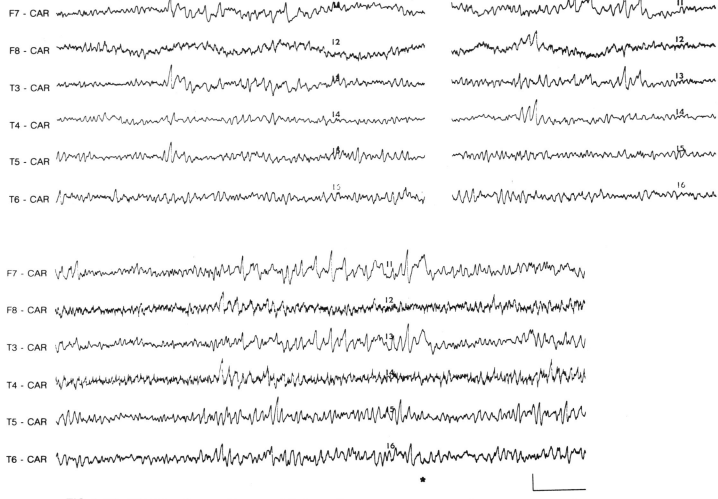

FIG. 3–64. Wicket spikes and temporal theta on the common average reference. 74 years. Once again, gradations between prominent apiculate waves at F7 and T3 and lower-voltage, more innocent-appearing forms occur in association with theta activity at F7 and T3. Again, we would not consider such activity to be definite left temporal spikes. The 400 msec wave (*asterisk*) occurring after the longest sequence of such forms and the intermittent slowing at F7 and T3 earlier in that sequence suggest focal dysfunction in that area, but this does not necessarily mean it is potentially epileptogenic. A sleep recording may distinguish between wicket spikes and abnormal temporal spikes, as only anterior temporal spikes may appear in sleep. Calibration signal 1 sec, 100μV.

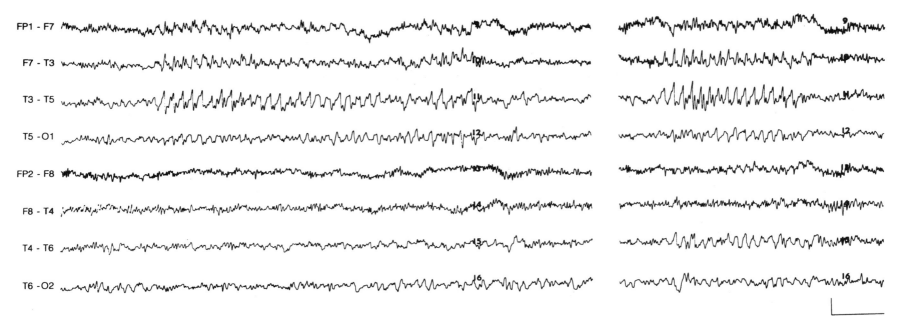

FIG. 3–65. Psychomotor variant. 18 years. Also known by the cumbersome term "rhythmic temporal theta bursts of drowsiness," these phenomena are long runs of sharply contoured, notched, 5–7 Hz waves which appear principally over the mid- or anterior temporal regions. A rhythm twice that of the dominant frequency is usually superimposed, as seen here. The apiculate portion may be slightly broader than that of wicket spikes, and the entire sequences may be more prolonged. However, the morphologies of these phenomena may merge. Calibration signal 1 sec, 50μV.

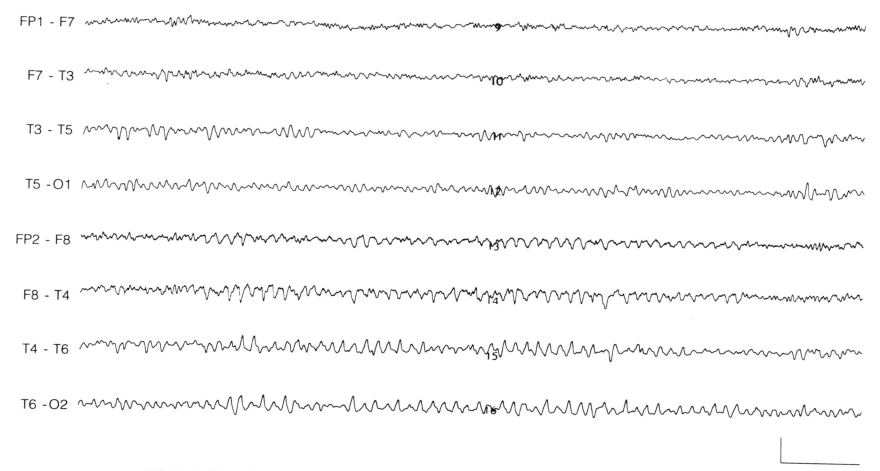

FIG. 3–66. Rhythmic psychomotor variant. 27 years. This tracing illustrates a more rhythmic morphology of psychomotor variant. The morphology does not change as the pattern proceeds; this distinguishes it from a focal seizure. Calibration signal 1 sec, 100µV.

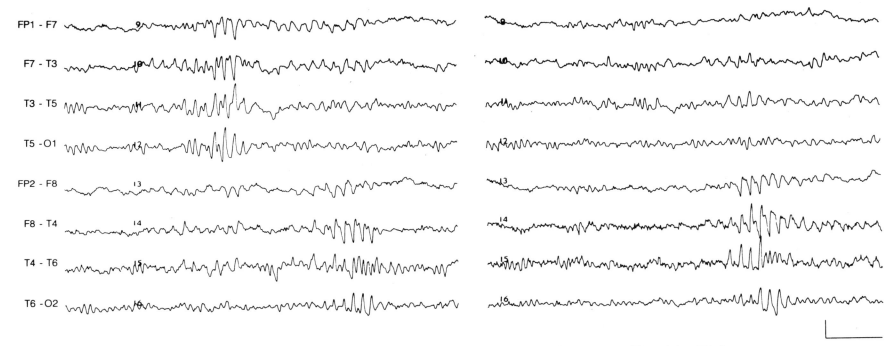

FIG. 3–67. Wicket spikes or psychomotor variant? 21 years. These apiculate waves at T3 and then T4 share morphological characteristics of each phenomenon. In any case, they are normal phenomena. Calibration signal 1 sec, 50μV.

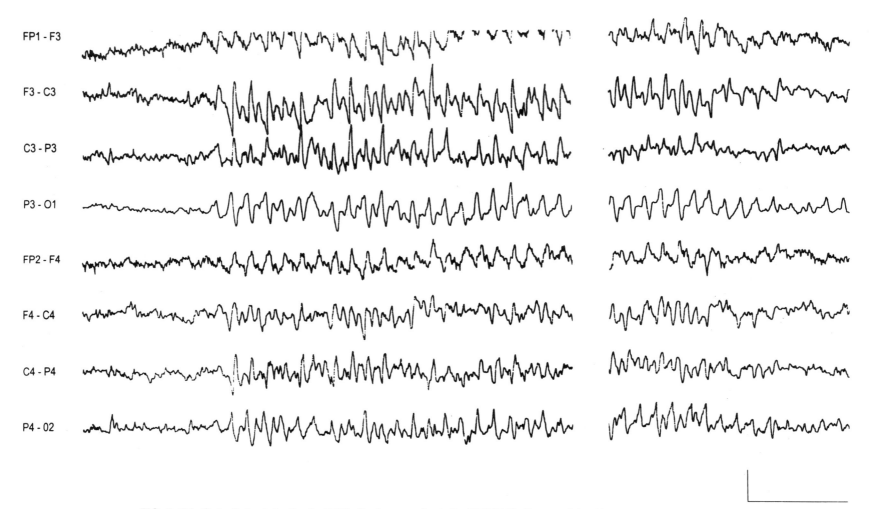

FIG. 3–68. Subclinical rhythmic EEG discharge of adults (SREDA). Sequential 6 Hz apiculate theta bilaterally, maximum at C3-P3. Calibration signal 1 sec, 50μV.

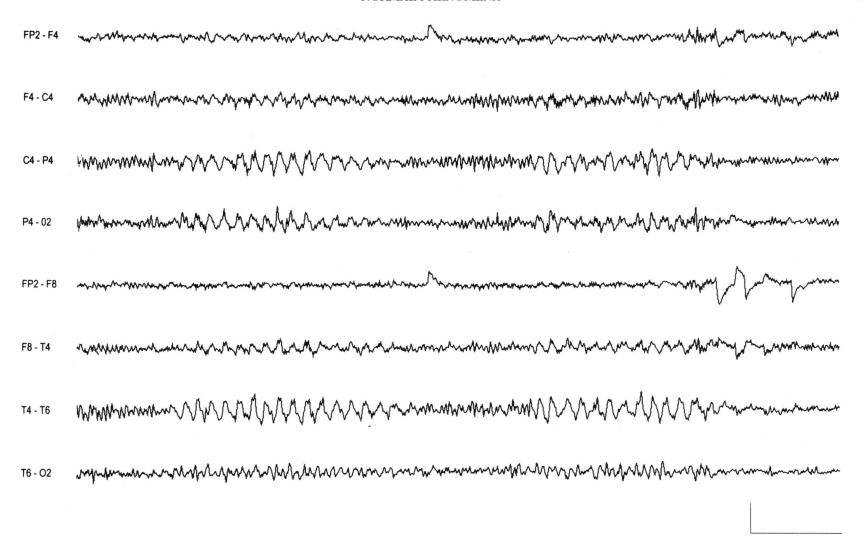

FIG. 3–69. SREDA at slow sweep speed. A speed of 15 mm/sec reveals the waxing and waning property of this phenomenon, seen here principally at the right parietal (P4) region spreading to the right posterior temporal oc-cipital region (T6, O2). Calibration signal 2 sec, 50μV.

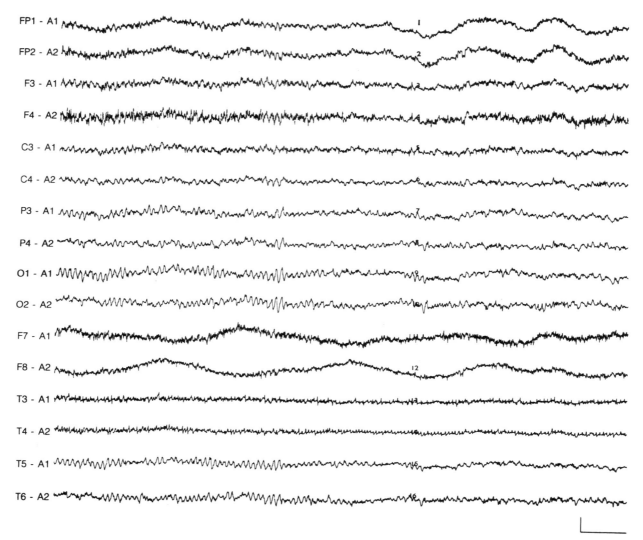

FIG. 3–70. Amorphous drowsy pattern. 62 years. Occasionally, no single EEG feature dominates the pattern: in this instance, theta, beta, muscle, and eye movement artifact all contribute. Slow lateral eye movements appear principally at F7,8, but involvement of A1,2 cause deflections in many other channels. Calibration signal 1 sec, 50μV.

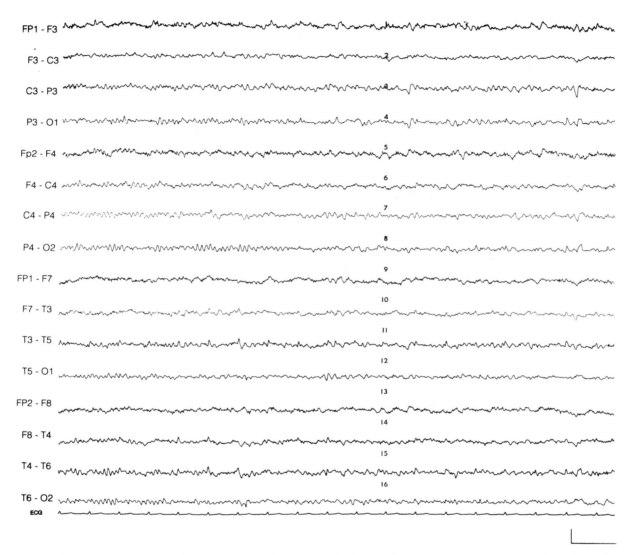

FIG. 3–71. Drowsiness with theta. 19 years. In some subjects, the dominant new wave form in drowsiness is diffuse theta activity. Before stating that a background activity is excessively slow for age, verify that transient drowsiness has not occurred. Scan the record for a more alert period and a higher background (alpha) frequency such as that of the first 5 seconds of this tracing. Calibration signal 1 sec, 50μV.

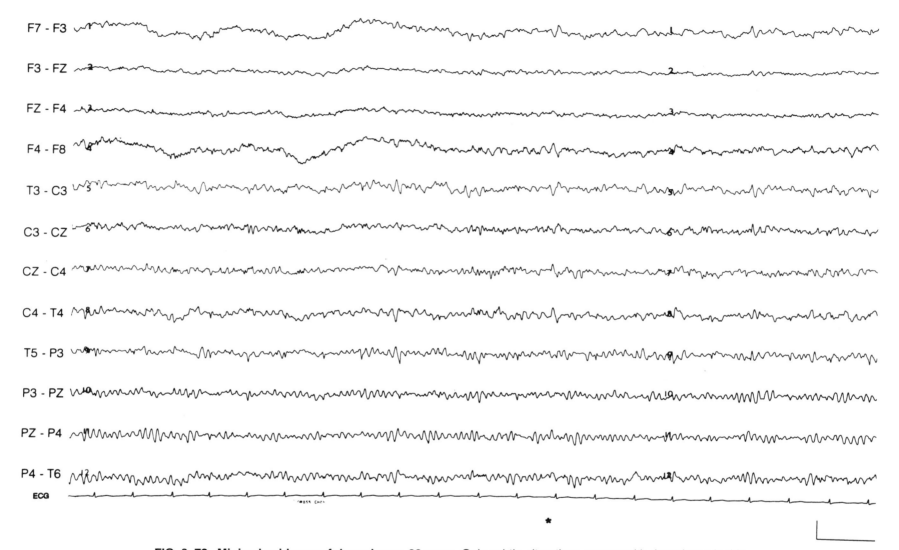

FIG. 3–72. Minimal evidence of drowsiness. 23 years. Only subtle alterations appear with drowsiness in this tracing: the blunt low-amplitude V-wave (*asterisk*), central-frontal theta activity, and slow eye movements are its evidence. Calibration signal 1 sec, 50μV.

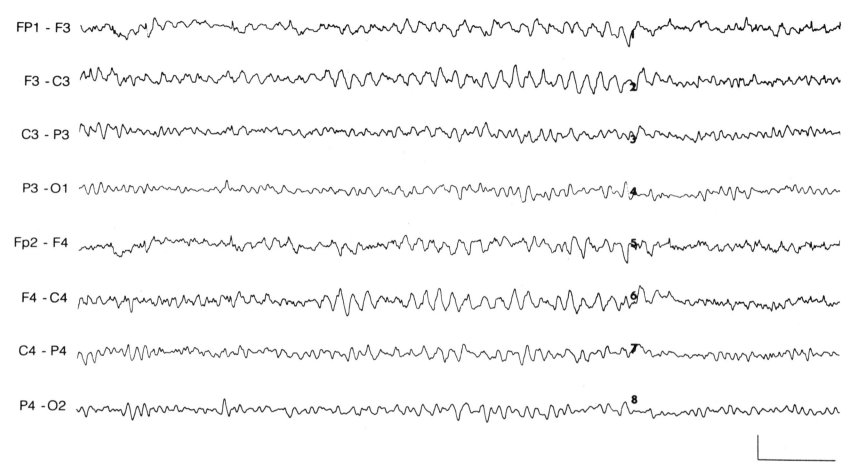

FIG. 3–73. Drowsiness with theta. 27 years. Prominent rhythmic 5–6 Hz theta may characterize drowsiness in some adults, as it commonly does in children. This is not an abnormality. Note the sudden return to wakefulness in the last 3 seconds. Calibration signal 1 sec, 50μV.

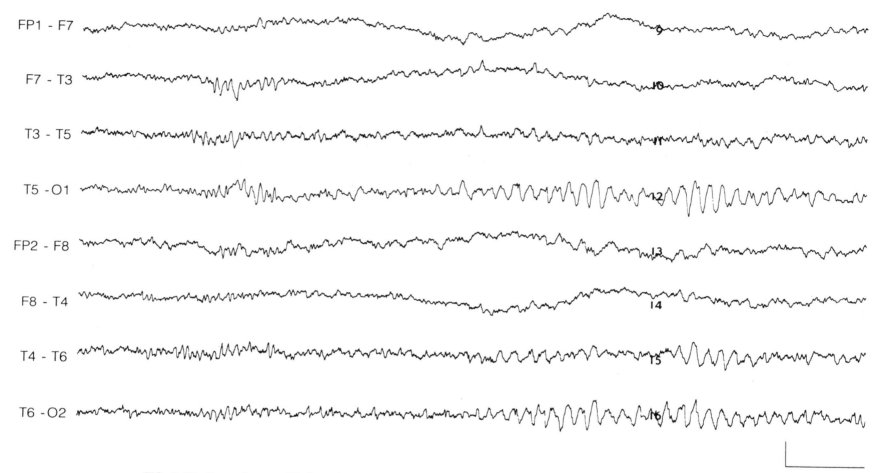

FIG. 3–74. Drowsiness with theta in a temporal montage. 34 years. In this instance, the theta appears posteriorly, replacing an amorphous beta-dominated background. The horizontal nature of the slow eye movements is indicated by the out-of-phase deflections involving the inferior frontal leads (F7, F8). Calibration signal 1 sec, 50μV.

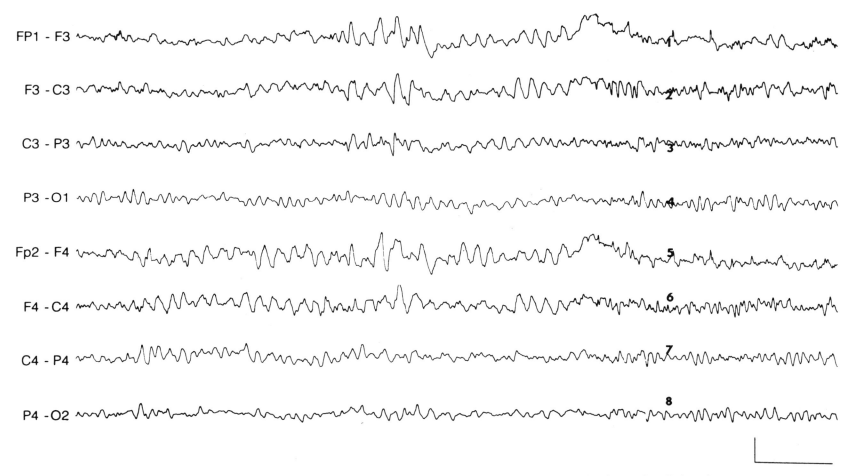

FIG. 3–75. Drowsiness with moderately bursting theta. 27 years. This is an example of occasionally bursting theta in drowsiness. It is unlikely that this constitutes an abnormality, and it may be simply a remnant of the burst pattern of drowsiness of childhood described by Kellaway and Fox (11). Alpha returns in the last few seconds, signifying arousal. Calibration signal 1 sec, 50μV.

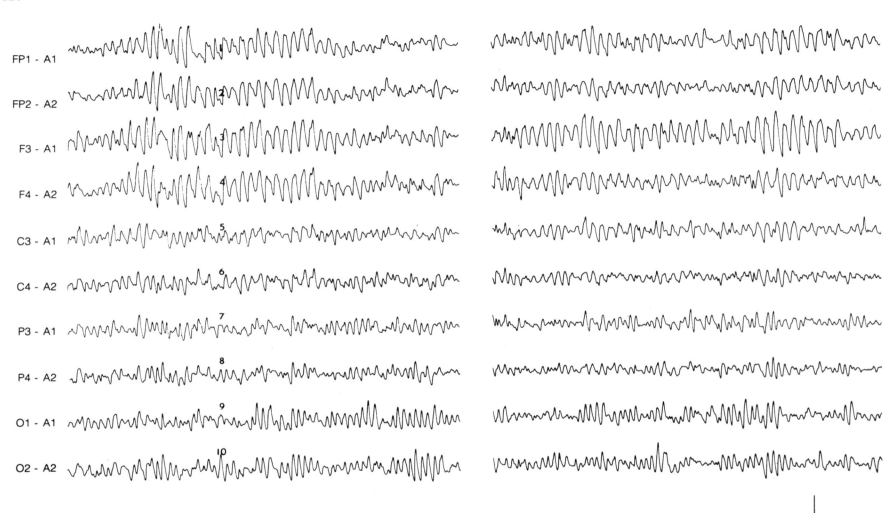

FIG. 3–76. Symmetrical and asymmetrical theta in drowsiness. 17 years. Normal phenomena, which usually appear bilaterally and symmetrically, may also normally appear asymmetrically; this is without clinical significance if no other background abnormality appears. The first segment illustrates symmetrical theta activity anteriorly, and the second segment depicts equally normal but asymmetrical rhythmic theta of drowsiness. Calibration signal 1 sec, 150μV.

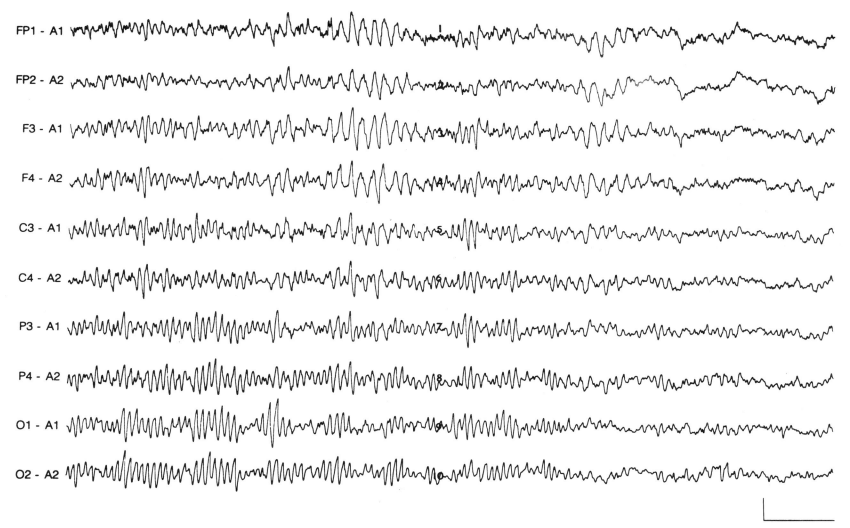

FIG. 3–77. Drowsiness and the ear reference montage. 20 years. Sinusoidal theta occurs in a burst before alpha activity recedes. Calibration signal 1 sec, 70μV.

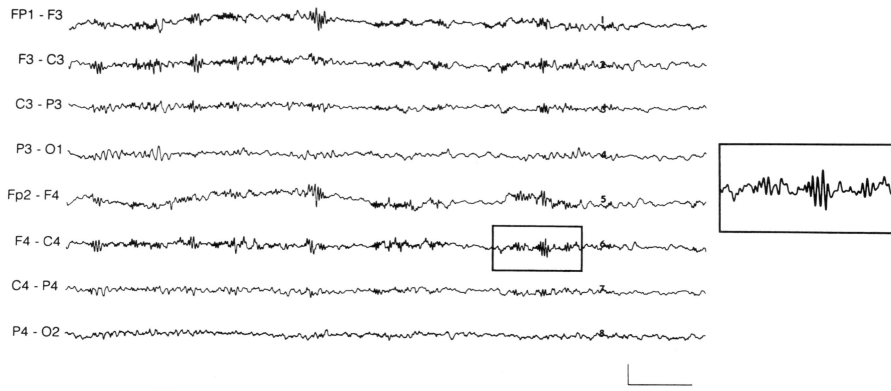

FIG. 3–78. Drowsiness and bursting beta. 41 years. Beta activity can appear in alarming bursts during drowsiness. Some components of each burst are apiculate; yet, these are not polyspikes, in which all components are usually apiculate and are followed by a slow wave. The morphology of beta bursts is depicted in the *square*. Calibration signal 1 sec, 70μV.

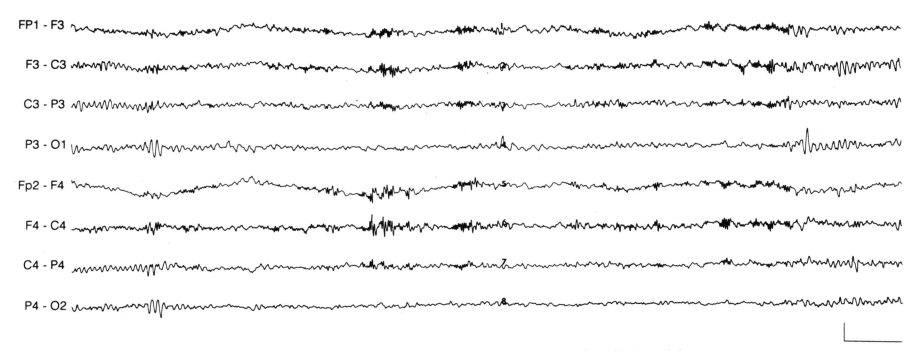

FIG. 3–79. Drowsiness. 41 years. Replacement of alpha with theta, augmentation of beta, and slow eye movements all characterize drowsiness. Note the return to alertness near the end of the tracing. Calibration signal 1 sec, 100μV.

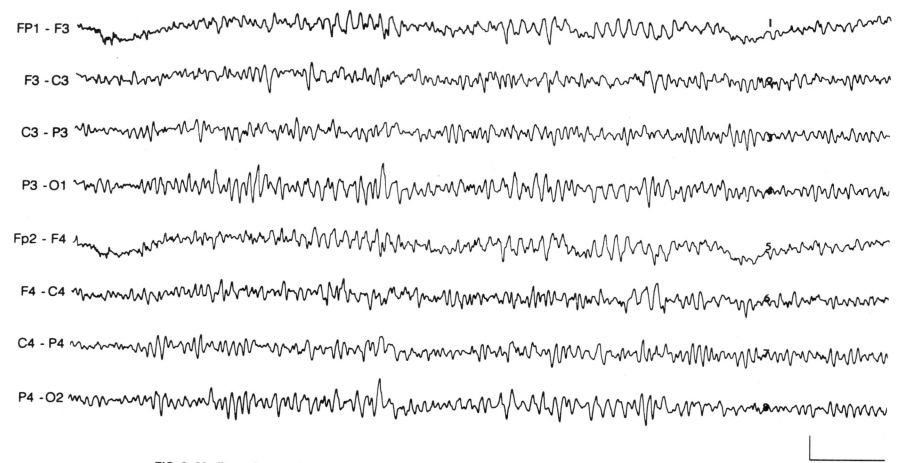

FIG. 3–80. Drowsiness with beta and theta. 20 years. Beta and theta augment together to create an irregular sequence of often apiculate waves in this segment. Note the partial preservation of ongoing alpha activity, upon which the beta and theta are superimposed. Calibration signal 1 sec, 70μV.

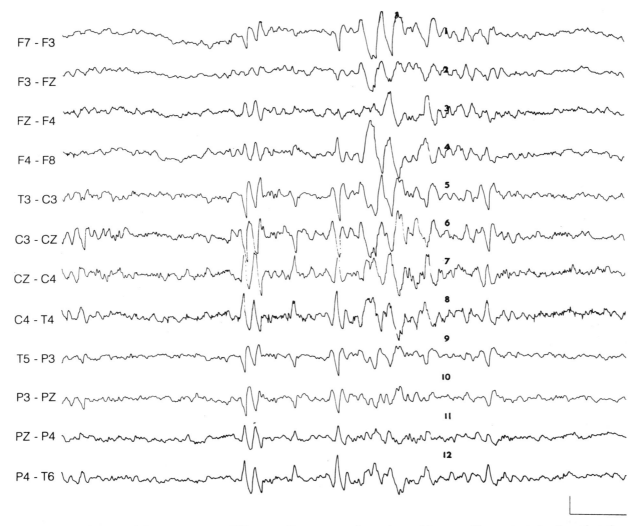

FIG. 3–81. Sequential vertex waves ("V-waves") on coronal montage. 34 years. The main deflection of each wave is electronegative, which is often preceded or followed by an electropositive phase. The morphology varies even within a burst, as seen here. Ongoing higher frequencies of the central region may become superimposed upon the V-waves, creating a "notch" appearance resembling spikes. Calibration signal 1 sec, 70μV.

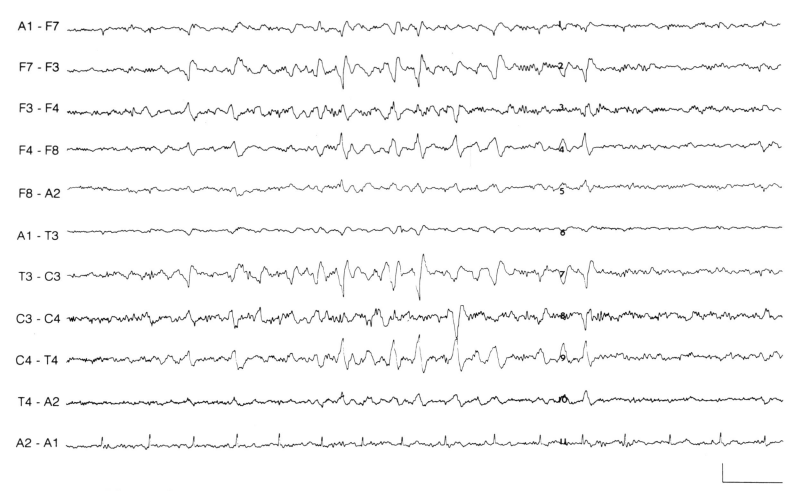

FIG. 3–82. Sequential V-waves in youth. 16 years. Even a reduced sensitivity (100 μV/10mm) fails to diminish the sharply contoured morphology of V-waves, which is their characteristic in youth. The location and morphology vary within this V-wave burst, as is usual. Calibration signal 1 sec, 100μV.

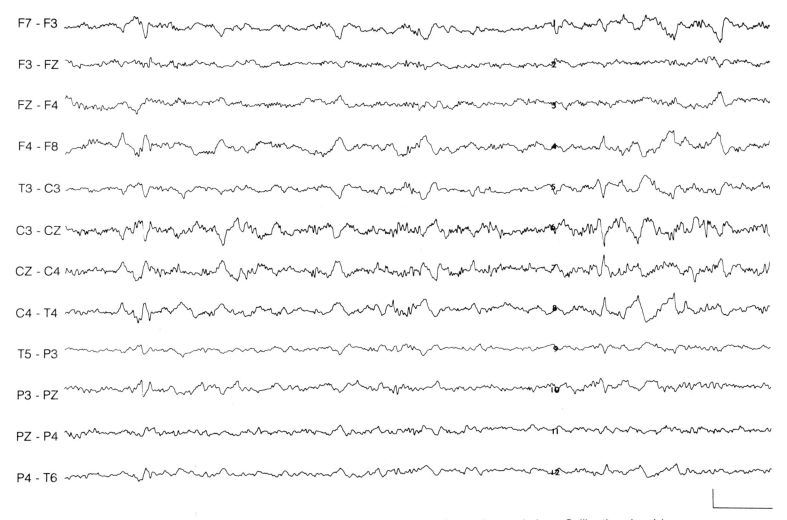

FIG. 3–83. Varieties of V-waves. 21 years. V-waves may normally vary in morphology. Calibration signal 1 sec, 70μV.

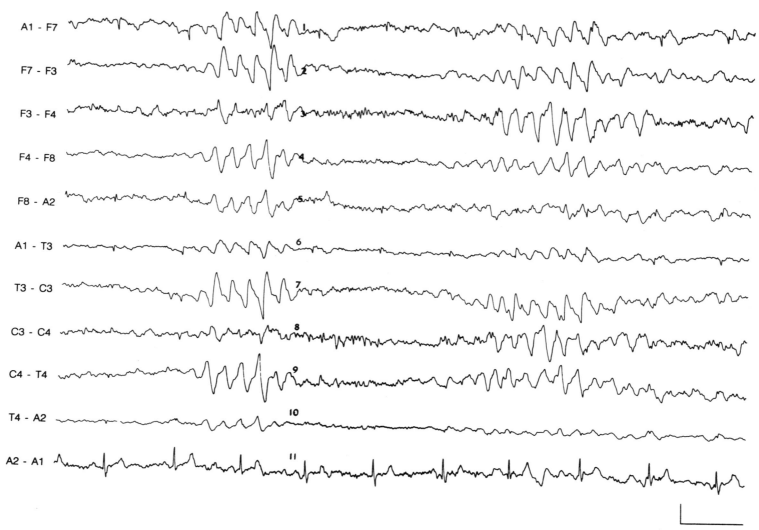

FIG. 3–84. V-waves. 33 years. Extension of V-waves to the central (C3,4) and frontal (F3,4) regions permits their recording in this coronal montage, which omits vertex leads. Their morphology may be simplified thereby. Note their appearance in bursts and that their principal polarity is electronegative, but that an alternating positive-negative-positive sequence appears. Central beta activity appears between such bursts. Calibration signal 1 sec, 50μV.

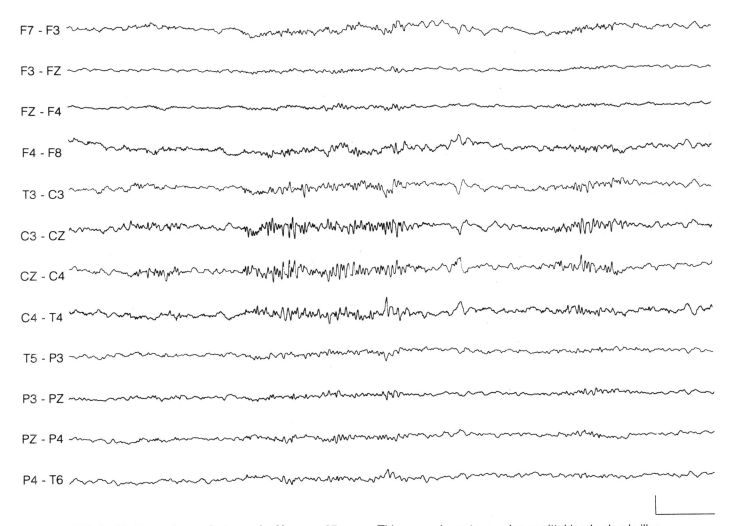

FIG. 3–85. Drowsiness, beta, and a V-wave. 25 years. This coronal montage using sagittal leads clearly illustrates augmentation of central beta activity and a V-wave. Calibration signal 1 sec, 70μV.

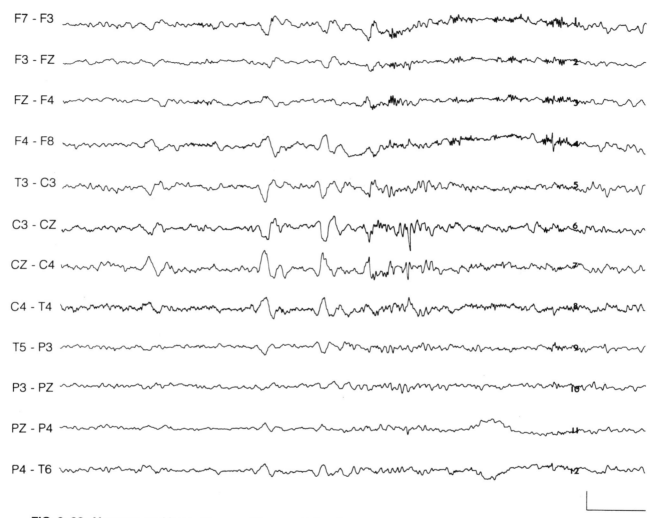

FIG. 3–86. V-waves and beta. 41 years. The sensitivity of 100 μV/10mm may have "blunted" the appearance of these V-waves. However, it did not blunt the spike-like appearance of accompanying central rhythms; this appearance results from a combination of wave forms and is not spikes, principally because no aftercoming slow wave appears. Note the electrode artifact at P4; electrode artifacts are usually electropositive, as in this instance. Calibration signal 1 sec, 100μV.

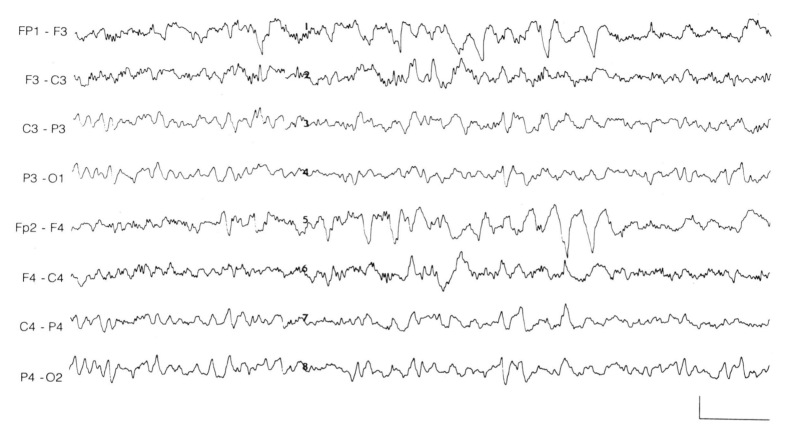

FIG. 3–87. Light sleep potentials on an anterior-posterior bipolar montage. 21 years. The broad anterior-posterior field of V-waves limits their expression on this montage. The primarily electronegative component is evident from the downward deflections in the Fp1-F3, Fp2-F4 derivations and from the simultaneous upward deflections in more posterior derivations. The moderate variability of V-wave morphology is a normal feature. Note the positive occipital sharp transients (POSTS) during most of this tracing. Calibration signal 1 sec, 70μV.

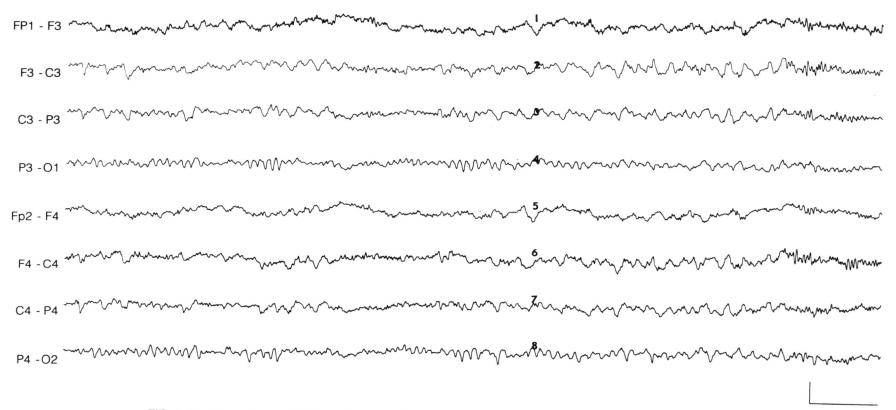

FIG. 3–88. Drowsiness with blunt V-waves. 42 years. The theta activity in this normal drowsy pattern is more apiculate than that of some earlier tracings. This likely results from the extension of sagittal V-waves to the parasagittal leads. Calibration signal 1 sec, 50μV.

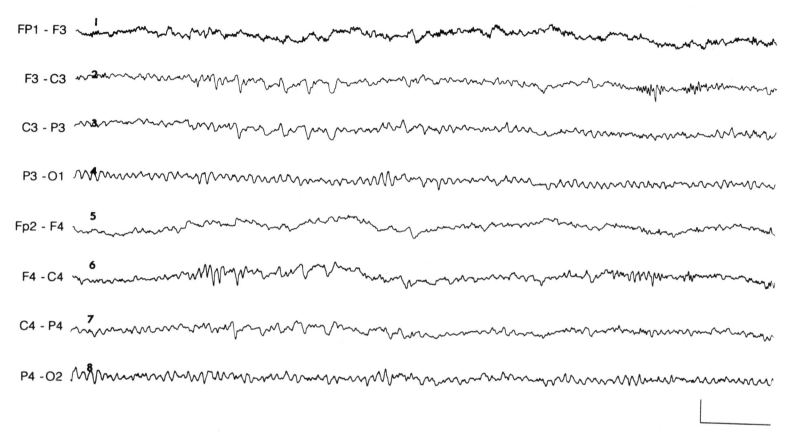

FIG. 3–89. Drowsiness with blunt V-waves. 42 years. V-waves are slightly more prominent in this tracing, in which a drowsy pattern appears superimposed on alpha activity. Alpha drop-out is often *not* the first electrographic manifestation of drowsiness. Calibration signal 1 sec, 50μV.

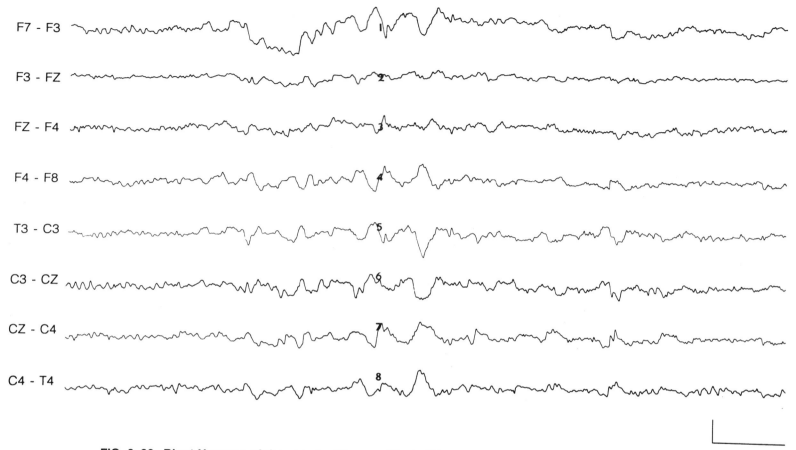

FIG. 3–90. Blunt V-waves of the elderly. 73 years. Blunted V-waves appear here. Without vertex leads, this phenomenon might appear as a 2 Hz "projected" phenomenon, with which it shares several characteristics. No significance can be ascribed to such blunt V-waves. Calibration signal 1 sec, 50μV.

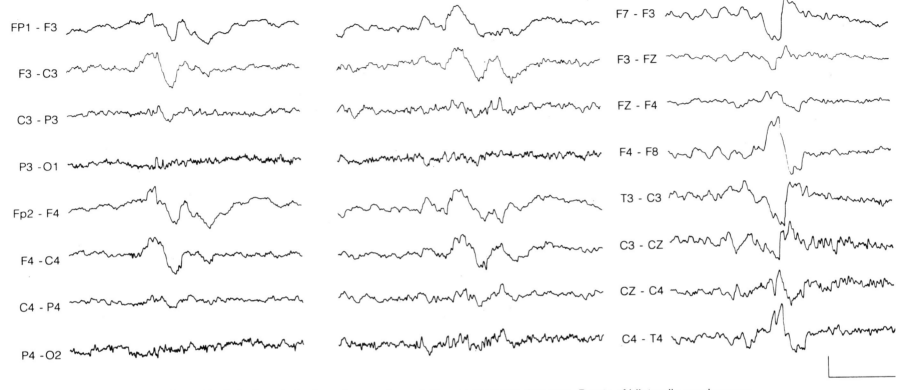

FIG. 3–91. Delta bursts in drowsiness of an adult over 60 years. 67 years. Bursts of bilaterally synchronous delta lasting about 1 second may normally appear in light drowsiness at this age (4). The maximum quantity of such waves that can be considered normal is not clear, but their appearance in about 10% of the drowsy recording would be acceptable. The third segment illustrates their association with a vertex wave at Cz. Calibration signal 1 sec, 50μV.

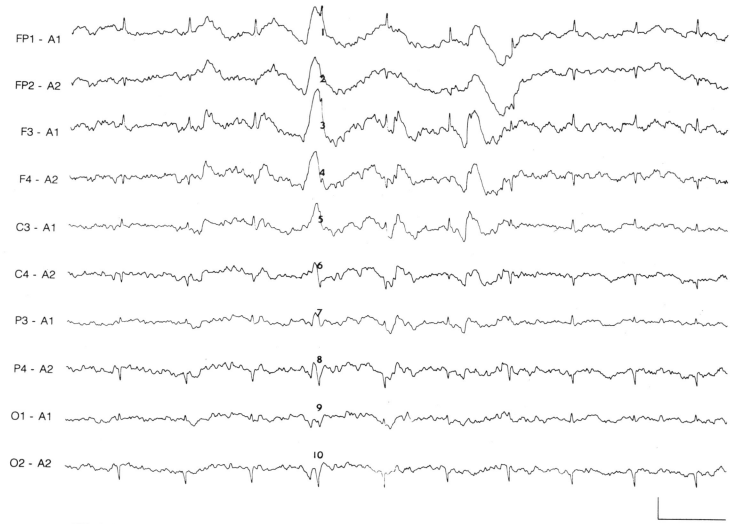

FIG. 3–92. Blunt V-waves on a referential montage. 73 years. The ear referential montage often best depicts diffuse wave forms. Unfortunately, the vertex leads were not employed in this run. The sporadic appearance of such rhythmic delta activity resembling frontally predominant V-waves could not be considered abnormal (12). The cardiac R-waves cause upward deflections in A1 derivations and downward deflections in A2. Calibration signal 1 sec, 50μV.

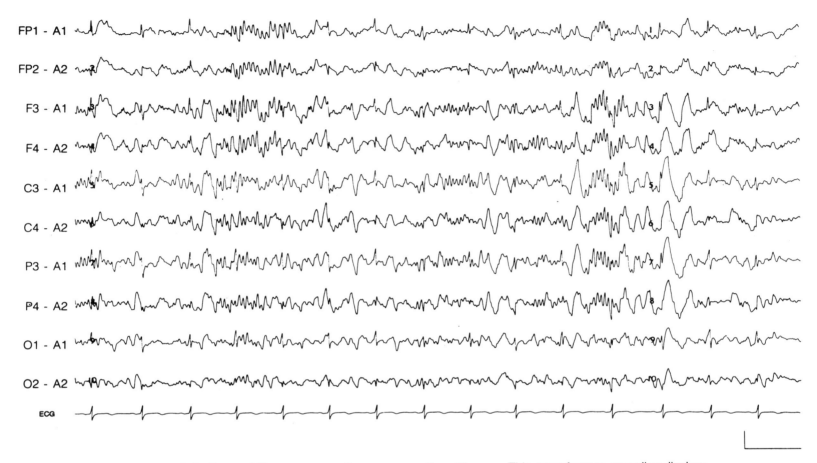

FIG. 3–93. Spindles and V-waves, ear reference recording. 39 years. This ear reference recording displays V-waves and spindles fully because of virtual lack of reference (A1, A2) involvement. The superimposition of ECG potential on V-waves creates a spike-wavelike picture in the third-to-last second. Calibration signal 1 sec, 50μV.

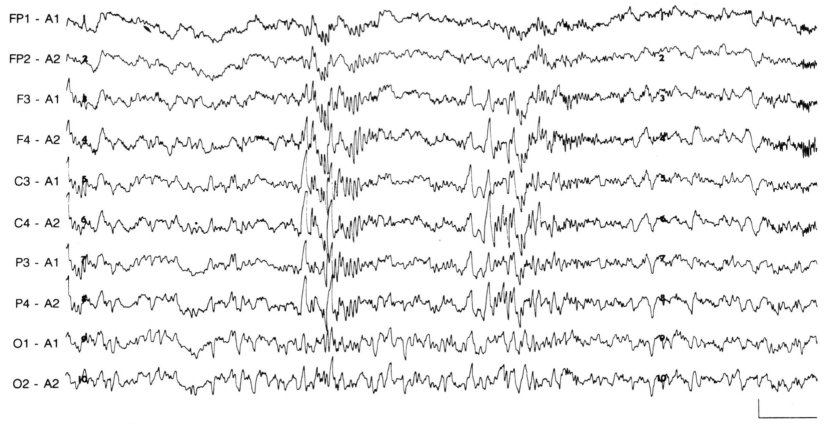

FIG. 3–94. V-waves, spindles and beta activity. 18 years. Partial or complete superimposition of these wave forms can create irregular, quite apiculate morphologies, as seen here. Notice the positive occipital sharp transients of sleep (POSTS) in the occipital derivations. Calibration signal 1 sec, 50μV.

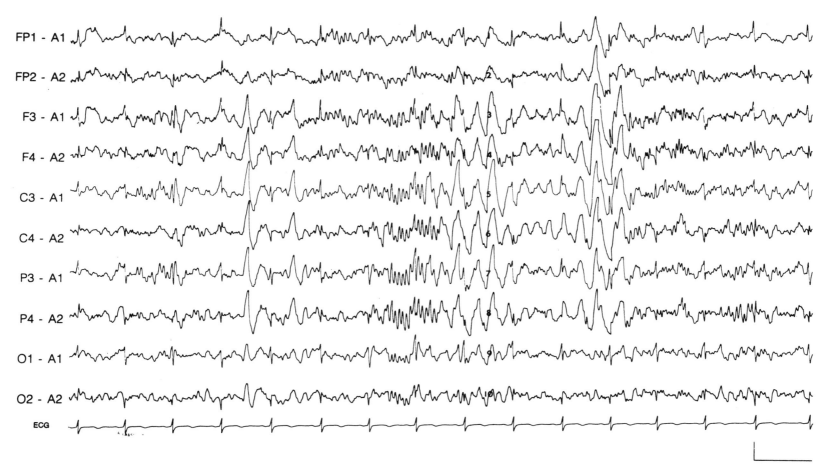

FIG. 3–95. V-waves, spindles and ECG artifact. 39 years. Prominent ECG artifact combines with V-waves to create a spike-wavelike appearance, underscoring the importance of ECG monitoring. Calibration signal 1 sec, 50μV.

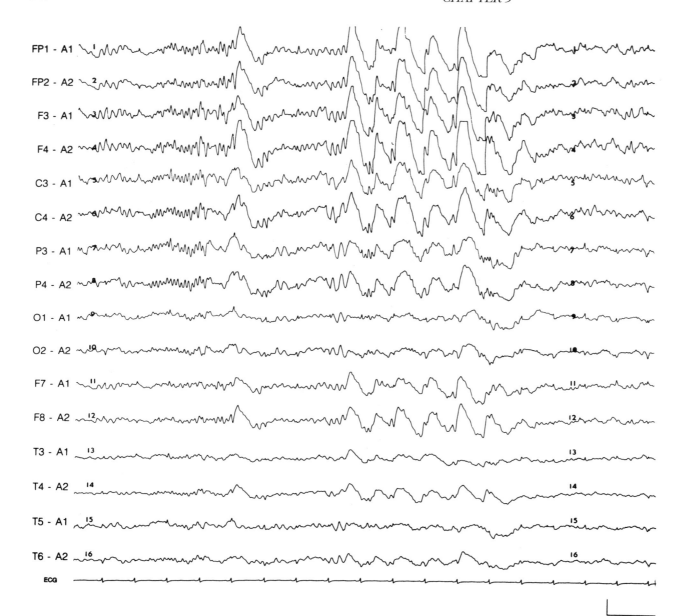

FIG. 3–96. Mitten pattern. 31 years. The combination of bursts of anterior rhythmic delta activity with relatively sharply contoured waves derived from the background activity may rarely create a complex appearing as a mitten pattern with the "thumb section" preceding. Although sharply contoured, this thumb section is considerably more blunt than the spike component of slow spike-wave discharges, the epileptiform pattern most closely resembling the normal mitten. Calibration signal 1 sec, 70μV.

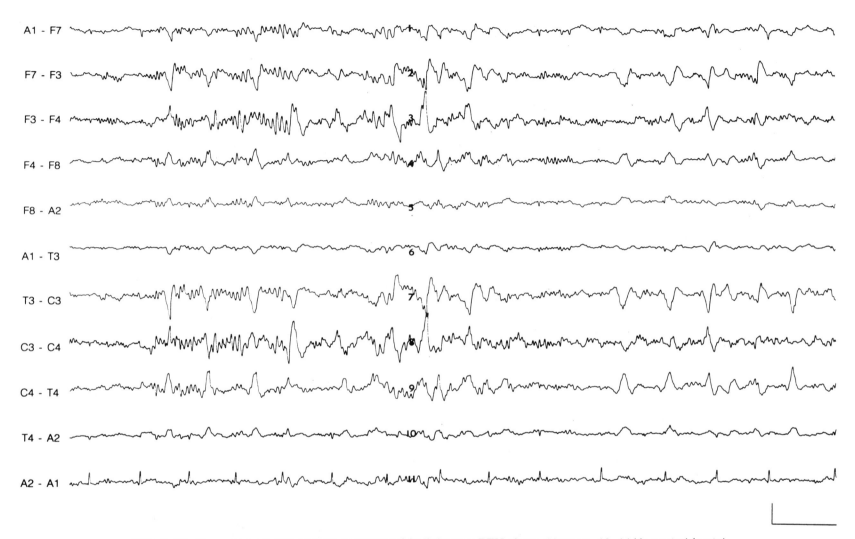

FIG. 3–97. V-waves and spindles (K-complexes) in light non-REM sleep. 16 years. 13–14 Hz central-frontal spindles are interspersed among some of the V-waves in this tracing constituting K-complexes, which appear in light sleep (12). Calibration signal 1 sec, 100μV.

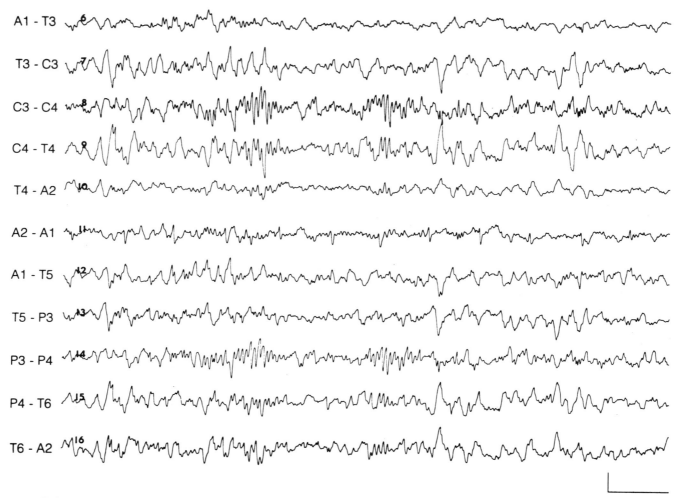

FIG. 3–98. V-waves and spindles in light non-REM sleep. 18 years. Sequential V-waves and irregularly shaped spindles appear principally in the central (C3,4) regions. Note the variation in the morphology of these normal V-waves and spindles. Calibration signal 1 sec, 50μV.

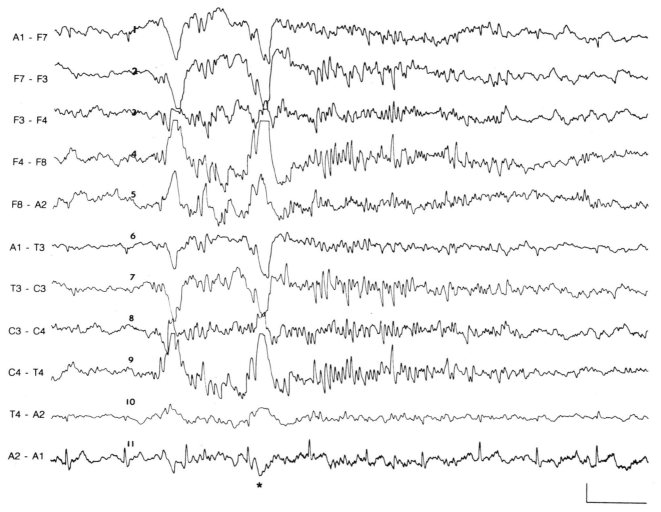

FIG. 3–99. Mittens and spindles of deep non-REM sleep. 35 years. High-voltage 400–500 msec waves centered near the vertex frontally and centrally may be notched in their ascending phase by a briefer, approximately 100–125 msec wave, creating a "mitten" pattern as seen here (*asterisk*). In this tracing, they are followed by irregular spindles which are not part of the mitten pattern. The greater frontal involvement of such vertex waves, the slightly slower frequency of the spindles, and the mitten pattern itself all attest to the deeper stage of sleep. Calibration signal 1 sec, 50μV.

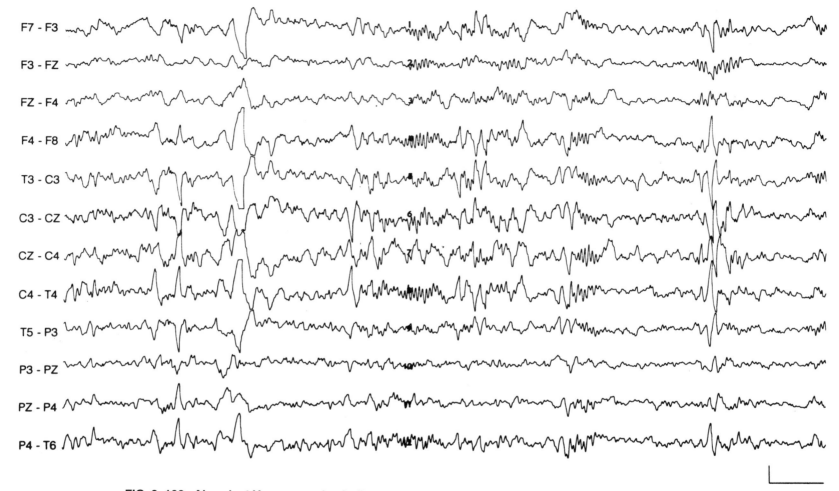

FIG. 3–100. Abundant V-waves and spindles. 19 years. The relatively high sensitivity (70 μV/10mm) has augmented the amplitude of these abundant V-waves and 14 Hz central frontal spindles in light non-REM sleep. The V-wave morphology varies from blunt to apiculate. Calibration signal 1 sec, 70μV.

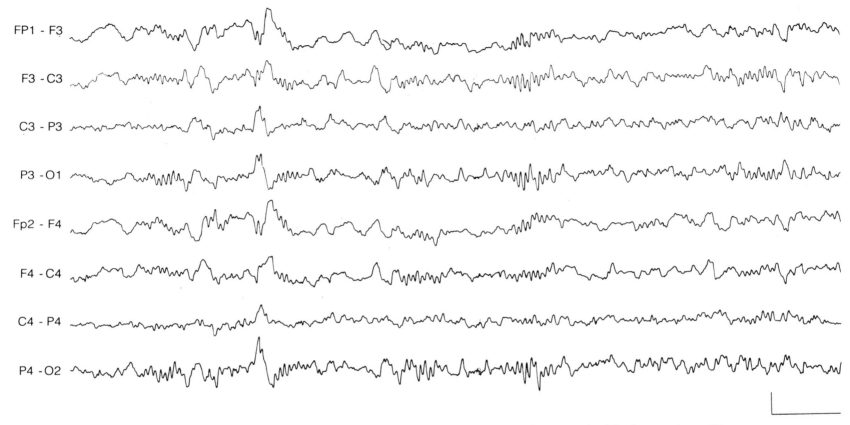

FIG. 3–101. V-waves and spindles in light non-REM sleep on an anterior-posterior bipolar montage. 67 years. The intermittent nature of spindles appears in this tracing with sporadic interspersed V-waves. In this light sleep tracing, the spindles appear principally in the central parietal (C3-P3, C4-P4) areas, from the nature of their phase reversals. Calibration signal 1 sec, 50µV.

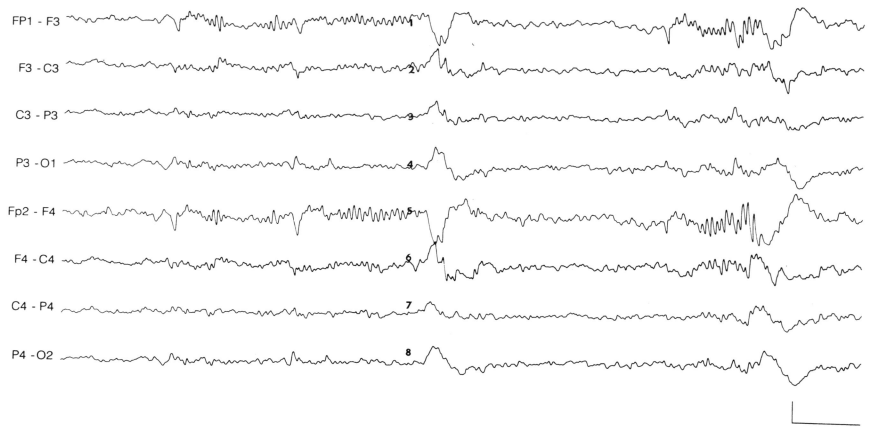

FIG. 3–102. Spindles and V-waves in light non-REM sleep on an anterior-posterior bipolar montage. 24 years. In this segment, also in light sleep, the spindles are expressed principally in the frontal regions (F3,F4). Calibration signal 1 sec, 50μV.

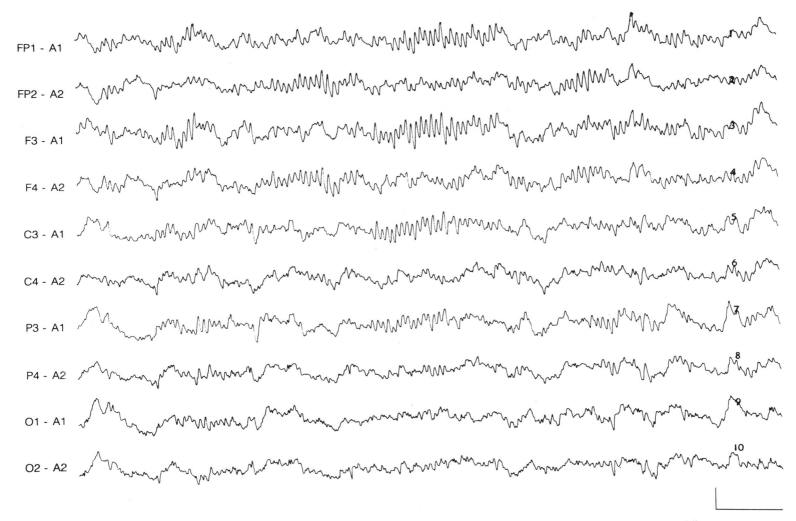

FIG. 3–103. Asynchronous normal sleep spindles. 81 years. Although sleep spindles usually occur in a bilaterally synchronous fashion, they may normally appear independently in either hemisphere, as noted here and by Gibbs and Gibbs (13). The overall quantity of spindles in this sample is normal. Calibration signal 1 sec, 50μV.

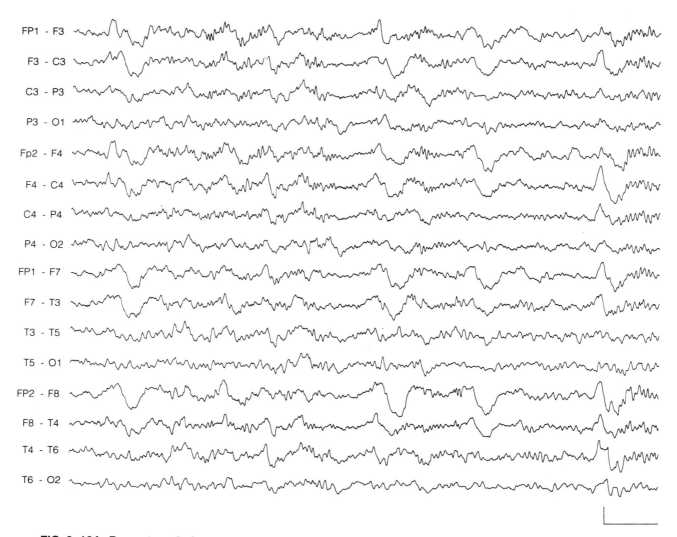

FIG. 3–104. Deep stage 3 sleep. 36 years. V-waves are less prominent in deep non-REM sleep (stage 3), which is dominated by diffuse delta and frontally predominant diffuse spindles. Calibration signal 1 sec, 70µV.

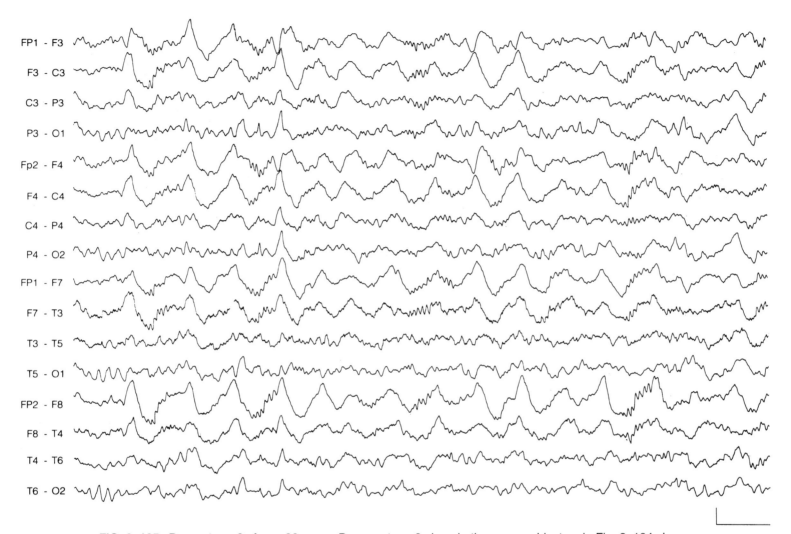

FIG. 3–105. Deep stage 3 sleep. 36 years. Deeper stage 3 sleep in the same subject as in Fig. 3–104 shows markedly augmented delta activity. The spindles have slowed to 11–12 Hz and appear principally frontally, although their field is diffuse. Calibration signal 1 sec, 70μV.

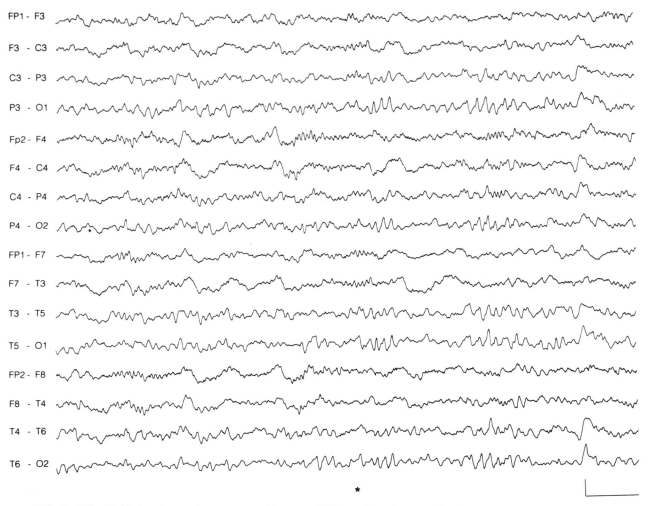

FIG. 3–106. Multiple sleep phenomena. 24 years. Diffuse delta, low-amplitude spindles, and blunt V-waves dominate this deep sleep tracing before the arousal stimulus (*asterisk*). After that, the delta attenuates slightly, and positive occipital sharp transients of sleep (POSTS) become prominent. Calibration signal 1 sec, 70μV.

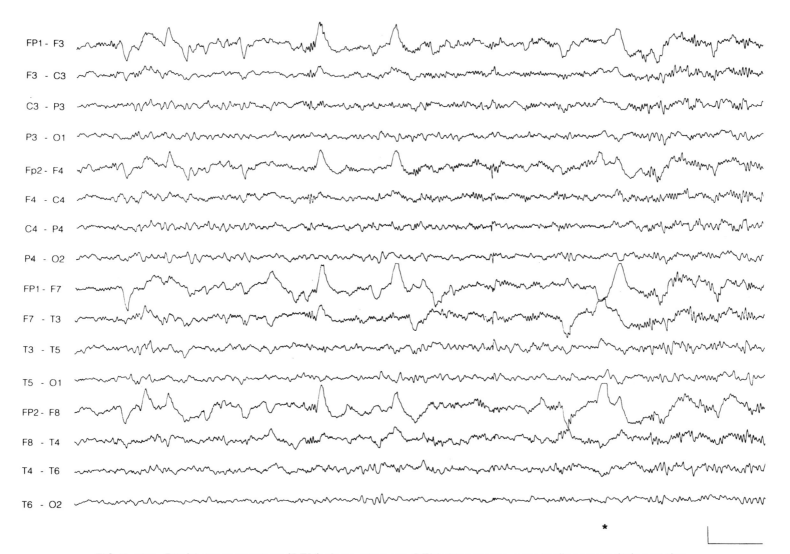

FIG. 3–107. Rapid eye movement (REM) sleep. 36 years. REM sleep may unexpectedly appear during routine recordings. As in this recording, a mixed frequency background occurs containing theta, beta, and minimal delta activity. Note the vertical rapid eye movements. A prominent rightward eye movement is also present (*asterisk*). Calibration signal 1 sec, 70μV.

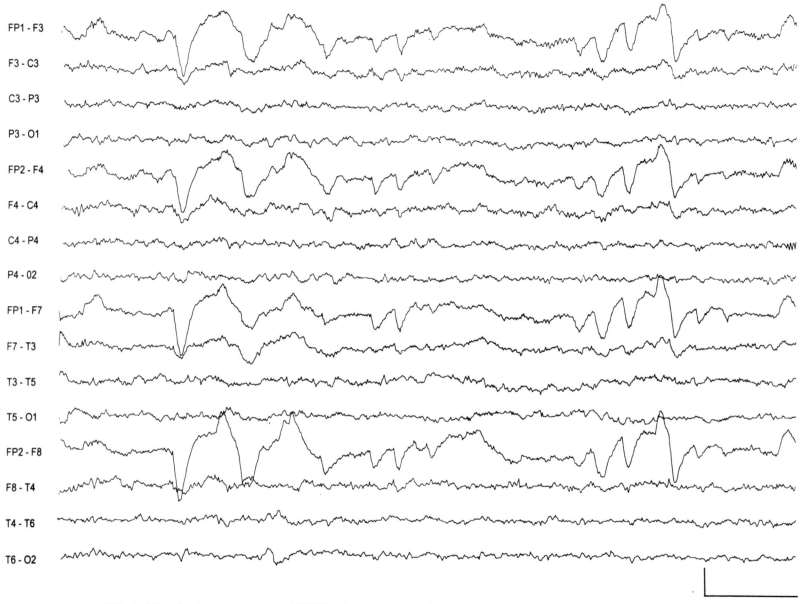

FIG. 3–108. Rapid eye movement (REM) sleep. 38 years. Bursts of synchronous vertical eye movements together with low-voltage continuous theta and minimal beta activity identify this epoch as REM sleep. Calibration signal 1 sec, 50μV.

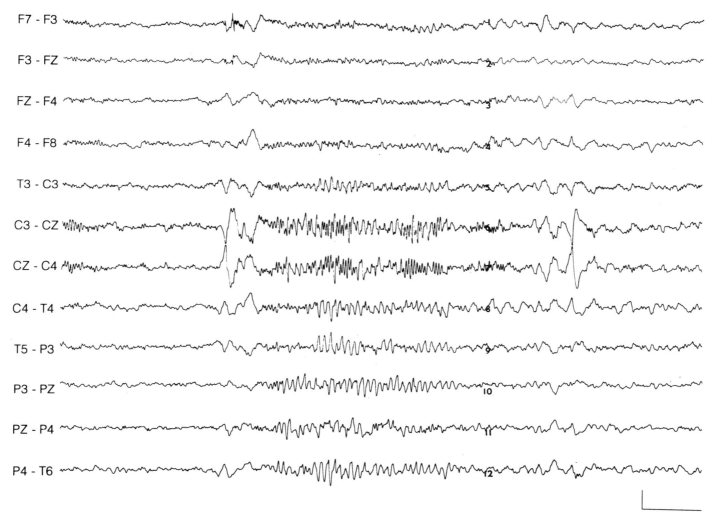

FIG. 3–109. V-waves in arousal and drowsiness. 19 years. Sharply contoured diphasic V-waves frame this brief arousal characterized by the reappearance of parietal alpha and central beta activity. All of these modifications are minimally reflected in the frontal leads. Calibration signal 1 sec, 50μV.

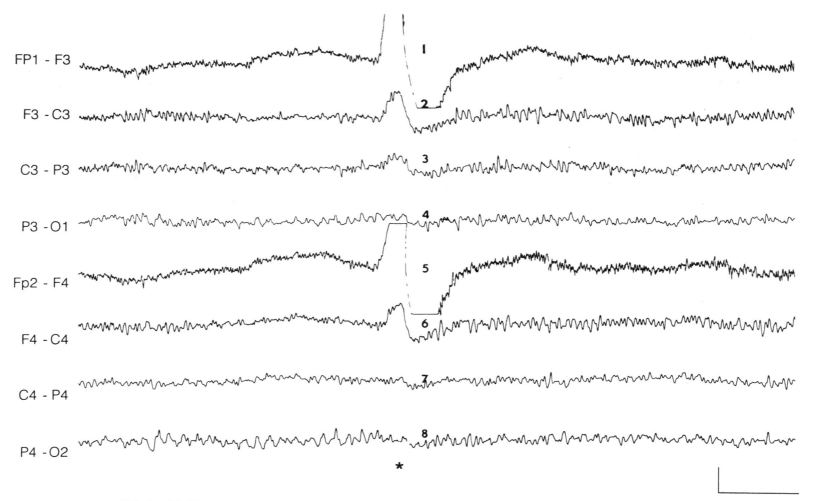

FP1 - F3

F3 - C3

C3 - P3

P3 - O1

Fp2 - F4

F4 - C4

C4 - P4

P4 - O2

FIG. 3–110. Normal drowsiness and alerting. 25 years. Eye opening, producing sudden electronegativity at the frontal polar (Fp1,2) and superior frontal (F3,4) derivations, is associated with enhanced quantity of diffuse beta and some attenuation of 6–7 Hz posterior rhythms of the drowsy epoch preceding this event. No abnormality appears; this quantity of beta and theta is well within normal limits. Calibration signal 1 sec, 50μV.

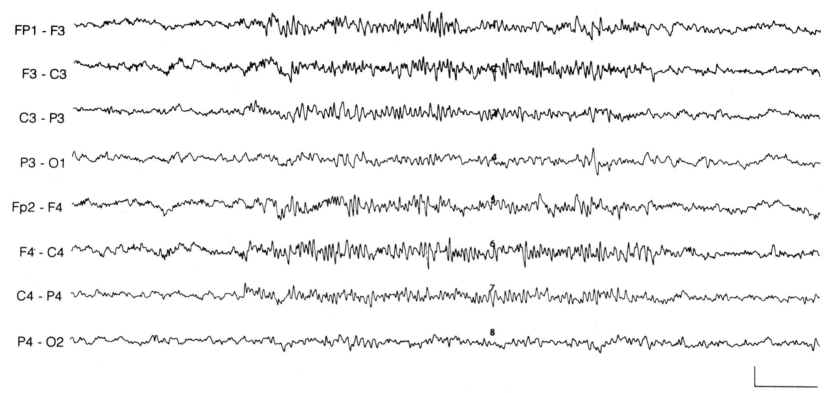

FIG. 3–111. Brief arousal from drowsiness. 23 years. Brief arousal in this instance is characterized by a sudden increase in 12–15 Hz waves diffusely for about 6 seconds, after which drowsiness returns. Calibration signal 1 sec, 50μV.

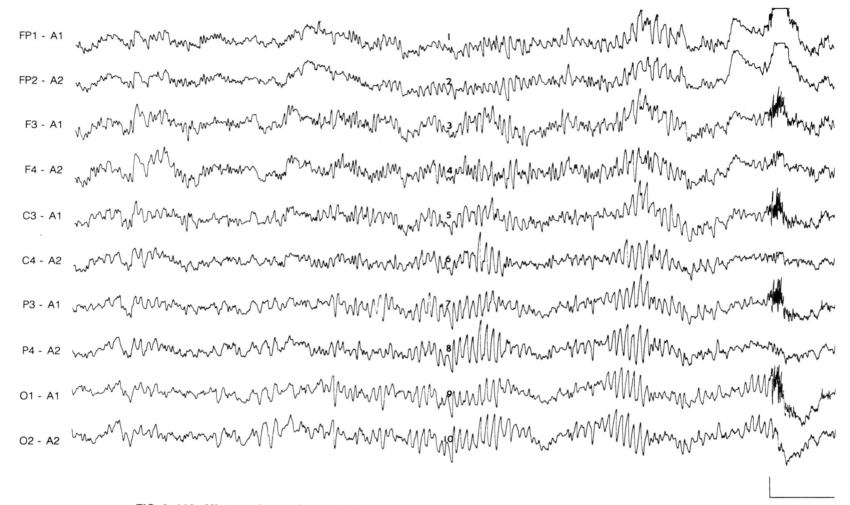

FIG. 3–112. Mixture of wave forms during arousal. 21 years. As seen in some other examples of arousal, activity in the alpha range appears in bursts posteriorly but is also present in frontal derivations (Fp1,2 and F3,4) in association with beta activity. Many factors may contribute to the diffuse underlying delta activity, including head movement, vertical and horizontal slow eye movements, and even glossokinetic potentials. Swallowing likely produced the burst of muscle potentials in the last second. Calibration signal 1 sec, 70 μV.

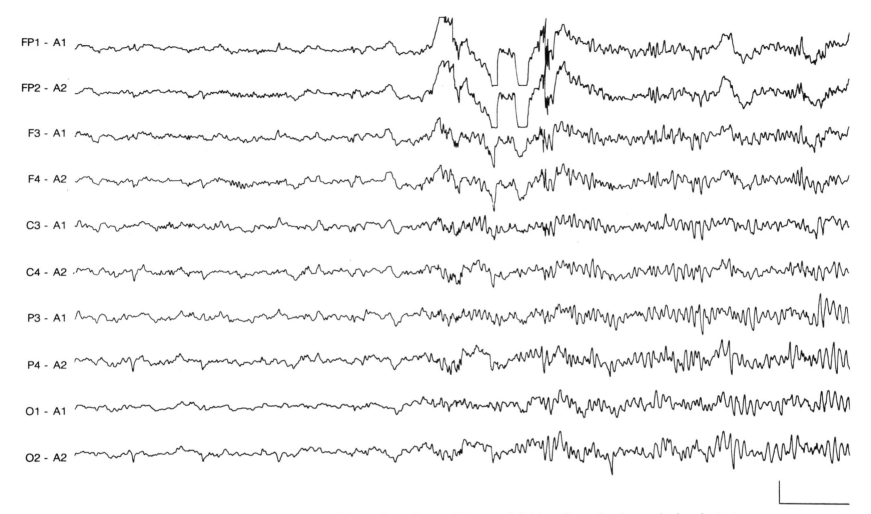

FIG. 3–113. Instantaneous arousal from drowsiness. 16 years. A light auditory stimulus evoked an instant change from diffuse theta and beta of drowsiness to an alpha-dominated awake pattern without intervening slow waves. The potentials recorded in the frontal polar leads represent eye opening to the auditory stimulus, then eye blinks with some frontal muscle artifact. Calibration signal 1 sec, 70μV.

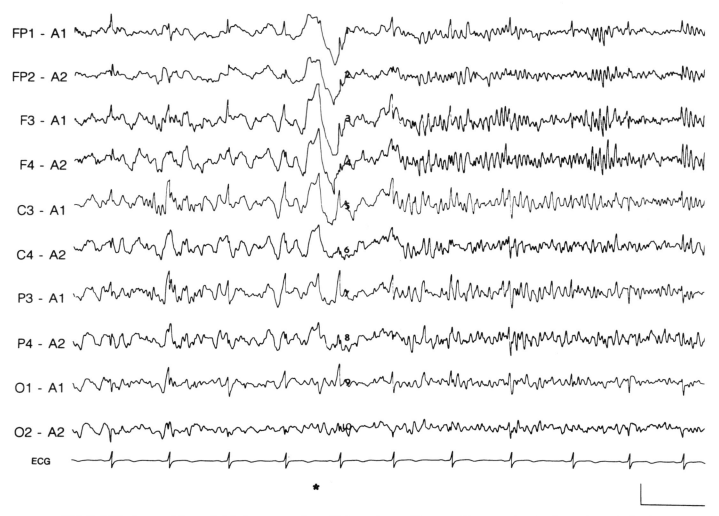

FIG. 3–114. Arousal from light sleep on referential montage. 39 years. From moderate sleep characterized by sleep spindles and V-waves, arousal is signaled by a single high-voltage frontally dominant, 600 msec slow wave (*asterisk*) followed by a wakefulness pattern including 8 Hz and 12–15 Hz activity. Calibration signal 1 sec, 50 μV.

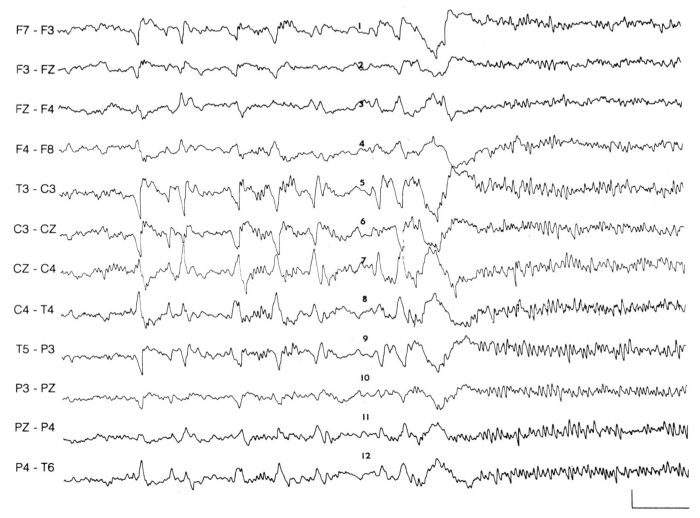

FIG. 3–115. Arousal from light sleep. 22 years. Sequential V-waves with interspersed spindles characterize the sleep stage here. Arousal is characterized by a single 600 msec high-voltage wave which is considerably less sharply contoured than are the V-waves. This is immediately followed by 11–12 Hz activity in the central parietal regions, characteristic of wakefulness. Calibration signal 1 sec, 50μV.

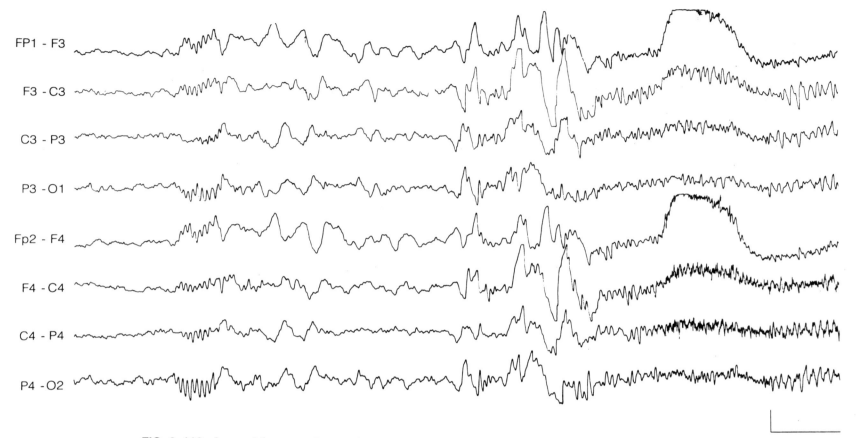

FIG. 3–116. Arousal from moderate sleep. 67 years. Arousal from moderate sleep is characterized by 2–3 high-voltage, frontally dominant slow waves lasting about 1 1/2 seconds, followed by a pattern characteristic of wakefulness. Calibration signal 1 sec, 50μV.

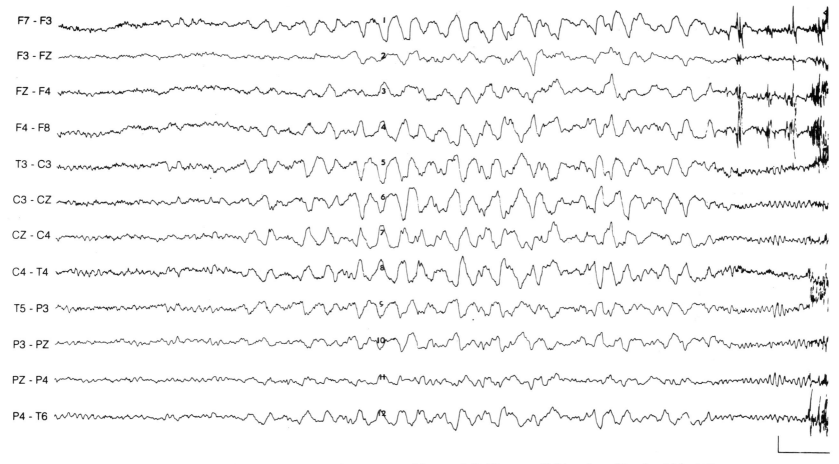

FIG. 3–117. Rhythmic waves in drowsiness-arousal in an adult. 76 years. Children from 3 to about 14 years commonly exhibit rhythmic 2–3 Hz waves diffusely in drowsiness and occasionally during arousal. Although this pattern declines precipitously in the teenage years, its sporadic persistence in normal adults has been documented (14). Alternatively, one could view this pattern as sequential very blunted vertex waves. This electrographic curiosity cannot be clearly labeled abnormal as there is an abrupt transition from this pattern to normal background activity (*note the last 2 seconds of the tracing*). Moreover, this pattern is preceded by normal background activity. We are unaware of any abnormal, intermittent rhythmic delta activity (IRDA), which appears in an otherwise completely normal EEG. Calibration signal 1 sec, 50μV.

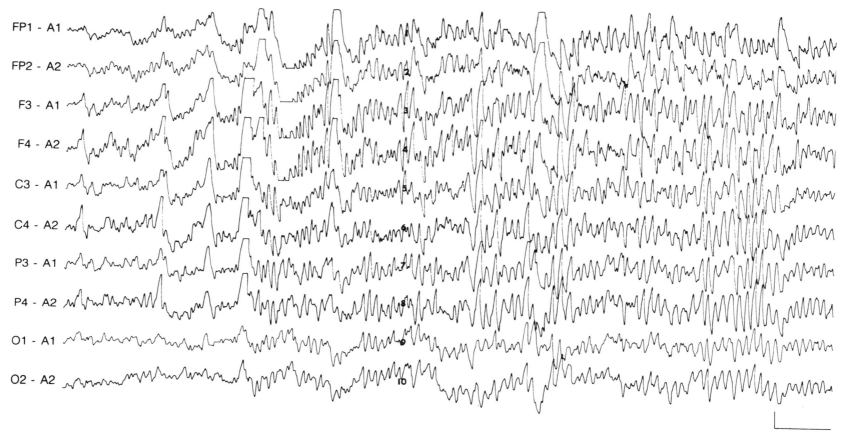

FIG. 3–118. Abnormal arousal. 22 years. Although a brief burst of delta or theta activity may be considered within normal limits in arousal from moderately deep sleep, these rhythmic 7 Hz and 4–5 Hz diffuse waves persist too long to be considered normal for this age (15, 16). Calibration signal 1 sec, 70μV.

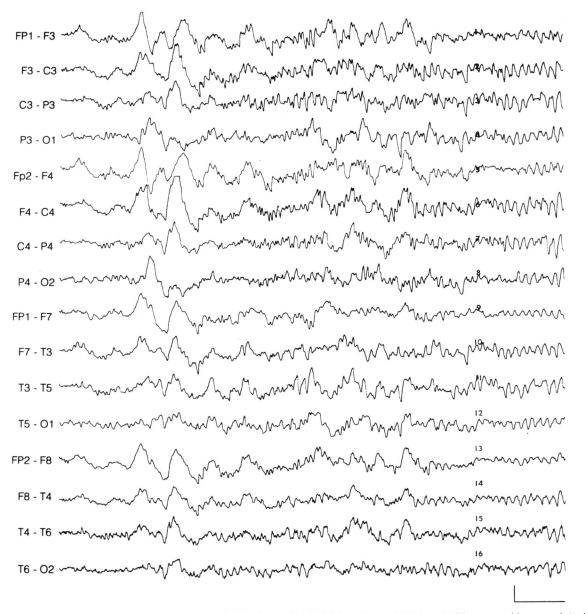

FIG. 3–119. Abnormal arousal. 71 years. Following an initial high-voltage delta burst, this arousal is associated with a mixture of delta and theta waves, the latter at many frequencies. The prolonged duration of such delta and theta and their very gradual replacement by awake rhythms constitute the abnormality. Calibration signal 1 sec, 50μV.

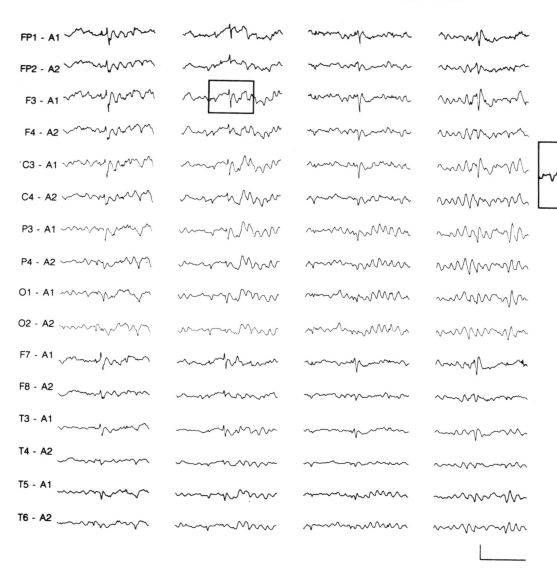

FIG. 3–120. Small sharp spikes (SSS). 41 years. Small sharp spikes (SSS) (benign epileptiform transients of sleep) are well expressed by ear referential montages (A1, A2). There is partial cancellation between the active ear reference and the posterior leads, but the field is broad, like that of other normal apiculate waves. These diphasic or monophasic spikes have an abrupt ascending limb but an even steeper descending slope, with a relatively small aftercoming slow wave. Unlike epileptogenic spikes, there is no disruption of the background activity. Although these SSSs appear principally in the left hemisphere, note the moderate involvement of homologous regions of the right. The enlarged square depicts the typical morphology of the small sharp spike. Calibration signal 1 sec, 70μV.

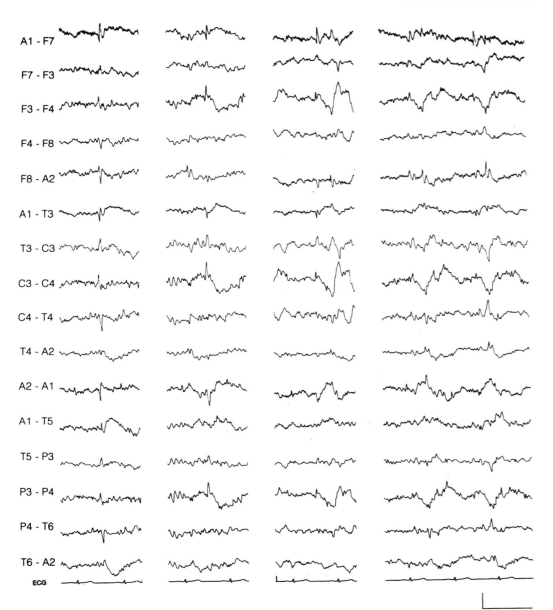

FIG. 3–121. Small sharp spikes on coronal montage. 60 years. The transverse dipole field of SSS enhances their expression by coronal montages, where they may be confused with abnormal anterior temporal spikes. The widespread field including occasional deflections in derivations crossing the midline (F3-4, C3-4, P3-4), the relative cancellation in posterior temporal-ear derivations (A1-T5, T6-A2), the characteristic diphasic very apiculate morphology, and the lack of disruption of background activity all serve to distinguish these from anterior temporal spikes. Anterior temporal spikes (not depicted here) almost equally involve A1 and F7 but involve T5 only minimally. Calibration signal 1 sec, 50μV.

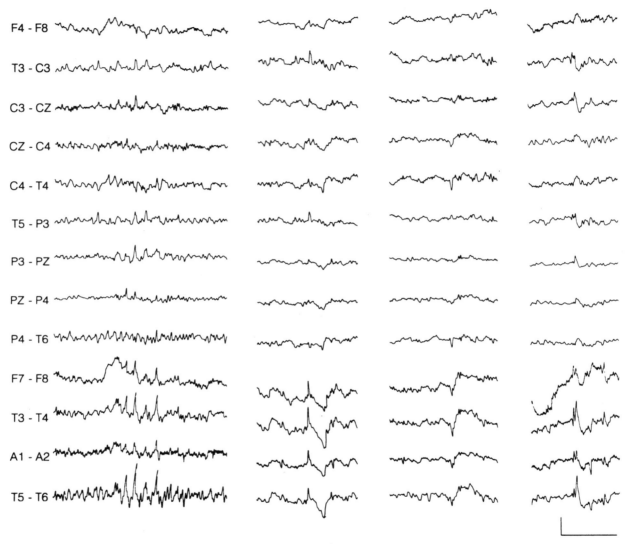

FIG. 3–122. Small sharp spikes, coronal montage and interhemispheric derivations. 39 years. The widespread gradual slope of SSS may create minimal deflections in bipolar coronal linkages but moderate deflections in interhemispheric derivations, because of the interhemispheric dipole. These principles are illustrated here. Calibration signal 1 sec, 50μV.

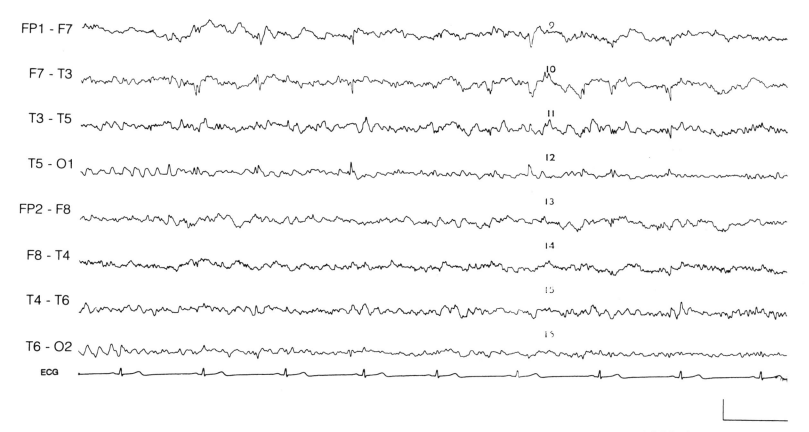

FIG. 3–123. Small sharp spikes on anterior-posterior bipolar montage. 29 years. Properties of SSS, depicted previously, prepare one for the most likely encounter—on the commonly used anterior-posterior bipolar montage. Their distinct morphology, widespread field, prominent involvement in the midposterior temporal areas (T3 and T5 in this instance), and the lack of a prominent aftercoming slow wave or any disruption in background rhythms distinguish these discharges from anterior temporal spikes. The left temporal intermittent delta activity in this example bears no relationship to the SSSs. Calibration signal 1 sec, 50μV.

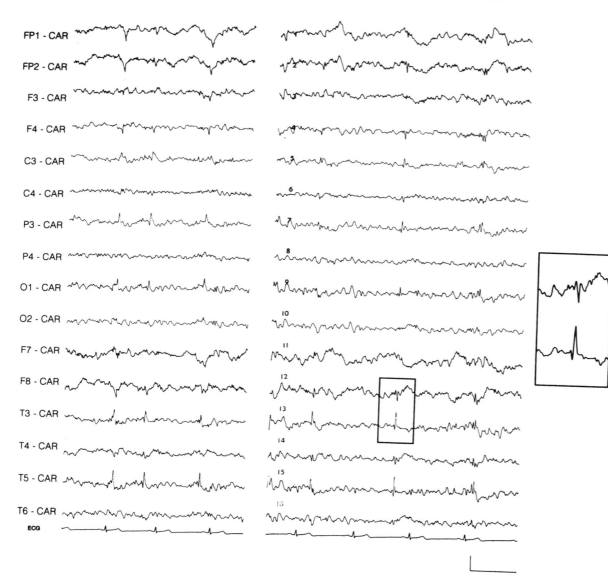

FIG. 3–124. Small sharp spikes and the common average reference. 29 years. The widespread field of SSS leads to their expression by the common average reference, and therefore they appear in most of its derivations. Although they appear principally at the left posterior temporal (T5) and left midtemporal (T3) derivations in these examples, they are out-of-phase (downward deflection) in the right hemisphere anteriorly. Such reversal of phase could represent either common average reference "contamination" or a broad field with principal electronegativity in the left posterior and positivity in the right anterior head regions. The enlarged section depicts the very steep slopes and apiculate points of the SSS. Calibration signal 1 sec, 50μV.

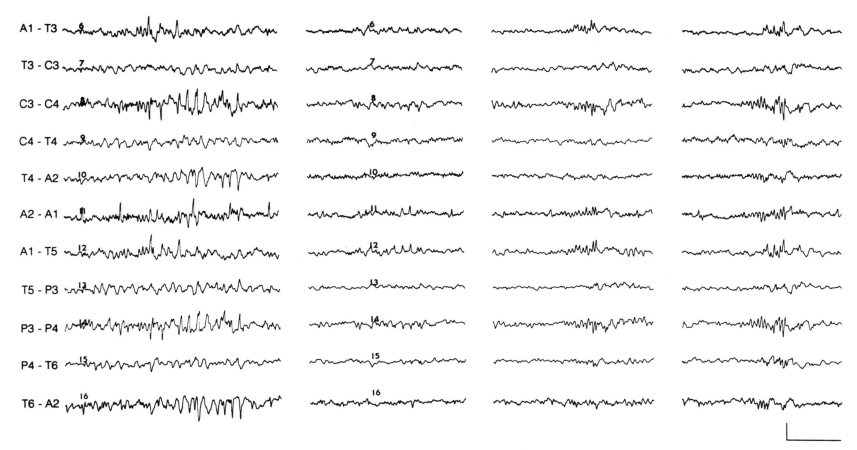

FIG. 3–125. 14 and 6 Hz positive spikes. 20 years. These segments depict the very apiculate nature and widespread fields of these phenomena, whose appearance sometimes merges with that of SSS and 6 Hz spike-waves. All of these are normal phenomena. Note that the 6 Hz feature predominates in the first two segments, whereas the 14 Hz morphology predominates in the 3rd and 4th tracings. The 14 and 6 Hz positive spikes are best illustrated on coronal montages such as this. Calibration signal 1 sec, 50μV.

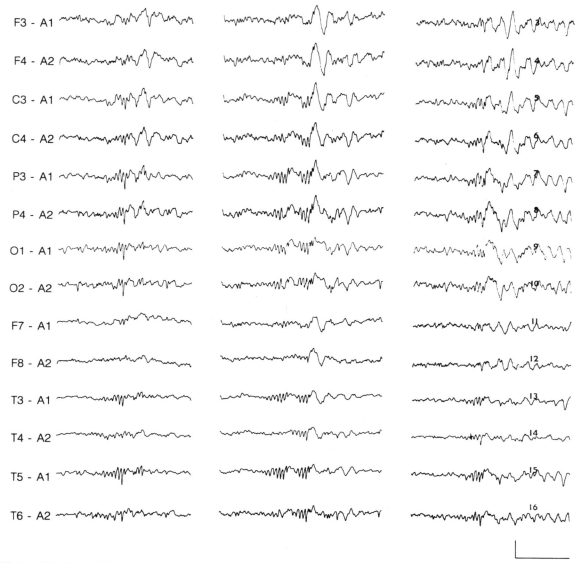

FIG. 3–126. 14 and 6 Hz positive spikes on ear reference montage. 25 years. These segments illustrate the diffuse nature of such electropositive phenomena. Lack of significant referential (A1, A2) contamination is evidenced by the minimal deflection in the Fp1-A1 and Fp2-A2 derivations, as this discharge appears principally in the posterior head (Fig. 3–125). Therefore, the downward apiculate deflections represent posterior electropositivity. When this discharge is followed by a prominent V-wave, as occurs in the 2nd and 3rd segments, the resulting complex resembles a polyspike-wave discharge. Calibration signal 1 sec, 70μV.

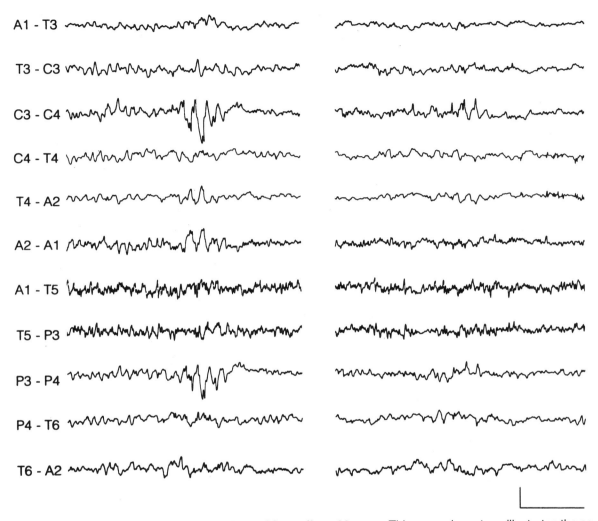

FIG. 3–127. 6 Hz spike and wave and 6 Hz positive spikes. 22 years. This coronal montage illustrates the co-existence of these two phenomena in the same recording as that described by Silverman (17). The burst in the left segment appears principally as a 6 Hz spike-wave discharge with a minimal electropositive spike component, whereas that in the right segment more resembles a 6 Hz positive spike. The relatively prominent spike at the C3-C4 derivation with minimal deflections in adjacent channels suggests a broad electropositive field in the right hemisphere with a possible coexisting electronegative field in the left hemisphere. Clinically innocent phenomena such as these often have broad fields. Calibration signal 1 sec, 50μV.

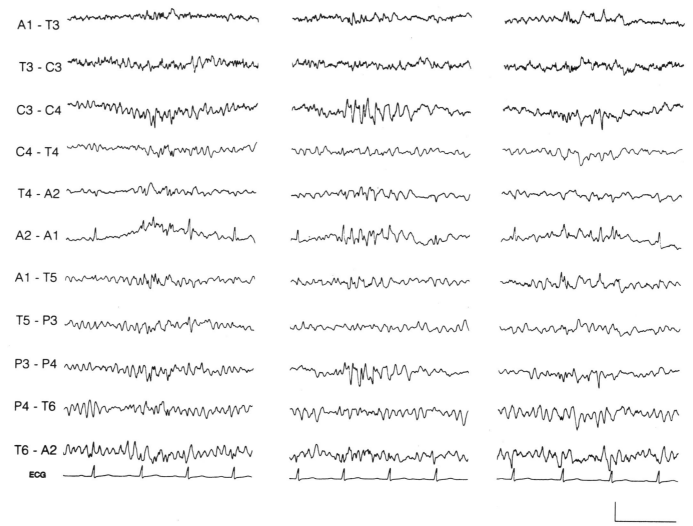

FIG. 3–128. 6 Hz spike-wave/positive spikes: incomplete expression. 23 years. These tracings illustrate the minimal appearance of such discharges, which are more prominent in earlier figures. Calibration signal 1 sec, 70μV.

Chapter 4

Focal Epileptiform Phenomena

Focal Spikes

- Apiculate wave forms.
- Distinct from "background."
- Interrupt background activity.
- Have more than one phase.
- Largest phase usually electronegative.
- Asymmetrical slopes.
- Involve more than one electrode position.
- Followed by slow wave.

Temporal Spikes (Figs. 1–6, 8, 9, 13–15, 20–24, 34)

- Major phase electronegative.
- Involve principally mandibular notch (M1), T1, F7, A1, T3 electrode positions.
- Occasional involvement of homologous contralateral (M2), T2, F8, A2, T4 and frontopolar (Fp1) regions.
- Sharply defined field, steep voltage gradients, inferolateral maximum; or broader field, gradual gradient, greater suprasylvian extension.
- Interspike variations in field are common.
- Associated with ipsilateral temporal delta and/or excess temporal theta.

Polyspikes (Figs. 13, 14, 32, 33, 56, 57)

- More apiculate than beta.
- Onset and offset abrupt.
- Delta waves may follow.

Occipital Spikes (Figs. 25–33)

- Electronegative.
- Eyes closed.
- Involve O1, O2, T5, T6.
- May require ECG monitor for identification.
- With or without loss of background (alpha).

Frontal Spikes (Figs. 39–48, 50–55)

- Usually electronegative.
- Occasionally widespread.
- Field may extend bilaterally.

Multifocal Spikes (Fig. 58)

- Three or more spike foci, with at least one in each hemisphere.
- Seizures in > 90%.
- Generalized tonic-clonic most common.
- Many have more than one type of seizure.
- Daily seizures common.

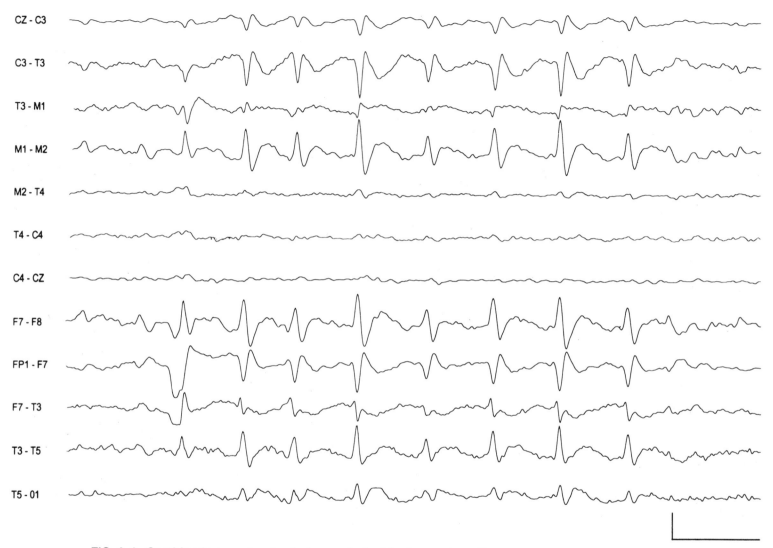

FIG. 4–1. Combined coronal and anterior-posterior bipolar montage illustrates temporal spikes. 38 years. The location of these frequent left temporal electronegative spikes is well depicted at M1 (left mandibular notch), T3, and F7 by this combined montage. The mandibular notch electrodes are placed 2.5 cm anterior to the tragus of the ear and immediately inferior to the zygoma (2). Calibration signal 1 sec, 200μV.

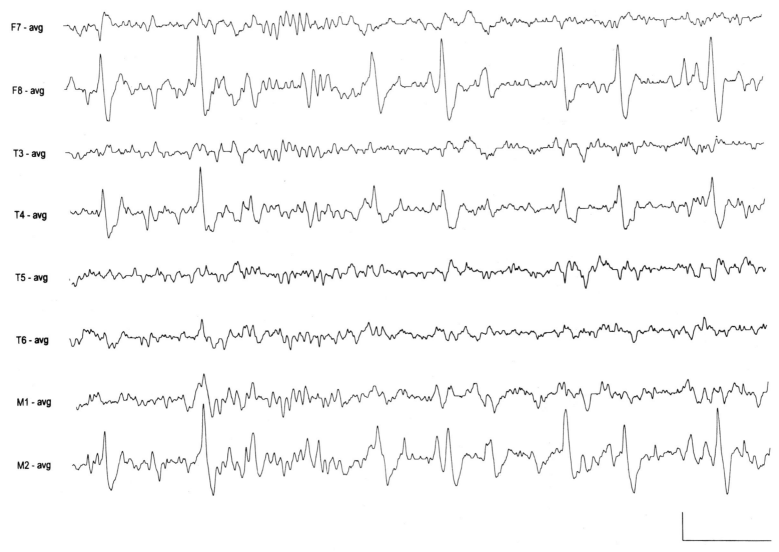

FIG. 4–2. Right anterior temporal spikes on common average reference montage. 35 years. A common average reference (CAR) clearly depicts the anterior mesial temporal distribution of spikes with lesions in this region, such as mesial temporal sclerosis. In this instance, spikes appear principally at the right anterior mesial temporal (F8, M2) positions with moderate spread to the right midtemporal region (T4). Such spikes in some patients appear principally at M2 and T4 with relatively less involvement of F8. The right posterior temporal region may become involved but should never be principally so. Note the minimal involvement of homotopic regions. Calibration signal 1 sec, 30μV.

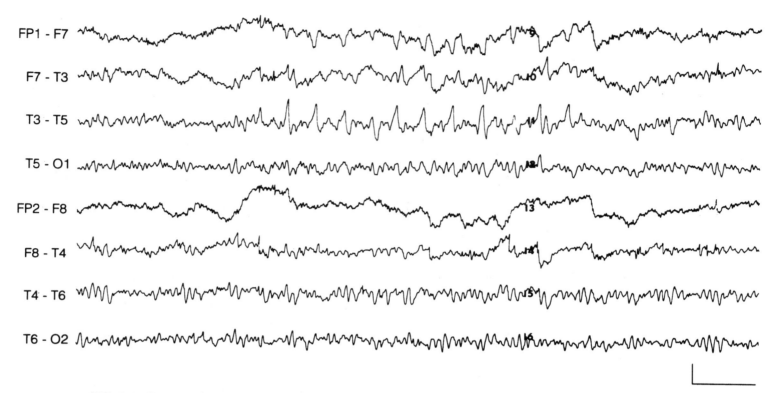

FIG. 4–3. Sequential left temporal spikes. 17 years. As noted in some previous tracings, combinations of background wave forms may produce morphologies similar to those seen in this sequence of spikes. However, two aspects of these discharges suggest that they are not superimpositions of background wave forms: (a) their distinct morphology, and (b) their stereotypy. Identification of apiculate waves as spikes depends upon these two factors—distinction from background rhythms and resemblance to other wave forms that are clearly spikes. Calibration signal 1 sec, 50μV.

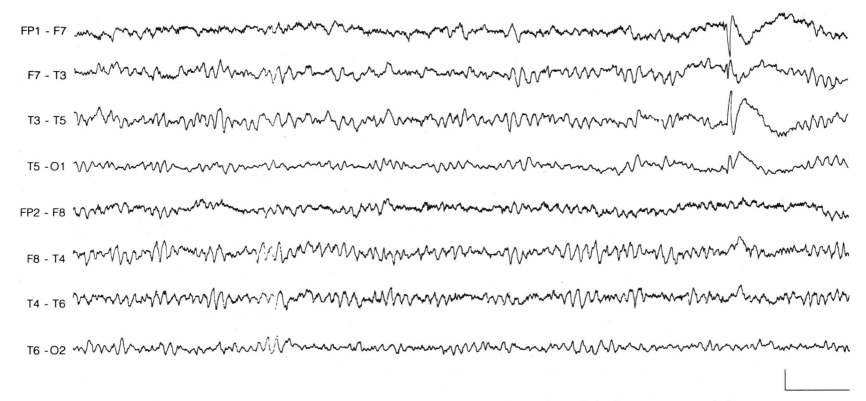

FIG. 4–4. Temporal spike with abnormal background. 63 years. Abnormal temporal spikes are accompanied by focal background abnormalities. Hyperventilation here elicited 3–5 Hz low- to medium-voltage waves in the left anterior-midtemporal region (F7-T3) and rare low-voltage delta activity in the same area. Note the normal right temporal background activity; the only alteration is a mild fluctuation of its amplitude and some slow eye movements. Calibration signal 1 sec, 50μV.

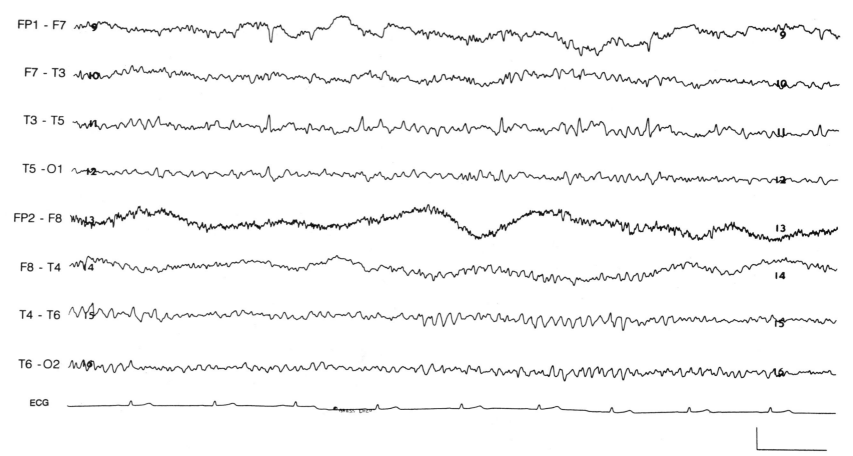

FIG. 4–5. Left temporal spikes. 36 years. The brevity and lack of prominent aftercoming slow waves of these left anterior-midtemporal (F7-T3) spikes create a morphology resembling small sharp spikes (SSSs). However, their discrete distribution, their presence during wakefulness, and the associated background abnormalities at F7-T3 all suggest that these are abnormal temporal spikes. Note the slow lateral eye movements which complicate the assessment of background activity in the temporal regions but do not preclude such assessment. ECG potentials would not be this prominent on most scalp recordings, nor would they have this distribution. Calibration signal 1 sec, 70μV.

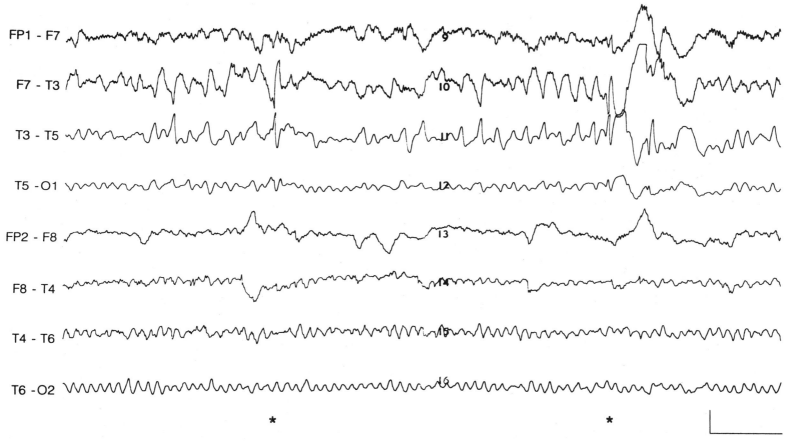

FIG. 4–6. Left temporal spikes and theta with skull defect. 24 years. Skull defects are commonly associated with sharply contoured wave forms, creating difficulties in identifying spikes. The negative potentials of nonepileptiform rhythmic waves at skull defects are commonly sharply contoured, as seen here. However, two of these apiculate forms (*asterisks*) clearly have steeper slopes and therefore sharper apices than the accompanying theta and can be identified as spikes. Calibration signal 1 sec, 100μV.

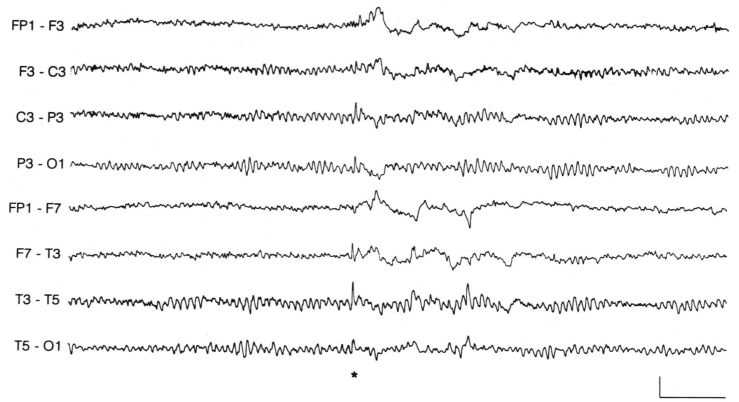

FIG. 4–7. **Small sharp spike while awake with a burst of lateralized delta.** 32 years. A phenomenon that traditionally belongs to one state may appear in another: this widely distributed discharge (*asterisk*) more resembles a small sharp spike than any other apiculate phenomenon. No "phase reversal" appears. Note its expression in most derivations. Its relationship to the left hemisphere burst of 1 Hz delta activity is not clear. Calibration signal 1 sec, 50μV.

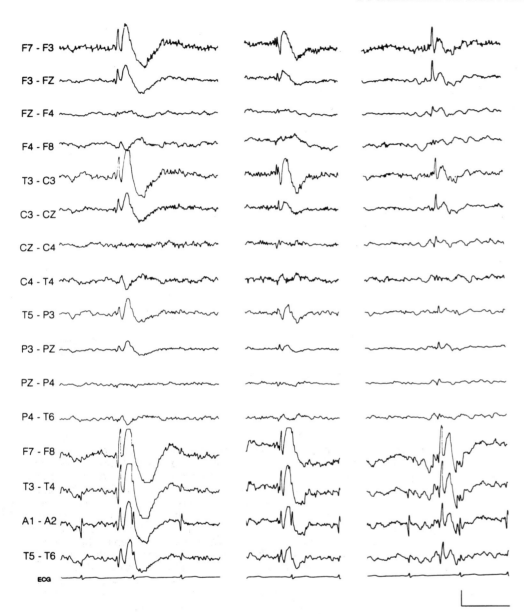

FIG. 4–8. Left temporal spikes on coronal montage. 49 years. Prominent, principally electronegative focal spikes at F7 and T3 with slight spread to A1 and T5. These abnormal anterior temporal spikes differ from small sharp spikes in that their field is more circumscribed, they are higher in voltage, and they have prominent aftercoming slow waves. The spread to F3 and C3 probably reflects volume conduction at the scalp. Calibration signal 1 sec, 50μV.

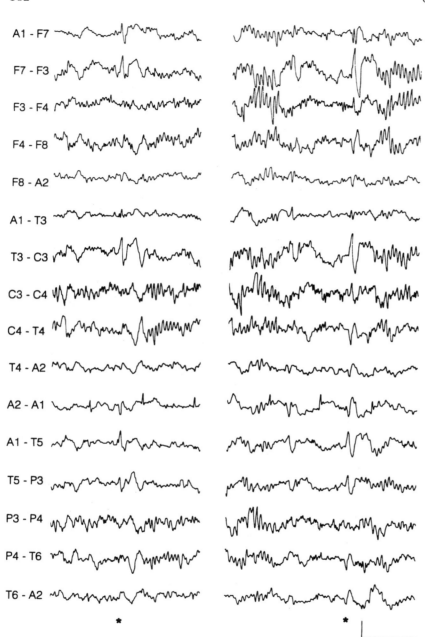

FIG. 4–9. Left anterior temporal spikes on coronal montage. 20 years. This coronal montage, including A1,2, is able to depict both the longitudinal and transverse extent of a temporal spike field (*asterisk*). Principal negativity occurs at A1-T3 electrode positions, as evidenced by the cancellation of potentials in that derivation, the downward deflection at A2-A1, and the upward deflection at A1-T5. The lower-amplitude upward deflection at A1-F7 suggests some involvement of F7, which is confirmed by the upward deflection at F7-F3. Prominent electronegativity at T3 is indicated by the upward deflection at T3-C3. For a spike of this voltage, as indicated by the prominent deflections at F7-F3 and T3-C3, the lack of a greater downward deflection at A2-A1 is surprising, as A1 is very electronegative. This suggests that crossfiring of this spike to A2 has created some negativity there. Downward deflections in right-sided derivations toward A2 are consistent with this, but such downward deflections may also indicate positivity at F4, C4, and P4. This distribution, in any case, resembles that of the type 1 spike described by Ebersole and Wade (18) suggestive of a mesial temporal origin. Calibration signal 1 sec, 50μV.

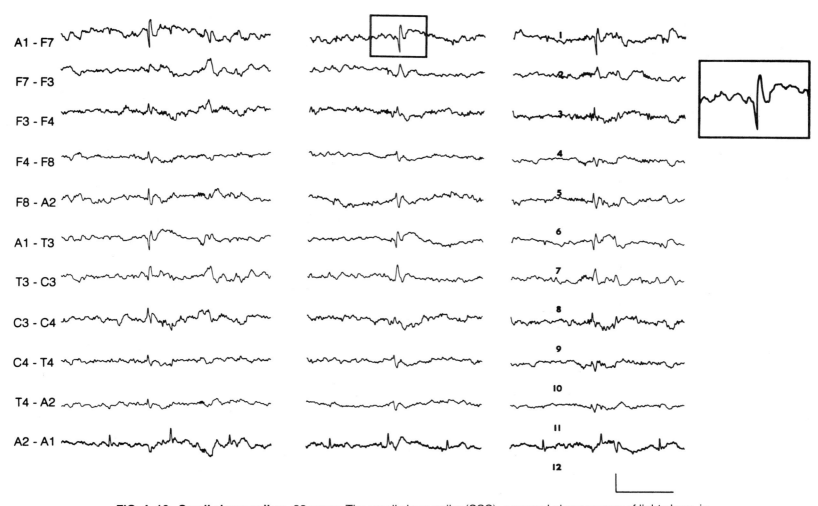

FIG. 4–10. Small sharp spikes. 32 years. The small sharp spike (SSS), a normal phenomenon of light sleep, is briefer than most abnormal anterior temporal spikes, has steep slopes, a relatively brief aftercoming slow wave, and a particularly wide field. This latter attribute is particularly well displayed by coronal montages, as seen here, in that the spike extends to the central, parietal, and frontal regions and well into the hemisphere contralateral to that of its principal expression. Calibration signal 1 sec, 50μV.

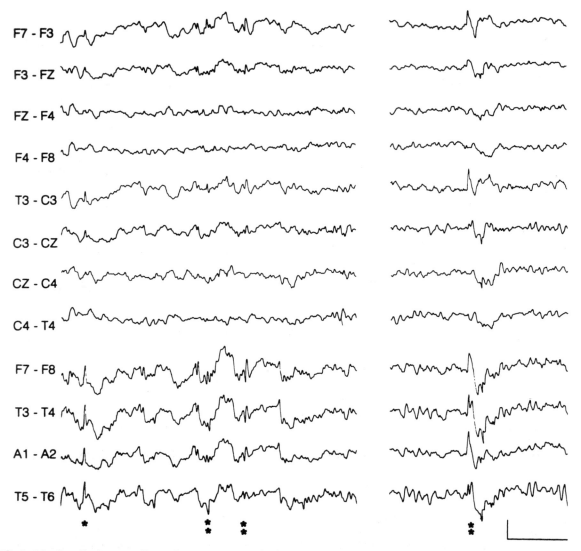

FIG. 4–11. Small sharp spikes of unusual morphology. 15 years. In the first (*left*) segment following a classi-cal small sharp spike (SSS) (*asterisk*) are several low-amplitude polyphasic potentials. Their field of distribution in the left hemisphere is diffuse, as evidenced by their low voltages on bipolar shorter-distance derivations and their better expression with interhemispheric derivations (*double asterisks*). The broad field, their brief duration, and the lack of a prominent aftercoming slow wave suggests their identification as variants of SSS. Unrelated left hemisphere delta appears. In the second (*right*) segment, a broad SSS (*double asterisks*), termed an "N-wave" by Reiher (19) appears. This complex consists of a diffuse, diphasic spike, then a wave, maximum in one hemi-sphere. This also is normal. Calibration signal 1 sec, 70μV.

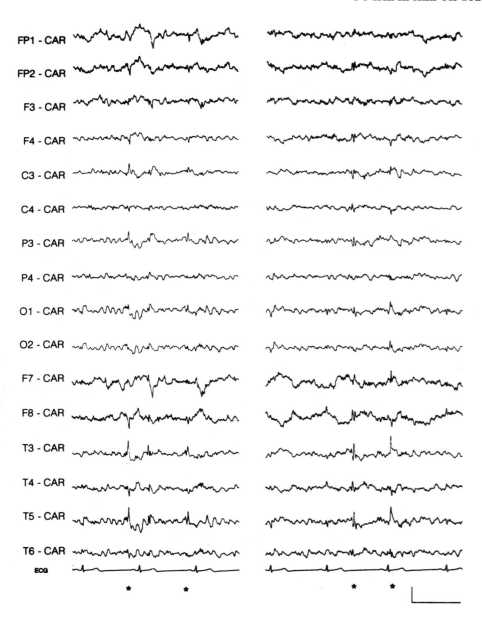

FIG. 4–12. **Small sharp spikes with the common average reference.** 29 years. The widespread field of these small sharp spikes (SSS) (*asterisks*) and their distinct, very sharp, and brief morphology with minimal to no aftercoming slow wave are all well depicted on the common average reference (CAR). CAR "contamination" from the widespread field causes SSS to appear in most channels. Anterior temporal spikes of this voltage would not appear on so many derivations of the CAR because their discrete field does not cause CAR "contamination." Calibration signal 1 sec, 50μV.

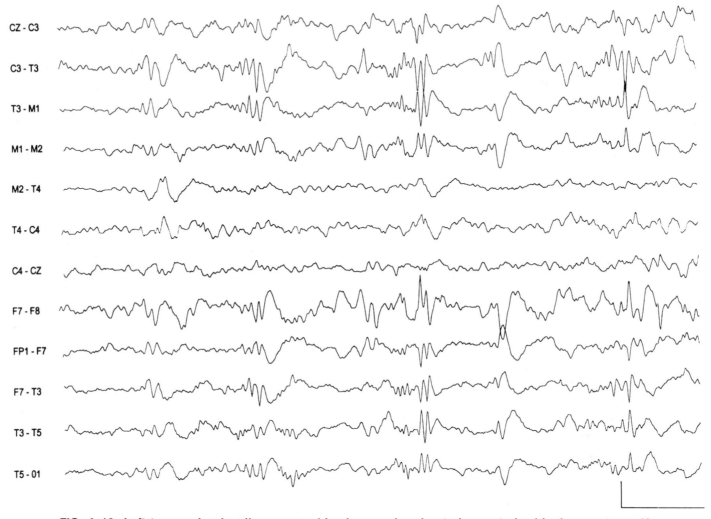

FIG. 4–13. Left temporal polyspikes on combined coronal and anterior-posterior bipolar montage. 40 years. Polyspikes may be slightly more difficult to recognize than single spikes as they do not emerge as starkly from the background activity. These appear principally in the left midtemporal (T3) region with contiguous spread to the left anterior inferior temporal area (F7, M1 [left mandibular notch]). Calibration signal 1 sec, 70μV.

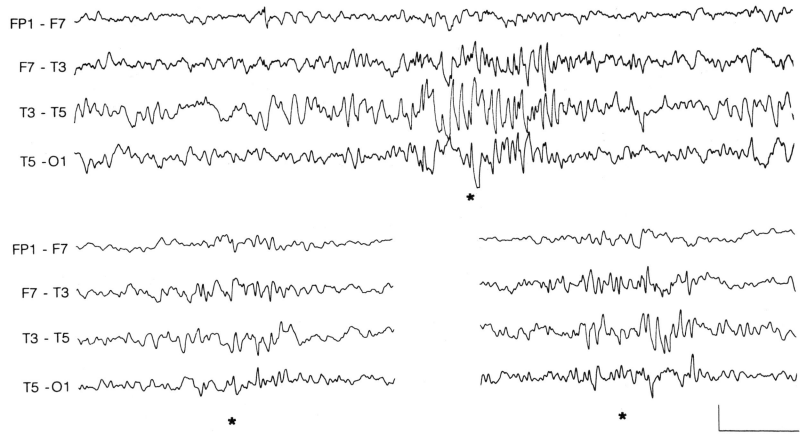

FIG. 4–14. Left temporal polyspikes. 37 years. Polyspikes may escape detection by the electroencephalographer because they blend more with the background rhythms than do single spikes, and no aftercoming slow waves may occur. These polyspikes (*asterisks*), appearing in light to moderate sleep, are progressively more difficult to detect going from the top tracing to the lower ones. The asterisks signify the center of each polyspike discharge. Calibration signal 1 sec, 70μV.

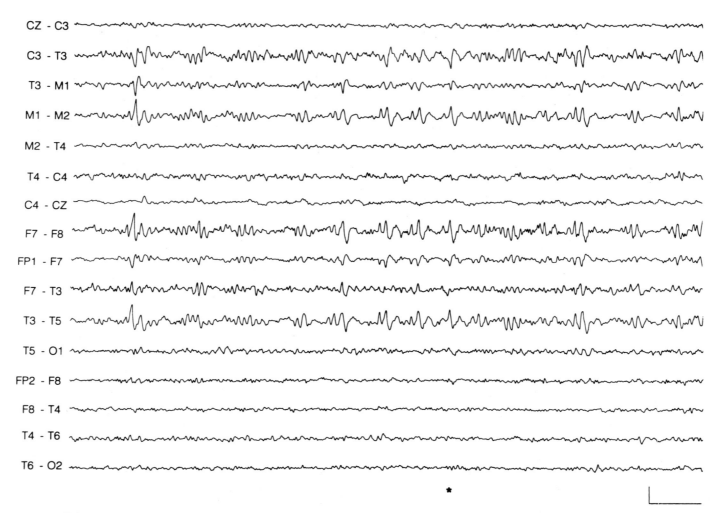

FIG. 4–15. Left temporal spikes and alphoid rhythm. 51 years. The phenomena in this and Figs. 4–16 and 4–17 range from the apiculate nature of left temporal spikes, seen principally in the left mandibular notch surface region (M1) with spread to the left anterior-midtemporal region (F7, T3), to the more rounded morphology of temporal alphoid rhythm in the same area. Such gradations between nonepileptiform and epileptiform phenomena create difficulties in interpretation. One approach is to maintain a relatively high threshold for spike identification and seek areas with unequivocal spikes (*asterisk*) before making positive identification. Calibration signal 1 sec, 70μV.

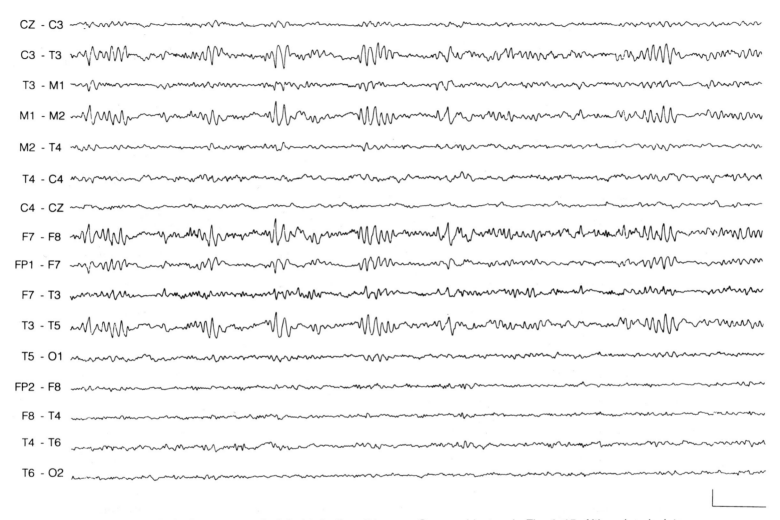

FIG. 4–16. Apiculate temporal alphoid rhythm. 51 years. Same subject as in Fig. 4–15. Although apiculate, the morphology of none of these waves is clearly distinct from the waxing and waning temporal alphoid rhythm. Calibration signal 1 sec, 70μV.

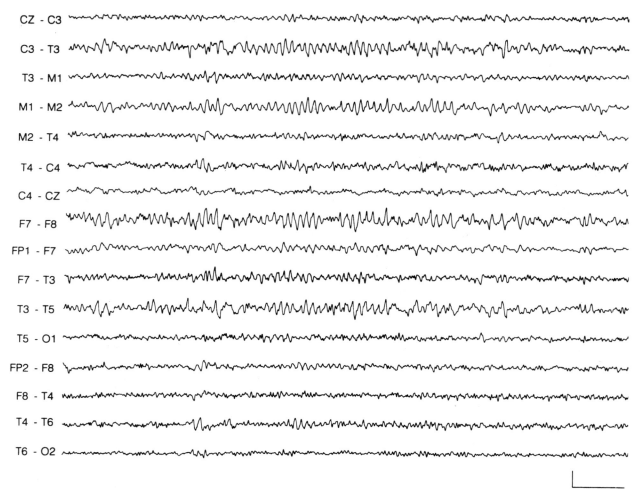

FIG. 4–17. Temporal alphoid rhythm. 51 years. Same subject as in Figs. 4–15 and 4–16. Even less apiculate example of temporal alphoid rhythm. Calibration signal 1 sec, 70μV.

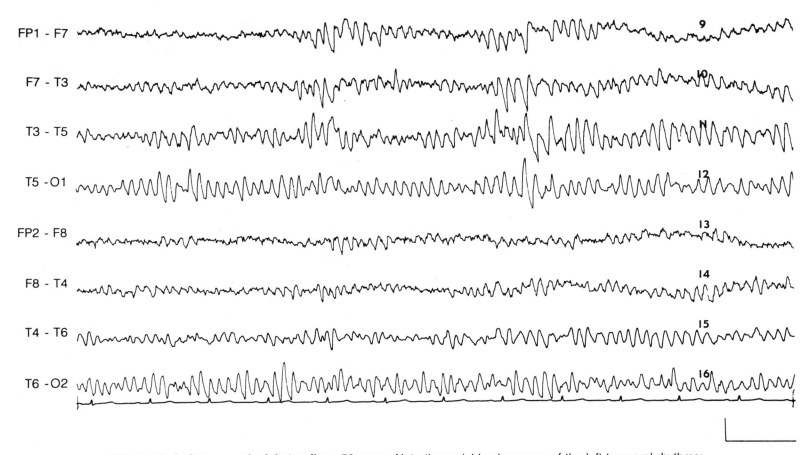

FIG. 4–18. Left temporal wicket spikes. 50 years. Note the variable sharpness of the left temporal rhythms; such wave forms can develop from an increase in the synchrony of ongoing background activity or the superimposition of background wave forms, that is, the left temporal theta and alphoid rhythm. Thus, such isolated sharpness can be expected from this background. Single wave forms of identical morphology could be considered spikes if several of a similar morphology appeared and if the background activity were more amorphous than rhythmic. In the latter case, such sharpness would not be an expected product of the background rhythms and would represent an epileptiform event—not the case here. Calibration signal 1 sec, 50μV.

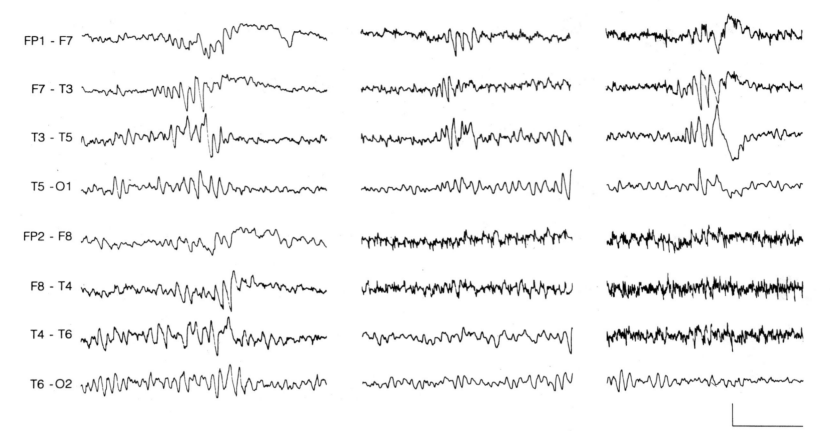

FP1 - F7

F7 - T3

T3 - T5

T5 - O1

FP2 - F8

F8 - T4

T4 - T6

T6 - O2

FIG. 4–19. Abrupt wicket spikes. 50 years. Probably occurring because of combinations of background wave forms (alphoid and theta), wicket spikes may emerge gradually as in Fig. 4–20 or may appear abruptly as occurs here. Although none of these waves could be considered a spike, the phenomena likely indicate excess temporal theta for age and state (wakefulness). Even though the most rightward example contains a slow wave, the preceding apiculate waves appear more as wicket discharges than anterior temporal spikes: even though their negative peaks are quite sharp, the wave forms could be considered (from their positive phases) as a burst of temporal alphoid (10 Hz) waves. Calibration signal 1 sec, 50μV.

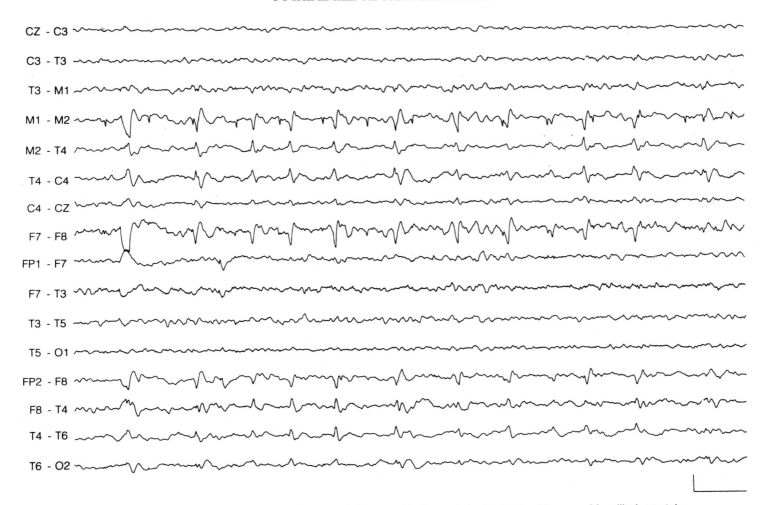

FIG. 4–20. Right anterior temporal spikes and the mandibular notch electrode. 36 years. Mandibular notch and anterior temporal electrode positions may depict temporal spikes better than the standard 10-20 System (2, 20). These stereotypic repetitive spikes appear principally at the mandibular notch electrode (M2) and at the inferior frontal-anterior temporal electrode (F8) with spread to the right midtemporal region (T4). Note their slightly greater amplitude on the coronal portion of this montage, involving M2, compared to the anterior-posterior portion. Right temporal delta activity accompanies these spikes. Calibration signal 1 sec, 70μV.

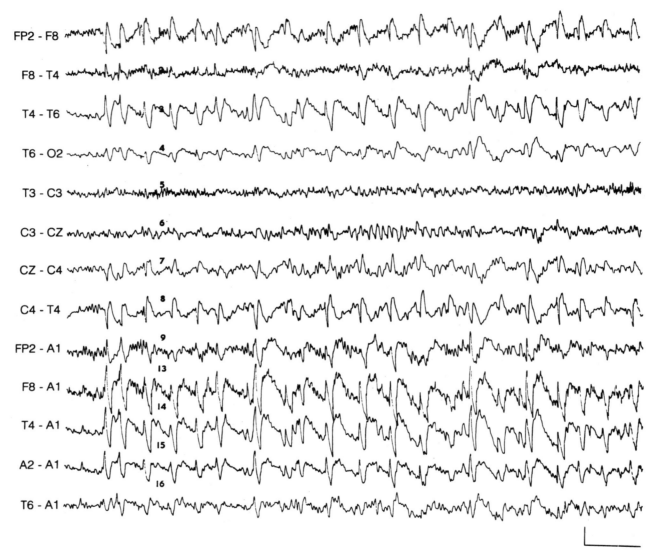

FIG. 4–21. Frequent right temporal spikes with a stereotyped field and morphology. 40 years. Simultaneous bipolar anterior-posterior and coronal montages with a referential montage to the contralateral ear illustrate principal involvement of F8 and T4 with moderate involvement of A2, a characteristic pattern of right anterior temporal spikes. Note the moderate spread to the right frontal polar region (Fp2) and the only slight spread to the posterior temporal region (T6). The prominent downward deflection in the C4-T4 derivation confirms the infra-Sylvian location of these spikes. Calibration signal 1 sec, 70μV.

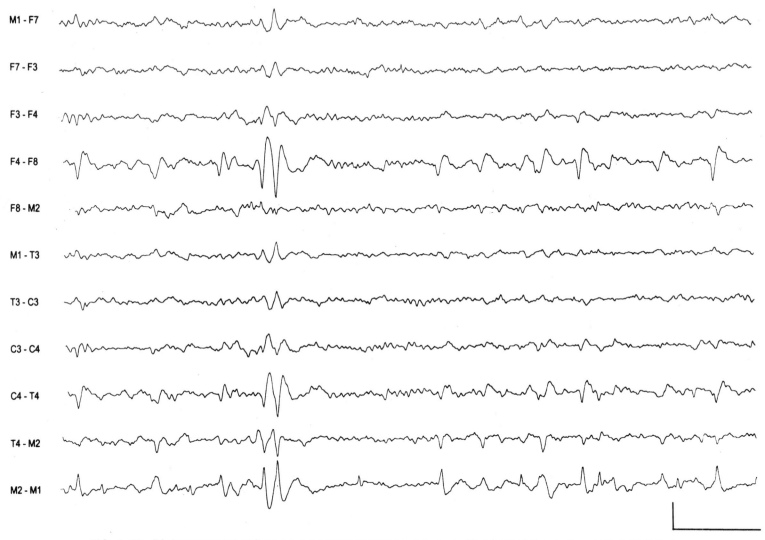

FIG. 4–22. Right temporal spikes on a coronal montage. 34 years. The field of these abundant right tempo-ral spikes is well depicted by this coronal montage, as intratemporal cancellation effects do not occur with these derivations. Thus, such spikes appear principally in the inferior-anterior temporal (M2-F8) region with moderate spread to the right midtemporal (T4) region. Note the slightly varying field of such spikes. Calibration signal 1 sec, 50μV.

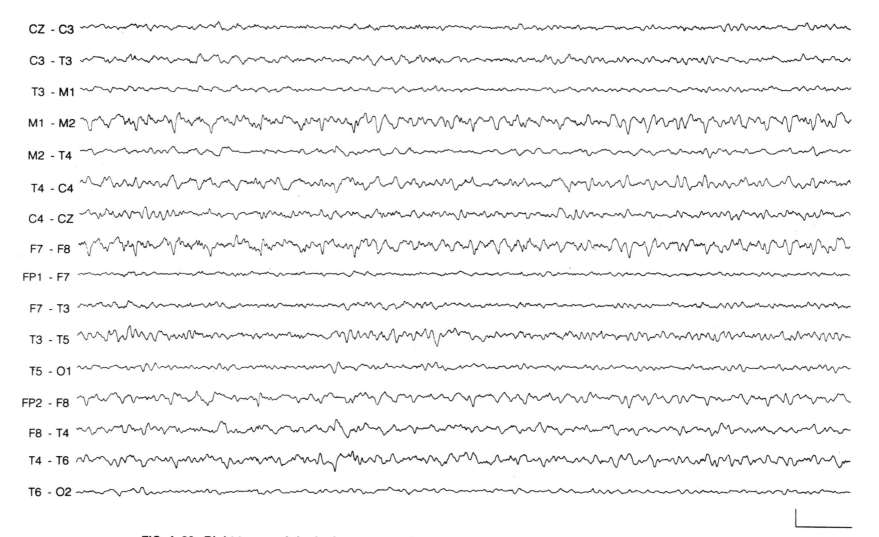

FIG. 4–23. Right temporal rhythmic waves and intermingled spikes. 36 years. Some patients with temporal lobe epilepsy have virtually continuous rhythmic to semi-rhythmic anterior temporal waves with intermingled spikes. Such patients may have continuous simple partial seizures with symptoms of fear or abdominal discomfort (21). Calibration signal 1 sec, 70μV.

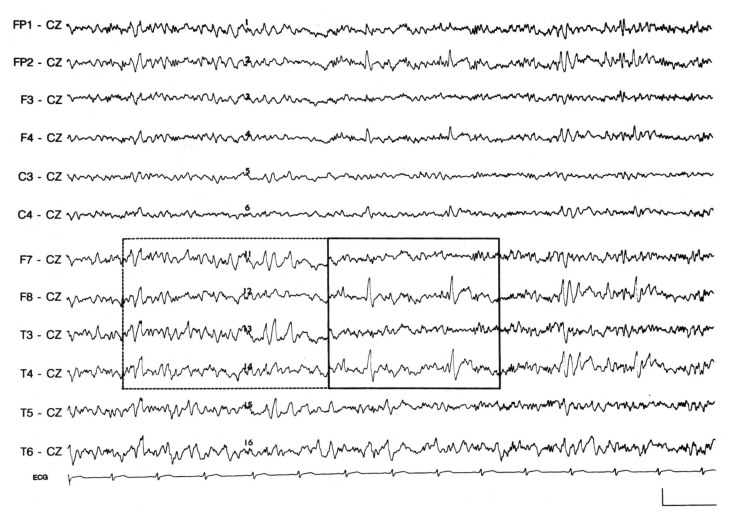

FIG. 4–24. Right temporal spikes and sharply contoured temporal theta. 35 years. This referential (Cz) montage illustrates the occasional difficulty of identifying temporal spikes because of the apiculate nature of much temporal lobe background activity (*dotted square*). The two definite temporal spikes (*solid square*) emerge clearly from the surrounding background activity and have aftercoming slow waves that are synchronous in the F8 and T4 positions. Note their spread to the frontal central areas (Fp2-C4), suggesting that they arise from the temporal neocortex (18). Calibration signal 1 sec, 70μV.

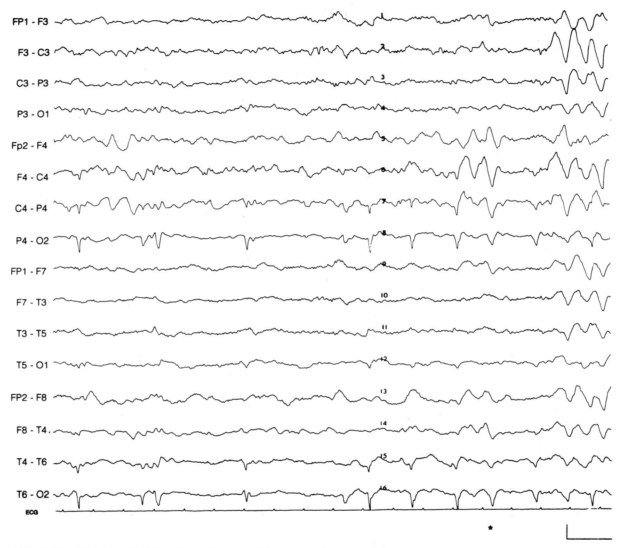

FIG. 4–25. Right occipital spikes. 52 years. The major phase of occipital spikes is almost always electronegative, as seen here. Propagation to the adjacent posterior temporal and parietal regions also commonly occurs, as
noted in the C4-P4 and T4-T6 derivations. The morphology of most of these spikes contrasts distinctly with that
of the background activity, but note the gradations of sharpness between obvious spikes and the apiculate waves
that constitute the nonspecific bursts toward the end of this segment (*asterisk*). Calibration signal 1 sec, 70μV.

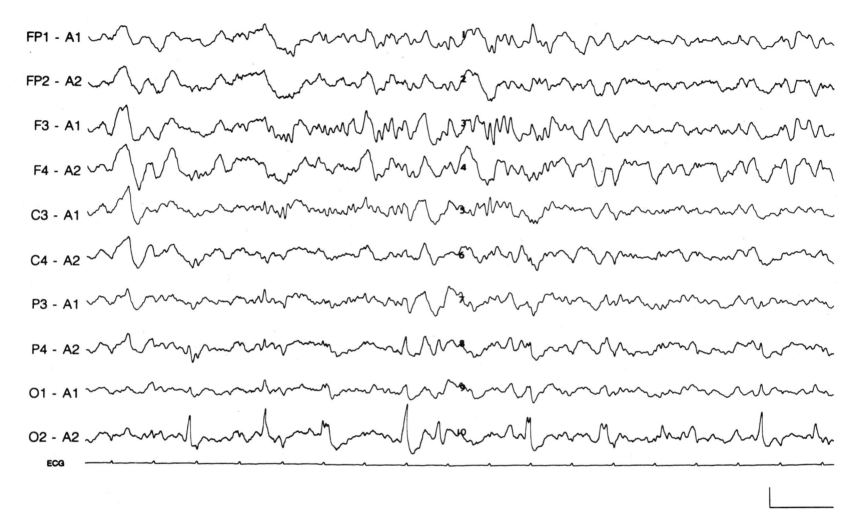

FIG. 4–26. Right occipital spikes and right hemisphere spindle reduction. 52 years. Same patient as in Fig. 4–25, in deeper sleep. The right occipital (O2) electronegative spikes persist, but more widespread right hemisphere dysfunction is revealed by the predominantly right-sided delta activity anteriorly and the reduction of spindles in the right hemisphere. In contrast, note the relative symmetry of the V-waves, which are more resilient to lesions. Calibration signal 1 sec, 70μV.

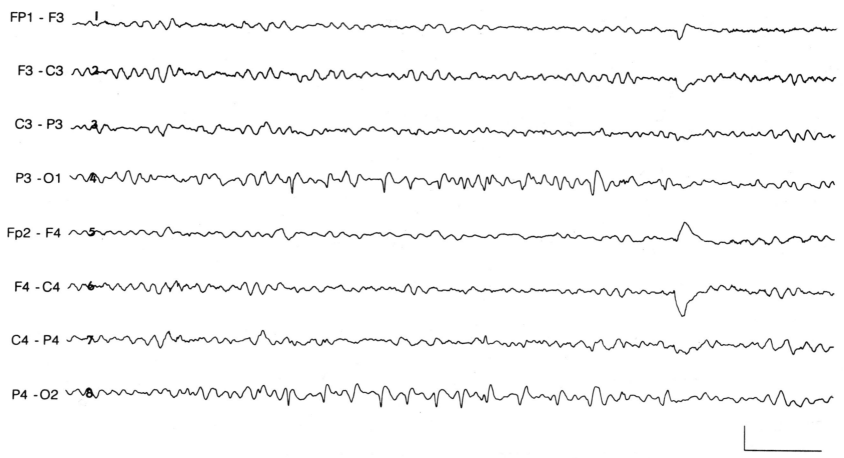

FIG. 4–27. Occipital spikes. 17 years. A very sharply contoured electronegative peak which distinguishes an occipital spike from other sharply contoured but more blunt posterior waves. ECG potentials are usually electropositive at O1, O2, as is the principal phase of lambda. Occipital spikes markedly attenuate with eye opening, whereas lambda are only present then. Occipital spikes commonly appear bilaterally, and a coronal montage would be required to distinguish the side of maximum voltage. Calibration signal 1 sec, 150μV.

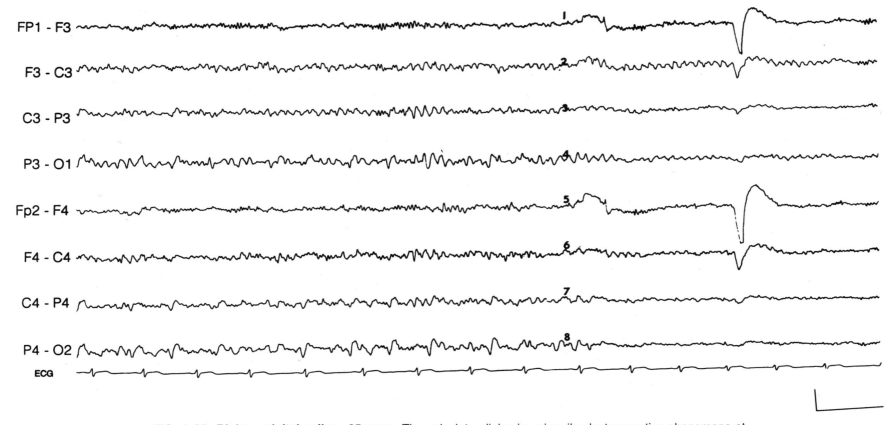

FIG. 4–28. Right occipital spikes. 35 years. The apiculate, diphasic, primarily electronegative phenomena at O2 with spread to P4 and minimal spread to O1 do not coincide with the ECG, are not lambda waves because the eyes are closed, and are not positive occipital sharp transients of sleep because of their polarity and because of the wakefulness. Therefore, they are a subtle expression of right occipital spikes. Note their abolition with slow eye opening as revealed by the low-amplitude electronegative frontal polar (Fp1, Fp2) wave with slight rightward deviation. Facile abolition by eye opening is a common feature of occipital spikes. Note that the 8 Hz background activity is better developed on the contralateral (left) side. Calibration signal 1 sec, 70μV.

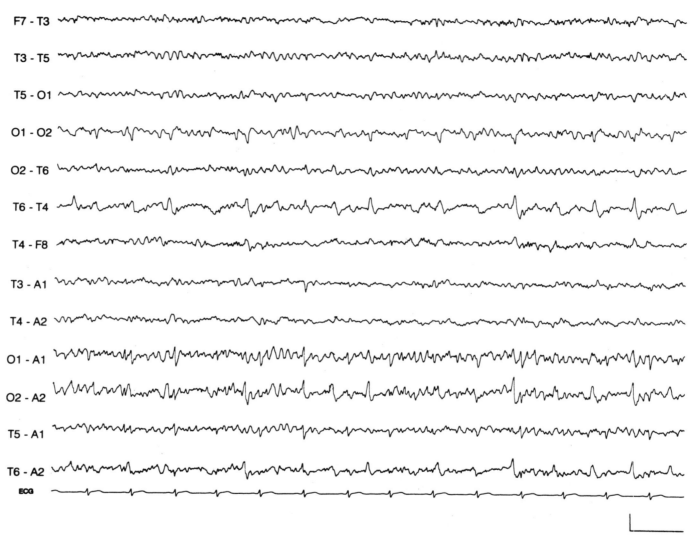

FIG. 4–29. Occipital spikes with posterior coronal and referential montages. 35 years. The often consider-able spread of occipital spikes to the ipsilateral posterior temporal region is depicted in this montage, where elec-trical cancellation between O2 and T6 occurs for most spikes. The usual lack of spread to the ipsilateral ear (A2 in this case) qualifies it as a reliable reference. Note the importance of ECG monitoring for posteriorly-situated and periodic epileptiform discharges. Alpha activity is lower-voltage on the right. Calibration signal 1 sec, 70µV.

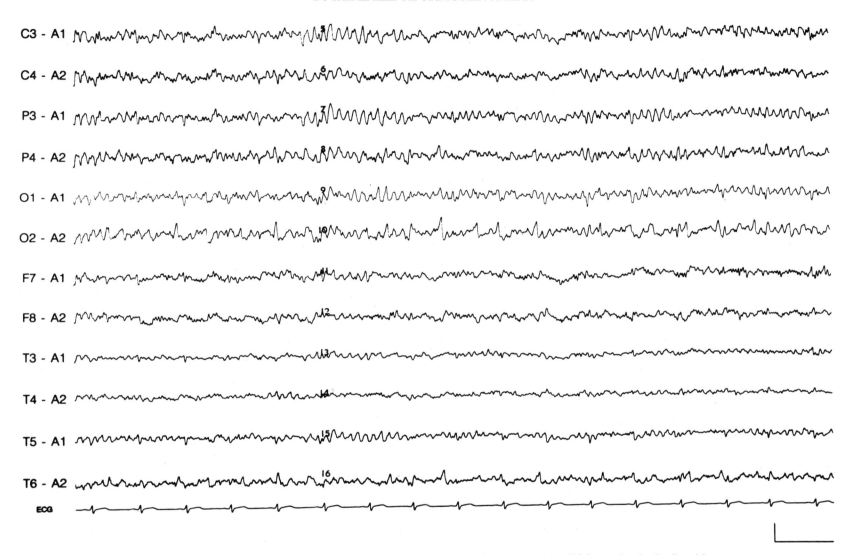

FIG. 4–30. Right occipital spikes. 35 years. The ipsilateral ear reference and the ECG monitor both allow identification of the apiculate wave forms in the right occipital-posterior temporal (O2,T6) area as spikes. With the eyes closed during wakefulness, these phenomena could not be either lambda or positive occipital sharp transients of sleep (POSTS), and their appearance only randomly coincides with the ECG. However, low-voltage ECG potentials appear at O1 and T5. Background activity is slower at O2 and T6 compared to O1 and T5. Calibration signal 1 sec, 70μV.

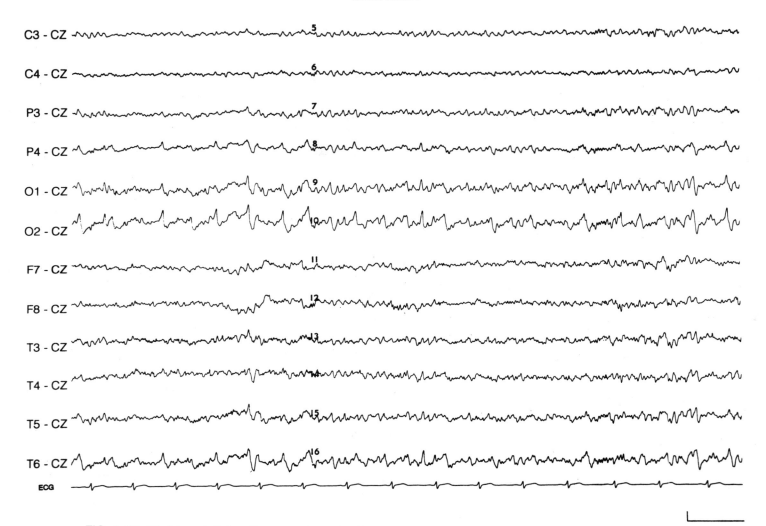

FIG. 4–31. Right occipital spikes on referential (Cz) montage. 76 years. The lack of Cz involvement in posterior and temporal spike fields qualifies it as a reliable reference. Same awake recording as in Fig. 4–30 showing higher-amplitude and frequent right occipital (O2) spikes with spread to the right posterior temporal (T6), right parietal (P4) and left occipital (O1) regions. The same differential diagnostic considerations as those described for Fig. 4–30 apply. Calibration signal 1 sec, 70μV.

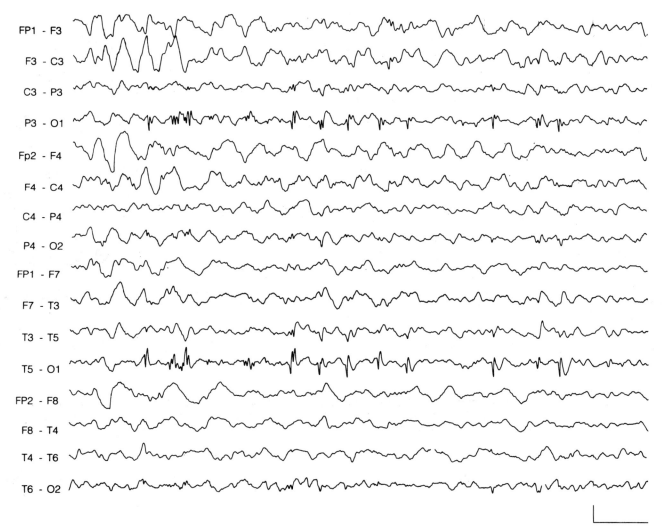

FIG. 4–32. Occipital spikes and polyspikes in sleep. 15 years. Abundant occipital spikes and polyspikes may appear only in non-REM sleep, as seen in the left occipital (O1) region. Note the slight spread to the left posterior temporal (T5) region and minimal spread to the left parietal (P3) and right occipital (O2) areas. Calibration signal 1 sec, 100μV.

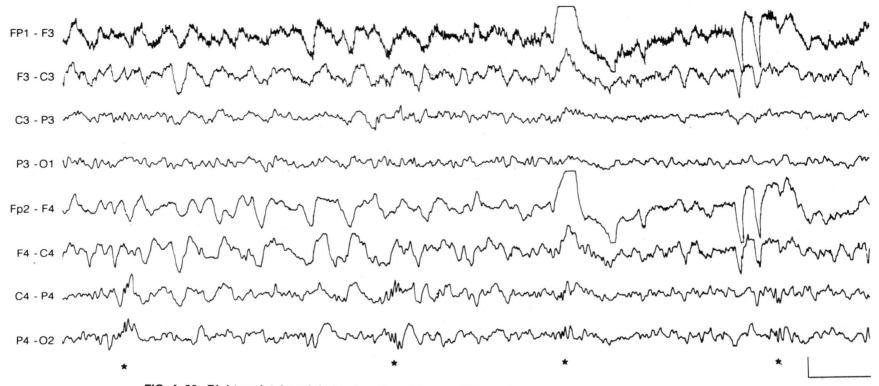

FIG. 4–33. Right parietal occipital polyspikes. 63 years. Diffuse abnormalities such as the right hemisphere-accentuated delta may partially obscure lower-amplitude focal abnormalities such as these right parietal (P4, O2) polyspikes (*asterisks*). Calibration signal 1 sec, 50μV.

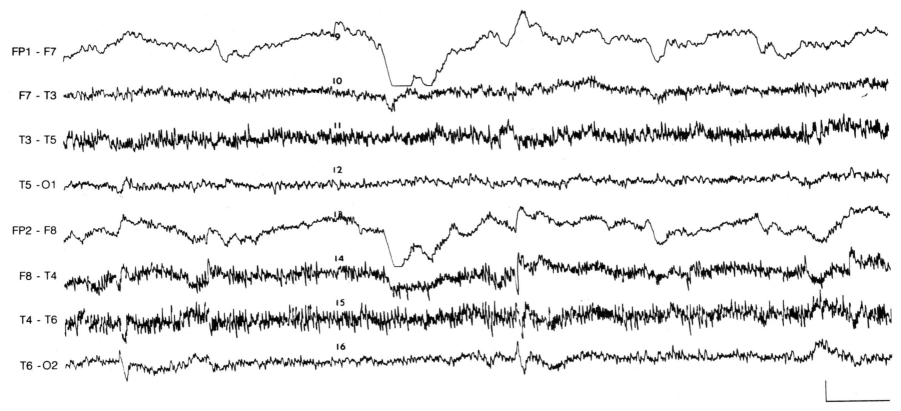

FIG. 4–34. Right temporal spikes, delta, and artifact as part of a larger field. 76 years. Despite continuous bitemporal muscle artifact, intermittent right midtemporal (T4) spikes appear which spread to the right posterior temporal region (T6). Intermittent 500–800 msec right temporal delta waves appear. It is likely that more persistent delta activity exists, but this is difficult to discern with the artifact. Full depiction of this field requires the parasagittal portion (next illustration). Calibration signal 1 sec, 70μV.

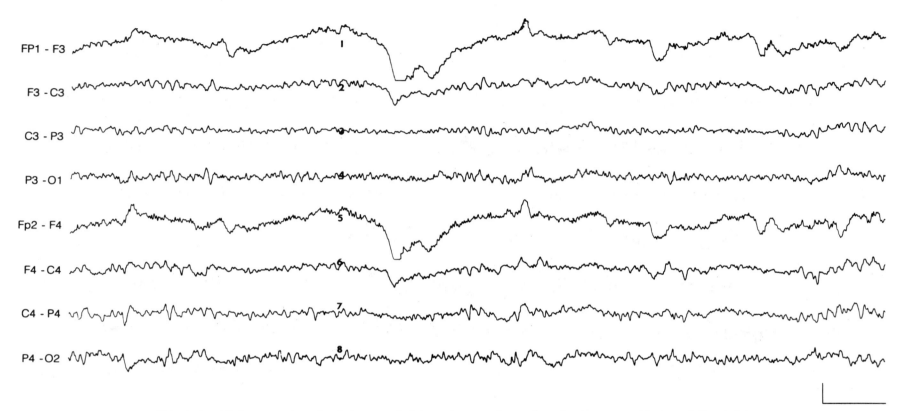

FIG. 4–35. Right central parietal theta and delta. 76 years. Recording simultaneous with that of Fig. 4–34 shows bursts of 5–6 Hz and 2 Hz waves in the right central parietal (C4, P4) region. Calibration signal 1 sec, 70μV.

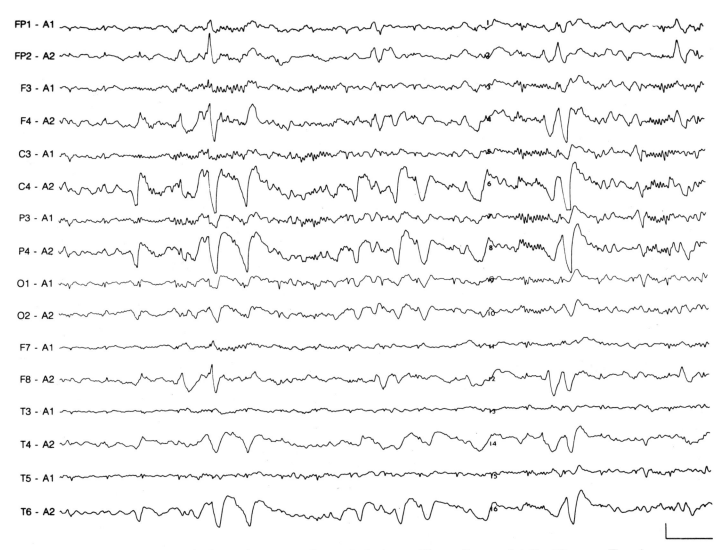

FIG. 4–36. Right hemisphere electronegative and electropositive spikes and delta. 26 years. The electronegative spikes and portions of spikes appear principally as upward deflections at the right frontal polar (Fp2), inferior frontal (F8), and superior frontal (F4) derivations of this ipsilateral ear reference montage. The electropositive components appear principally as downward deflections at the right central (C4) and right parietal (P4) derivations. Delta activity appears principally in the right central, parietal, and midposterior temporal (T4, T6) derivations. That the right ear (A2) electrode is not principally involved in the electropositive spikes and delta phenomena is indicated by the lower-amplitude deflections in the Fp2, F4, and O2 derivations: if A2 were "active," this pattern of amplitudes would imply principal involvement of the right inferior temporal, right occipital, and right frontal regions—a most unlikely circumstance. Often, the contribution of a reference electrode to the expression of a phenomenon can be gleaned by careful analysis. Note the reduction of spindles in the right hemisphere, further evidence of its dysfunction. Calibration signal 1 sec, 100μV.

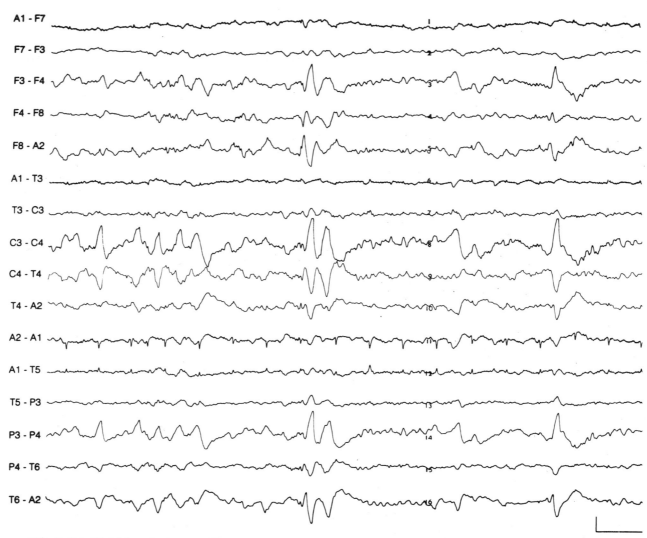

FIG. 4–37. Right hemisphere spikes on a coronal montage. 26 years. Same recording as in Fig. 4–36 and similar spike distribution: the initial negative components are virtually confined to the right frontal (F8,F4) region, and the positive components are more posterior and widespread. Their strictly unilateral location, their high amplitude from the parietal to the frontal region, and the accompanying delta disqualifies these discharges from being V-waves. Concurring with Daly (22), we see no distinction between spikes and sharp waves, recognizing that gradations of duration exist. Calibration signal 1 sec, 100µV.

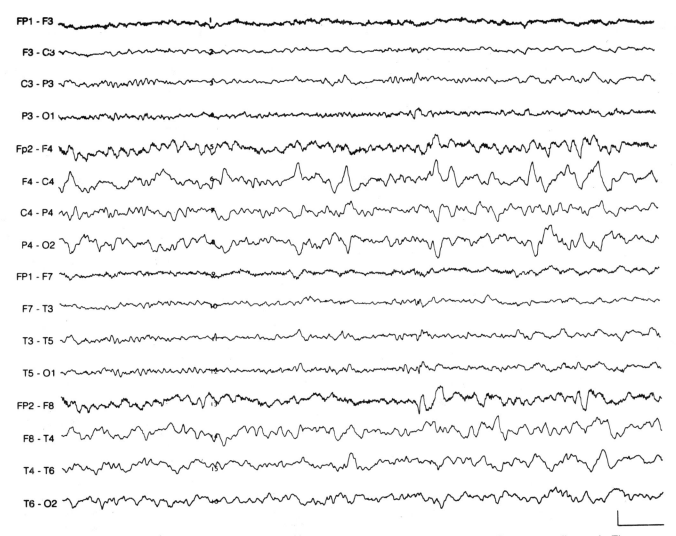

FIG. 4–38. Electropositive right central parietal spikes in wakefulness. 26 years. Same recording as in Figs. 4–36 and 4–37. Electropositive right central parietal (C4, P4) spikes and right hemisphere delta. Notice the very limited propagation of these phenomena to the homologous regions of the left hemisphere. Same distribution of electropositive events as in Figs. 4–36 and 4–37. Calibration signal 1 sec, 70μV.

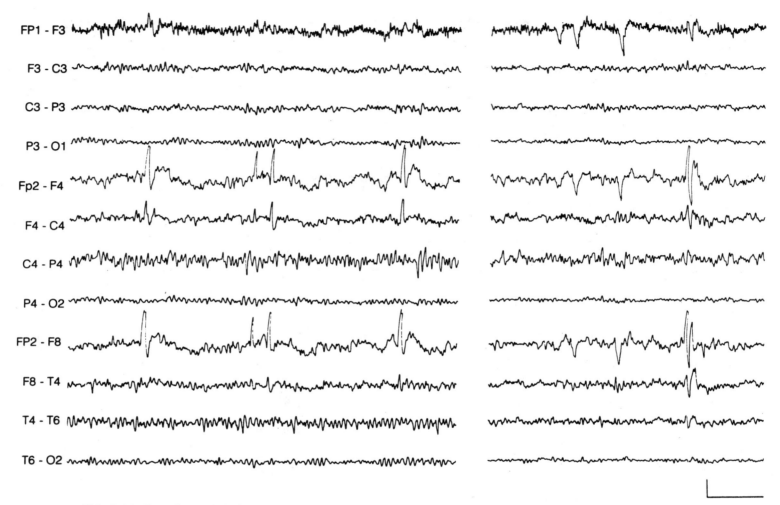

FIG. 4–39. Prominent right frontal spikes and delta. 41 years. There should be little difficulty in identifying the right frontal polar (Fp2) location of both the spikes and the delta activity although the spikes spread more to the right superior frontal region (F4) than does the delta. Note the 15 Hz breach rhythm at the C4-P4 derivation and minimally at the F4-C4 derivation. The second (*right*) segment illustrates the distinct bifrontal polar (Fp1, Fp2) electropositive deflection of eye movements and the initial electronegative deflection of the Fp2 spike. Calibration signal 1 sec, 50μV.

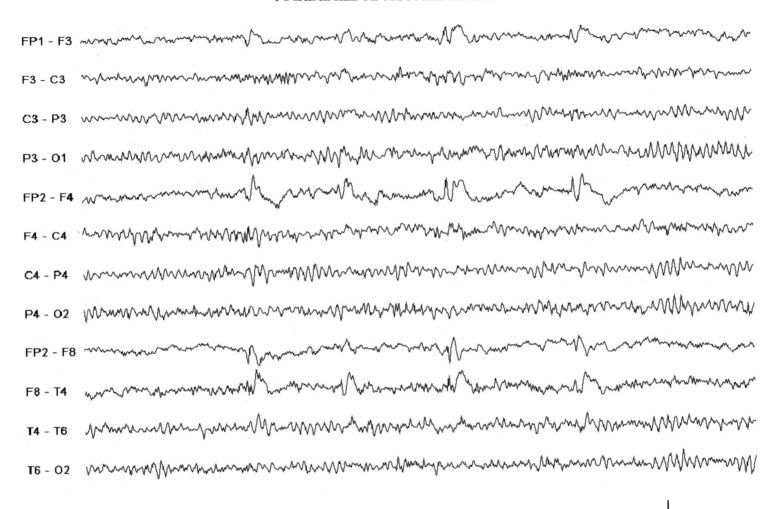

FIG. 4–40. Right frontal spikes. Right frontal polar inferior frontal (Fp2, F8) spikes are depicted on this bipolar montage. Prominent deflection in the F8-T4 derivation would be unusual with an anterior temporal spike, where cancellation in that derivation would have occurred. Calibration signal 1 sec, 50μV.

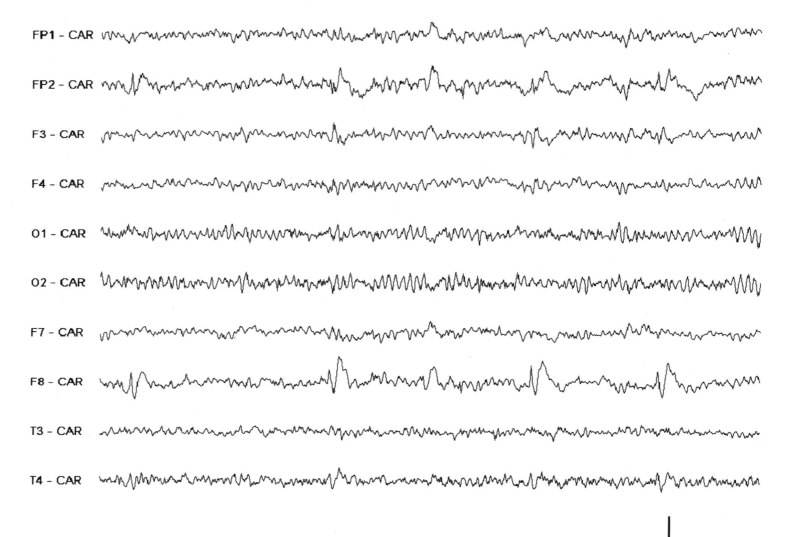

FIG. 4–41. Frontal spikes with common average reference (CAR). Common average reference (CAR) of these same spikes illustrates the principal right inferior frontal (F8) involvement with spread to the right frontal polar (Fp2) region and only minimal temporal (T4) spread. This confirms further that the F8 position can represent inferior frontal as well as anterior temporal phenomena. Calibration signal 1 sec, 50μV.

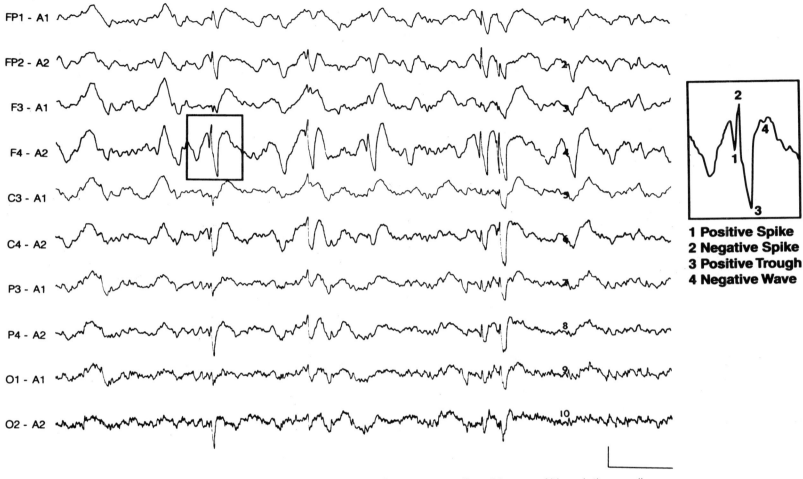

FIG. 4–42. Right hemisphere spikes on an ear reference recording. 20 years. Although these spikes appear principally in the right superior frontal region (F4) with spread to the right central (C4) and other regions, their morphology—a brief spike, then a comparatively large electropositive trough and following wave—resemble more that of a unilateral spike-wave complex than spikes from a focal lesion. Note the larger field of the electropositive trough (3) and following electronegative wave (4) than that of the spike (1, 2). The larger amplitude of the spike-wave at the F4-A2 derivation compared to other parasagittal derivations virtually excludes the possibility of significant reference (A2) involvement. *Inset:* Components of a completely expressed focal spike: 1) initial positive phase, 2) negative phase, 3) positive trough, and 4) negative wave. Calibration signal 1 sec, 200μV.

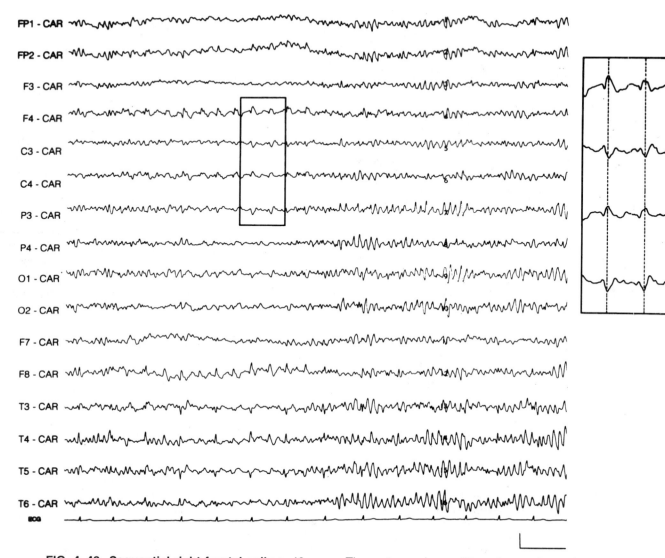

FIG. 4–43. Sequential right frontal spikes. 40 years. The metronomic repetition of some low-voltage spikes and their morphology both create an ECG-like appearance. These discharges are centered at F8 with spread to F4 and C4, with an apparent dipole with C3 and P3 as evidenced by the out-of-phase deflections (*inset*). T4 only rarely becomes involved. The other regularly repetitive apiculate waves are ECG artifacts. Calibration signal 1 sec, 50μV.

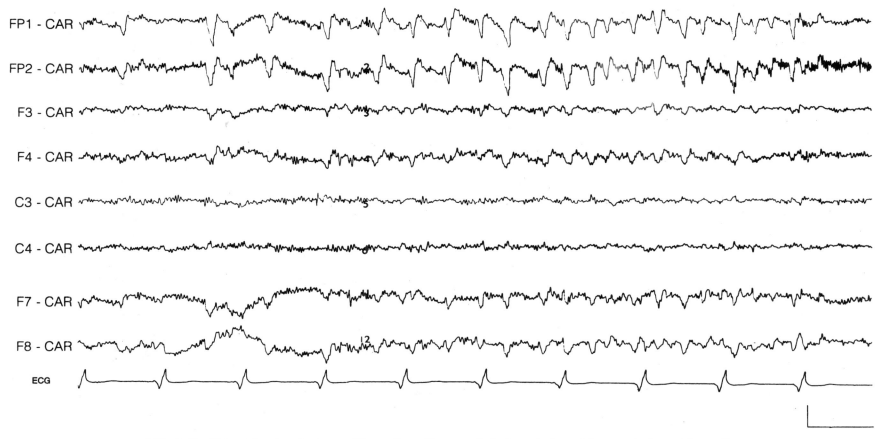

FIG. 4–44. Bifrontal polar electropositive spikes. 76 years. Both the polarity and the morphology of these discharges resemble eye blinks, but the only eye movements in this recording during drowsiness are slow lateral eye movements, as seen in the F7, F8 derivations in the 2nd to 4th seconds. The triphasic contour of some of these discharges would be distinctly unusual for eye blinks, as the initial negative component does not occur with eye blinks. Calibration signal 1 sec, 50μV.

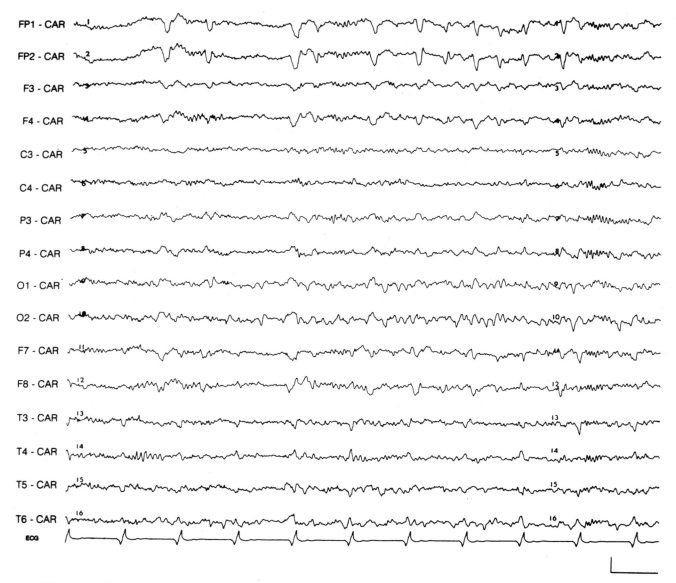

FIG. 4–45. Frontal polar spikes in non-REM sleep. 76 years. Same subject as in Fig. 4–44. The continued presence in non-REM sleep bifrontal polar (Fp1, Fp2) spikes gives further evidence that the potentials of the previous tracing were not eye movements. The greater out-of-phase deflections in the parietal and occipital derivations compared to posterior temporal derivations suggests an anterior-posterior dipole field. Note the spindles in the last part of the tracing. Calibration signal 1 sec, 50μV.

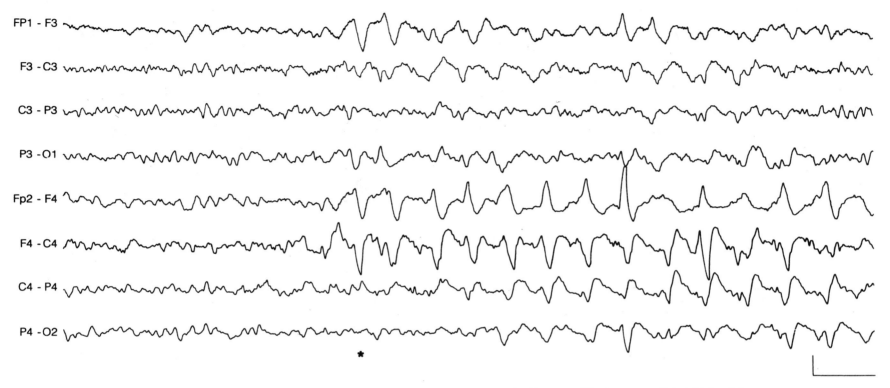

FIG. 4–46. Sequential right frontal broad spikes (sharp waves). 63 years. These sequential right frontal spikes have a variable field. Although some of the later discharges are clearly electropositive at F4, the first definitive discharge (*asterisk*) does not demonstrate a reversal of each phase, raising the possibility of a rapidly propagating focus from F4 to Fp2 (in a manner similar to the occipital-frontal lag of triphasic waves). Spikes later in the sequence extend more posteriorly to engulf the entire right hemisphere. Involvement of the homologous left regions occurs commonly with frontal spikes, and therefore the apiculate deflections at Fp1 do not indicate an additional focus there. The left hemisphere delta appears only when that of the right hemisphere is of high voltage, and therefore no definitely independent left hemisphere abnormality is demonstrated. A left ear reference montage or the common average reference (CAR) would depict the spike field better than this bipolar montage. Calibration signal 1 sec, 100μV.

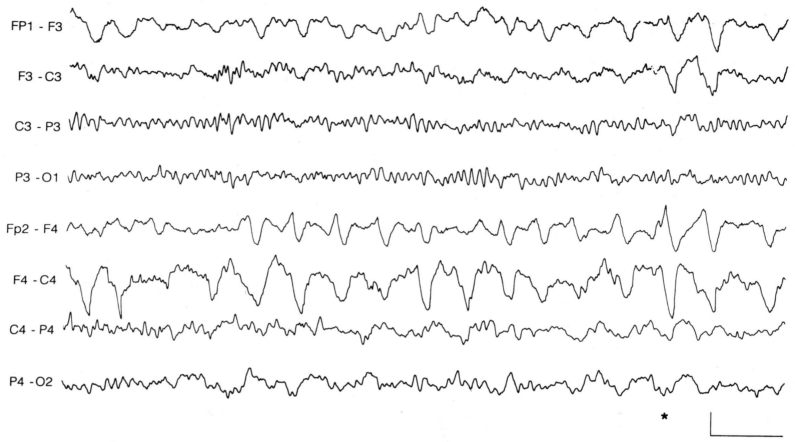

FIG. 4–47. Right frontal spikes and right hemisphere delta. 63 years. More than one type of epileptiform discharge appears in the right frontal region. The most frequent are electropositive broad spikes at Fp2-F4. Electronegative spikes, at Fp2 (*asterisk*), are occasionally superimposed upon such electropositive spikes. The diffuse right-sided delta activity and the loss of right-sided alpha activity reflect widespread right hemisphere dysfunction. Although some of these broad spikes have a triphasic contour, these are not "triphasic waves" because of their unilateral (right) predominance with a normal awake background activity in the left hemisphere. The low-voltage left frontal delta likely reflects spread from the frontally accentuated right delta, as each wave on the left has a counterpart on the right. Calibration signal 1 sec, 70μV.

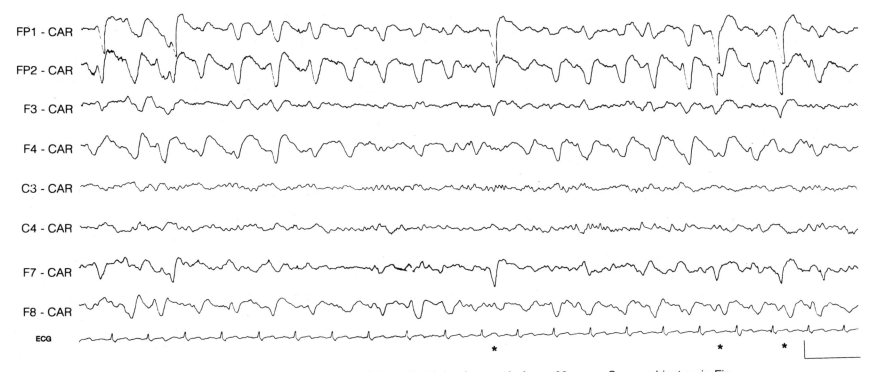

FIG. 4–48. Bifrontal spikes, maximum right, with triphasic morphology. 63 years. Same subject as in Fig. 4–47. Although these sequential primarily electropositive bifrontal polar (Fp2, Fp1) broad spikes resemble triphasic waves in their anterior location and morphology, their asymmetry and the normal left hemisphere background activity indicates that they are not triphasic waves. Eye blinks (*asterisks*) are distinguished by their location and morphology. Compare with Figs. 4–44 and 4–45. Calibration signal 1 sec, 100μV.

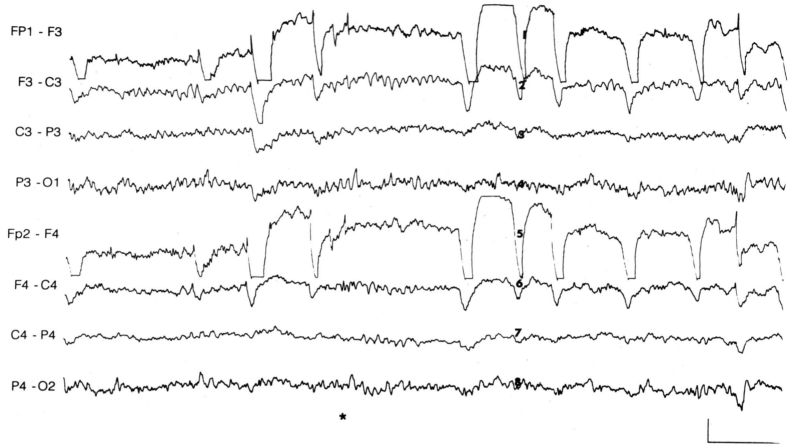

FIG. 4–49. Eye movements and periocular muscle potentials. 20 years. Derivations involving the frontal polar (Fp1, Fp2) leads demonstrate prominent eye blinks. Periocular muscle potentials precede some of the eye blinks or occur independently (*asterisk*). The electropositive sharply contoured potentials in the occipital (O1, O2) leads are lambda waves. Note the asymmetrical mu, a common feature of that wave form. Calibration signal 1 sec, 50μV.

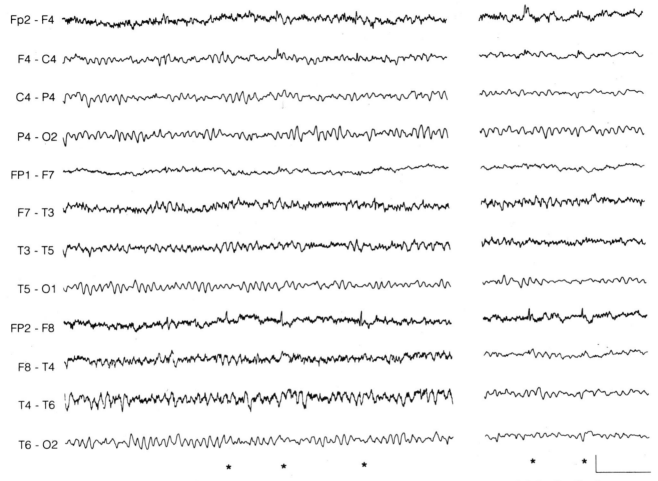

FIG. 4–50. Low-voltage right frontal polar spikes. 23 years. Usually, low-amplitude, very brief spike-like forms in the frontal polar leads are periocular muscle potentials. However, these (*asterisks*) are right frontal polar (Fp2) spikes. This should be suspected because of their spread to F4 as revealed by the F4-C4 derivation. These spikes did not propagate to Fp1, as revealed by the Fp1-F7 derivation, nor did they propagate to F3 (not shown). Calibration signal 1 sec, 50μV.

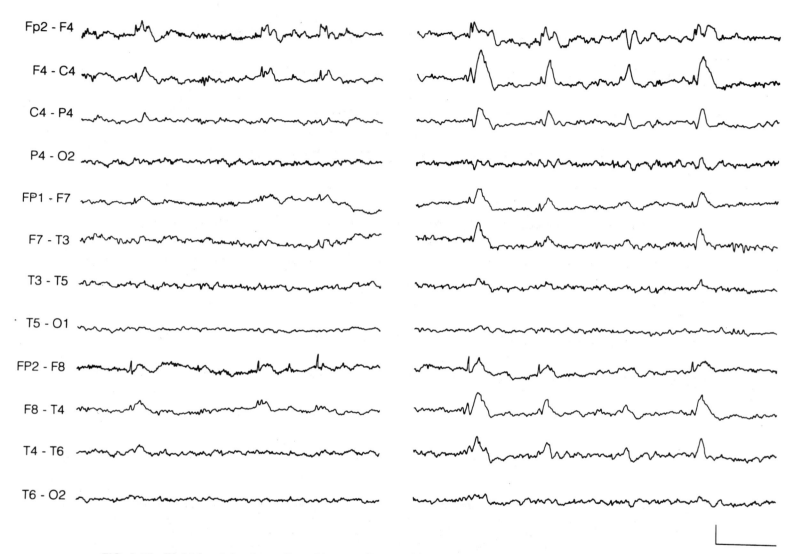

FIG. 4–51. Right frontal polar spikes. 23 years. Same subject as in Fig. 4–50. The amplitude and field of these spikes increase in drowsiness, and the accompanying slow waves become considerably more prominent. Some propagation to the left frontal region (Fp1, F7) is seen. Calibration signal 1 sec, 70μV.

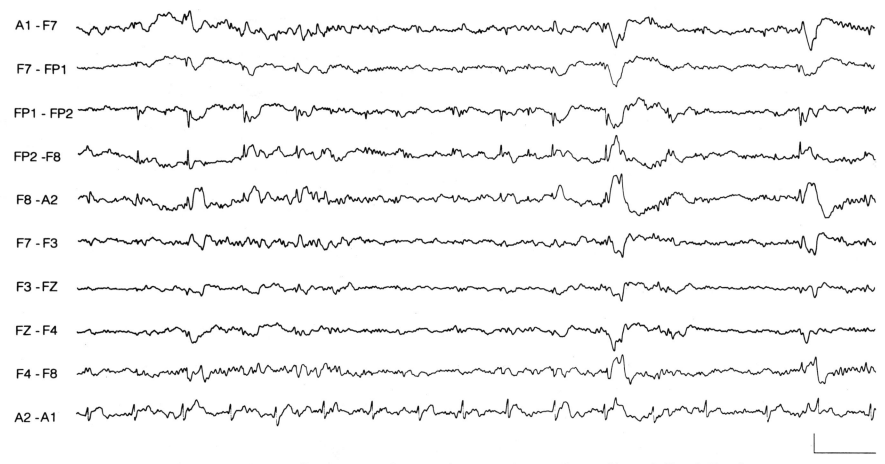

FIG. 4–52. Frontal polar spikes on an anterior coronal montage. 23 years. Same subject as in Figs. 4–50 and 4–51. This montage clearly depicts these spikes and their field as occurring in the right frontal polar region (Fp2), with slight spread to the right inferior frontal region (F8) and the left frontal polar region (Fp1). Note the value of an ECG monitor as provided by the ear leads (A2-A1) in distinguishing these spikes, of nearly metronomic repetition, from cardiac potentials. Calibration signal 1 sec, 70μV.

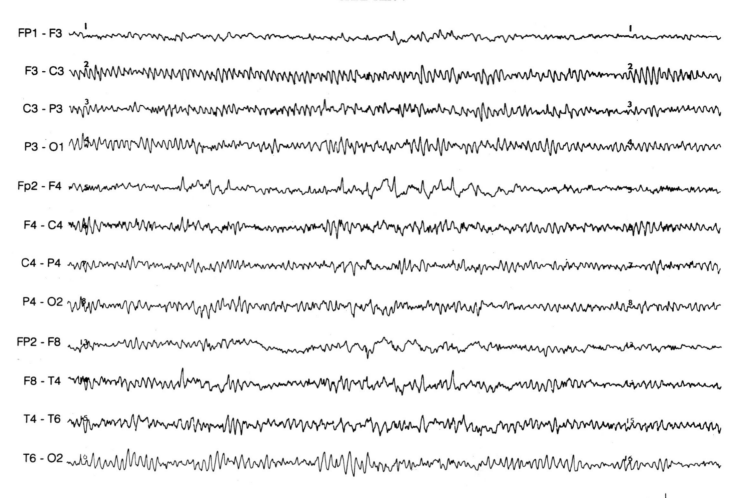

FP1 - F3

F3 - C3

C3 - P3

P3 - O1

Fp2 - F4

F4 - C4

C4 - P4

P4 - O2

FP2 - F8

F8 - T4

T4 - T6

T6 - O2

FIG. 4–53. Right frontal polar-inferior frontal spikes. 40 years. These right frontal polar–right inferior frontal (Fp2-F8) spikes appear in the Fp2-F4 and F8-T4 derivations with electrical cancellation at the Fp2-F8 derivation for most of the spikes. One of them appears principally at F8. Note the slight propagation of spikes to Fp1, and the 2 Hz right frontal delta activity which accompanies the spike series. Calibration signal 1 sec, 70μV.

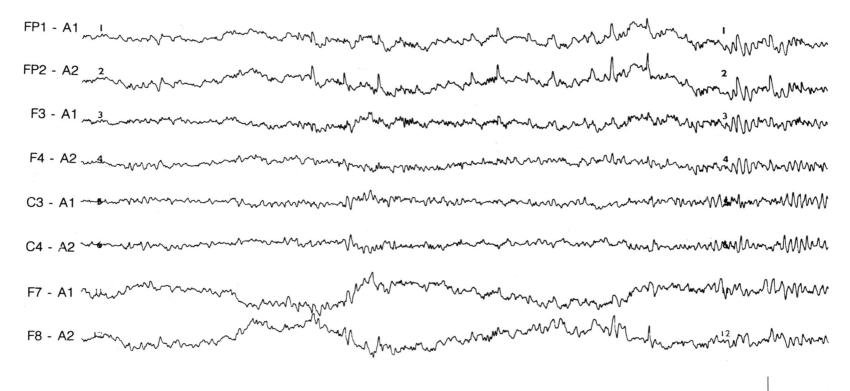

FIG. 4–54. Right frontal polar spikes on ear reference montage. 40 years. Same subject as in Fig. 4–53. The right frontal polar (Fp2) location of these spikes is evident with moderate spread to the left frontal polar (Fp1) region. Sporadic spread to the right inferior frontal region (F8) can be seen, even though the inferior frontal regions (F7, F8) are involved in eye movements. The ear reference (A2) is not involved in a frontal spike field. Calibration signal 1 sec, 70μV.

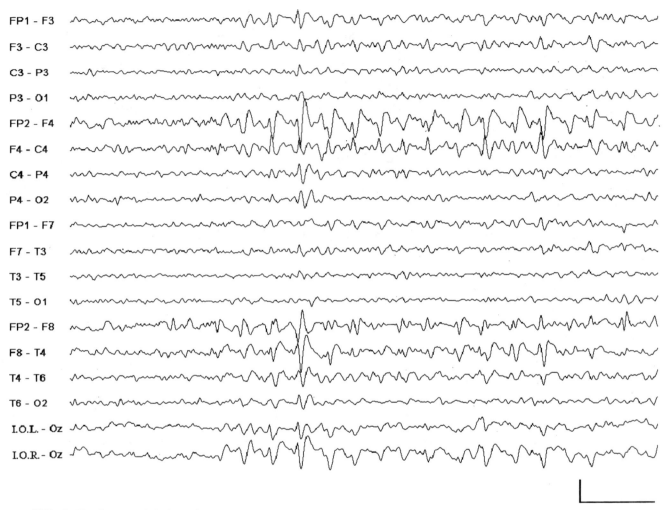

FIG. 4–55. Sequential right frontal spikes extending to infraorbital region. Although used to monitor extraocular movements, infraorbital leads may record potentials involving the anterior frontal regions. These derivations suggest a dipole with principal negativity at the right superior frontal region (F4) and principal positivity at the right frontal polar region (Fp2, IOR). A referential recording would clarify this further. IOL, infraorbital left; IOR, infraorbital right. Calibration signal 1 sec, 50μV.

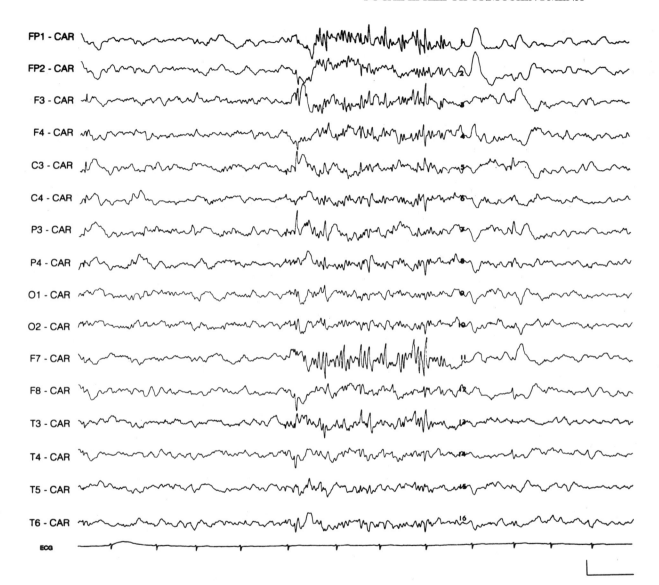

FIG. 4–56. Regionally accentuated polyspikes. 14 years. Involvement of the common average reference (CAR) by a phenomenon limits the confidence with which one may assess its regional distribution using the CAR. CAR "contamination" is revealed by the quantity of the phenomenon seen in a derivation distant from the site of principal involvement. Thus, these polyspikes appear principally at F7 with prominent spread to Fp1 and moderate spread to F3. Their minimal expression in the O2-CAR derivation indicates negligible CAR involvement. The progressive voltage decline of right hemisphere polyspikes going posteriorly suggests that such potentials, often of phase opposite to left hemisphere polyspikes, represent part of an interhemispheric dipole instead of CAR "contamination." Note the incongruency between the localization of the initial spike in the left parietal central (P3, C3) region with that of the succeeding polyspike discharge. Light sleep recording. Calibration signal 1 sec, 150μV.

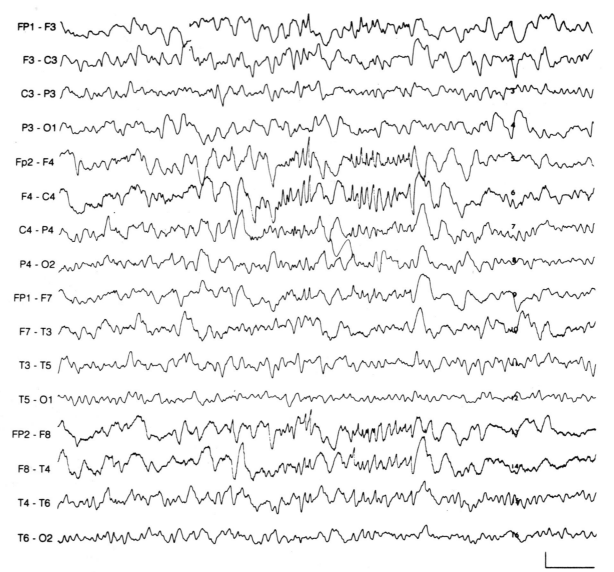

FIG. 4–57. Right frontal polyspikes and diffuse delta activity. 19 years. The diffuse delta activity, slightly more in the right hemisphere, is suddenly interrupted by 7–9 Hz sequential spikes in the right frontal polar (Fp2) region with spread to the right superior frontal (F4) and right inferior frontal regions (F8). Note the slight propagation to the left frontal polar (Fp1) region. Such propagation to the homologous region of the contralateral hemisphere occurs commonly with frontal spikes. Calibration signal 1 sec, 100μV.

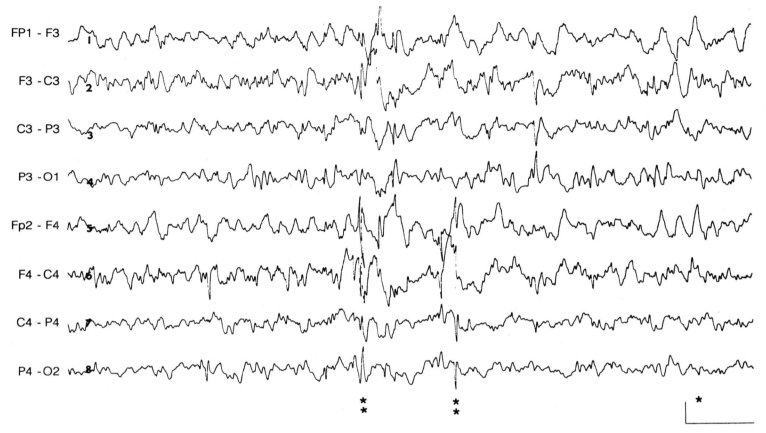

FIG. 4–58. Multiple independent spike foci. 14 years. Scrutiny of this tracing reveals spikes in multiple regions of each hemisphere, a phenomenon found principally in children and adolescents (5, 23). Over 90% of such patients have seizures, most of them frequently. The background activity contains some sharply contoured waves (*asterisk*) but these can be distinguished from the spikes (*double asterisks*) because of the shallower slopes and consequently more blunted peaks of the background activity. Calibration signal 1 sec, 100μV.

Chapter 5

Generalized Epileptiform Phenomena

Generalized Spike-Wave and Polyspike-Wave Complexes (Figs. 1–9, 11, 19, 24, 25, 35)
- Bilaterally synchronous spike-wave complexes with repetition rate of 2.5 to 4 Hz.
- Bursts begin and end abruptly.
- Repetition rate slows during long paroxysms.
- Maximum amplitude usually at F3, F4; occasionally posterior (P3,4; O1,2).
- Variable anterior-posterior extension.
- May be maximally or exclusively expressed in one hemisphere; such asymmetry shifts.
- Gradation between "generalized" and "focal" spike waves occasionally occurs.
- Incomplete forms are common.
- In sleep, repetition rate is slower, less regular.

Secondary Bilateral Synchrony (Figs. 12, 13)
- Focal or regional spikes leading directly to bisynchronous spikes and/or spike-waves.
- Focal interparoxysmal abnormality in same region.

Slow Spike-Waves (Fig. 5, 14)
- 1–2 Hz repetition rate.
- More abundant than 3 Hz spike-waves.
- Slow background.
- Bursts begin and end gradually.

6 Hz Spike-waves (Figs. 15–17)
- 5–7 Hz.
- Diffuse, posterior- or anterior-accentuated.
- Spike component is small, brief.
- Morphology of anterior-predominant form merges with 3 Hz spike-waves; possibly more epileptogenic than posterior 6 Hz spike-waves.

Burst of Polyspikes (Figs. 20–27, 29–34, 41, 42)
- Burst of spikes repeating at 10–25 Hz.
- Irregular discharge rate.
- Generalized, maximum frontally.
- 40–350µV.
- Duration 1–8 seconds.
- Tonic seizures or absence in association.
- May occur on eye closure.

Photoparoxysmal Response (Figs. 36–40, 43–46)
- Polyspikes, spike-waves.
- Spike repetition rate varies within burst and is unrelated to flash rate.
- May extend beyond flash stimuli.
- Diffuse with anterior or posterior maximum expression.
- Eye closure and eyes closed most easily elicit spike-waves.
- Most frequently induced by 15 flashes per second with eyes closed, 20 per second with eyes open.
- Threshold lowers with repeated flash stimuli.

Photomyogenic (Photomyoclonic) Response (Figs. 38, 47)
- Muscle potentials from facial muscle contractions, principally orbicularis oculi and frontalis.
- 50 msec latency.
- Principally with eyes closed.
- Increases gradually as flash continues; stops with flash.
- May coexist with photoparoxysmal response.

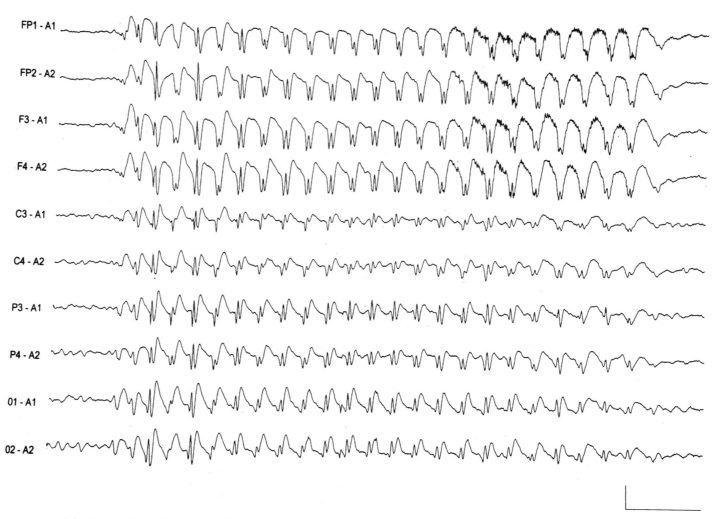

FIG. 5–1. 3 Hz spike-waves. 6 years. Sudden onset and termination of bilaterally synchronous spike-waves whose repetition rate slows slightly as the burst proceeds. Ultimately, the wave component becomes more prominent than the spike. Calibration signal 1 sec, 500μV.

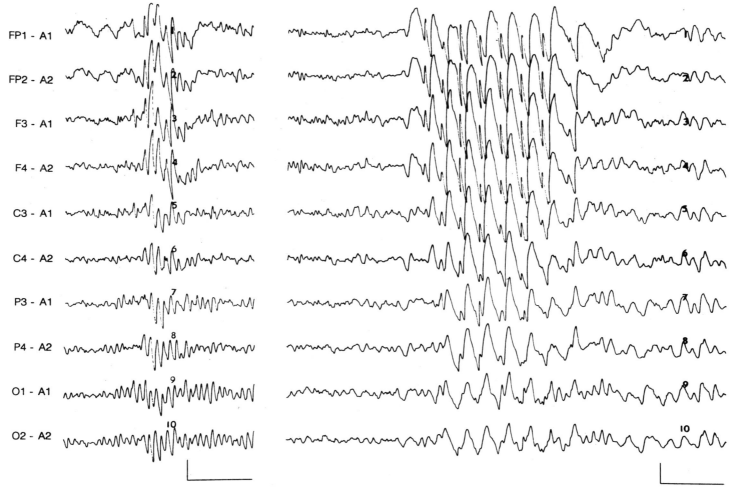

FIG. 5–2. A nonspecific burst and spike-waves. 17 years (*left*), and 18 years (*right*). Many records that ultimately demonstrate classical 3 Hz spike-wave discharges (*right*) will also contain less specific diffuse abnormal bursts (*left*). The occurrence of such a burst should indicate a more prolonged recording favoring ear referential montages which best depict generalized spike-waves. Hyperventilation or photic stimulation may elicit such spike-waves. Note the bisynchronous onset and offset of these spike-waves, and their gradual extension more posteriorly as the spike-wave sequence proceeds. Left calibration signal 1 sec, 150μV. Right calibration signal 1 sec, 200μV.

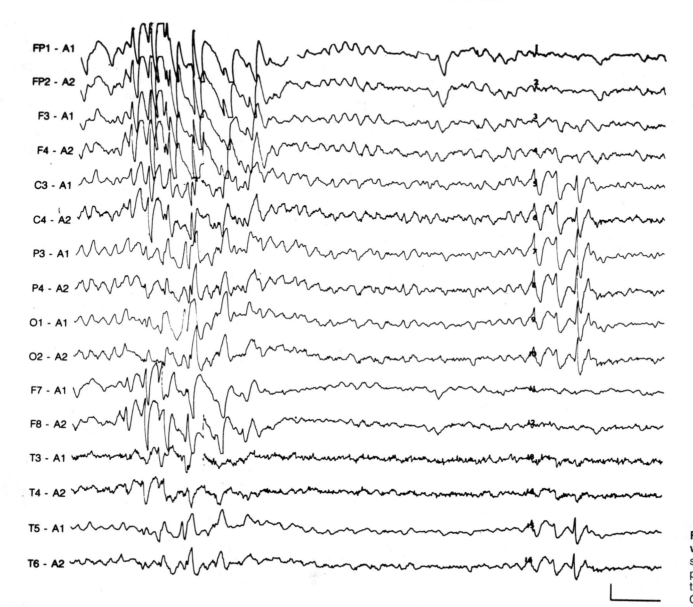

FIG. 5–3. The varying field of spike-waves. 29 years. In the initial burst, the spike-waves, initially 3 Hz then 2 Hz, appear principally in the frontal regions, whereas the subsequent burst is centered posteriorly. Calibration signal 1 sec, 100µV.

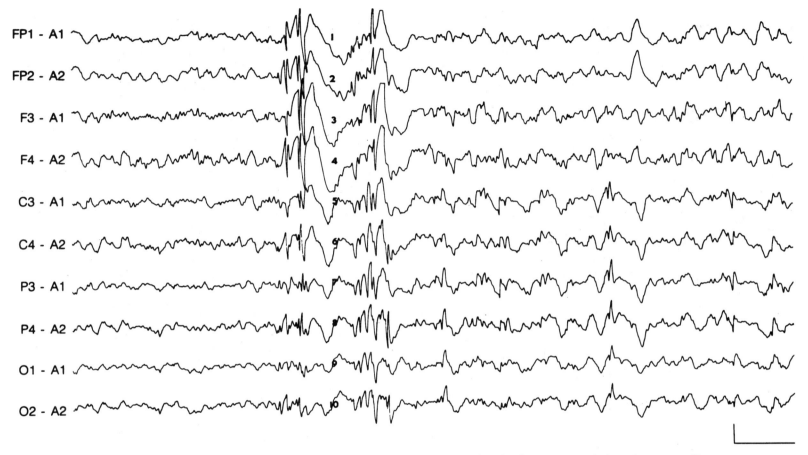

FIG. 5–4. Spike-waves that linger. 14 years. Although most generalized spike-waves end abruptly, some will continue in a less prominent fashion, as occurs here. Compare the 6 seconds following the prominent polyspike waves with the 3 seconds preceding them. Calibration signal 1 sec, 150μV.

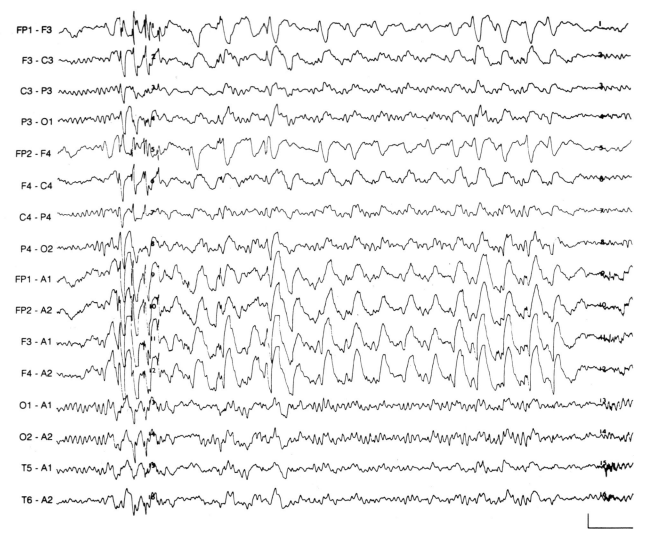

FIG. 5–5. 3 Hz spike-waves and slow spike-waves on bipolar and ear reference montages. 29 years. This sequence is unusual in that the 3 Hz spike-waves are immediately followed by 2 Hz slow spike-waves, although Bauer et al. (24) have found this combination in adults with slow spike-waves. Note how bisynchronous epileptiform discharges are better displayed on ear reference recordings than on bipolar montages. The lower-amplitude slow spike-waves in the center of the tracing are virtually not detectable by the bipolar montage. Calibration signal 1 sec, 70µV.

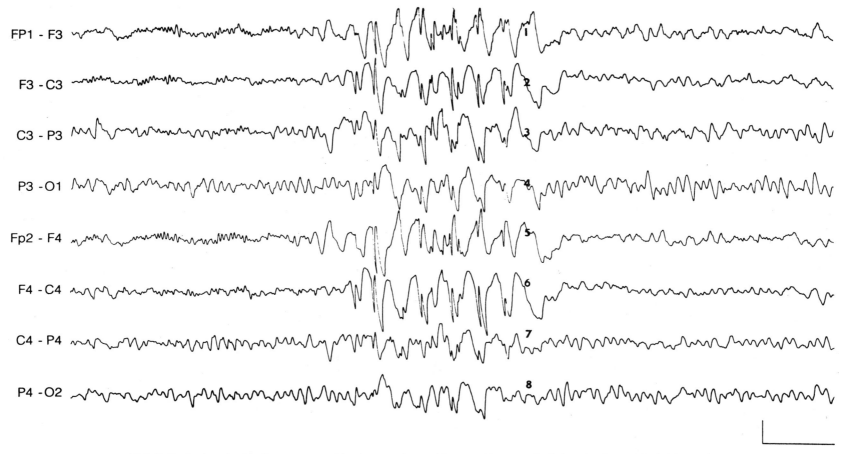

FIG. 5–6. A classical spike-wave on bipolar montage. 18 years. Because both inputs of most derivations of a bipolar montage lie within the spike-wave field, partial cancellation effects distort the regular and smooth morphology of the spike-wave discharge. Nonetheless, the onset, intraburst, and offset bisynchrony is evident. As expected, there are no abnormalities of background activity, although a slightly increased quantity of theta activity follows the discharges. Calibration signal 1 sec, 70μV.

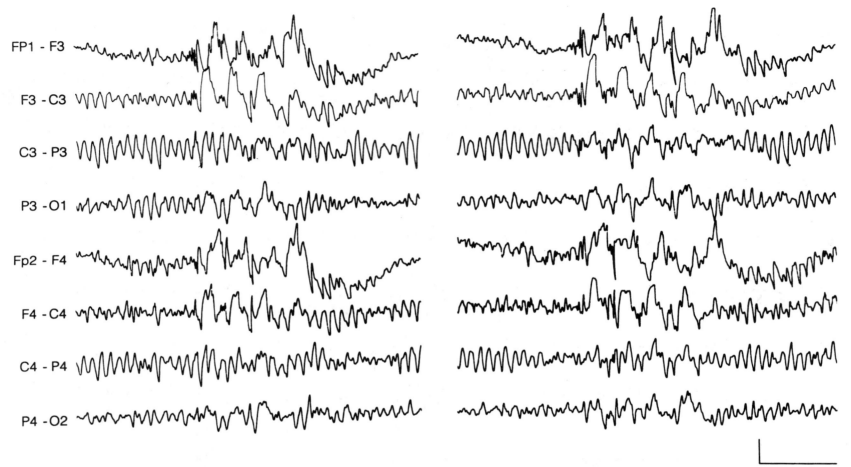

FIG. 5–7. 3 Hz spike-waves. 64 years. All of the components of spike-wave complexes described by Weir (25) are difficult to identify on a bipolar montage, particularly when the spike-wave complex competes with background activity, as appears here. Instead, one sees single or multiple spikes of variable morphology preceding 300 msec, rhythmic or semi-rhythmic waves and appearing in a frontally dominant, bilaterally synchronous manner without a focal onset or offset. By placing a ruler along the presumed electrical baseline (from the mean of activity prior to and after the spike-wave complex), one can discern a considerable positive component which represents the trough between the spike and the wave (26). Calibration signal 1 sec, 50μV.

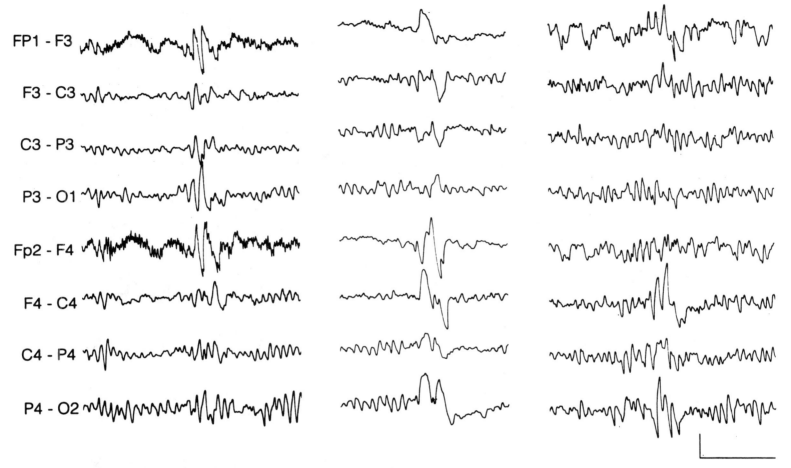

FIG. 5–8. Nonspecific bursts may herald spike-waves. 26 years (*left*), 16 years (*center*), 17 years (*right*). Bursts of 5–8 Hz high-voltage waves may occur in recordings containing bisynchronous spike-waves. These nonspecific bursts may be spike-waves whose spikes were undetected by scalp electrodes or were canceled in bipolar montages. Each of these segments contains some apiculate waves which are suggestive, but not definitely, spikes. If such nonspecific bursts occur and there is a clinical question of a generalized epileptic disorder, a more prolonged recording with "activation" by hyperventilation, sleep, or photic stimulation might clarify the situation. Left calibration signal 1 sec, 50µV. Center calibration signal 1 sec, 70µV. Right calibration signal 1 sec, 100µV.

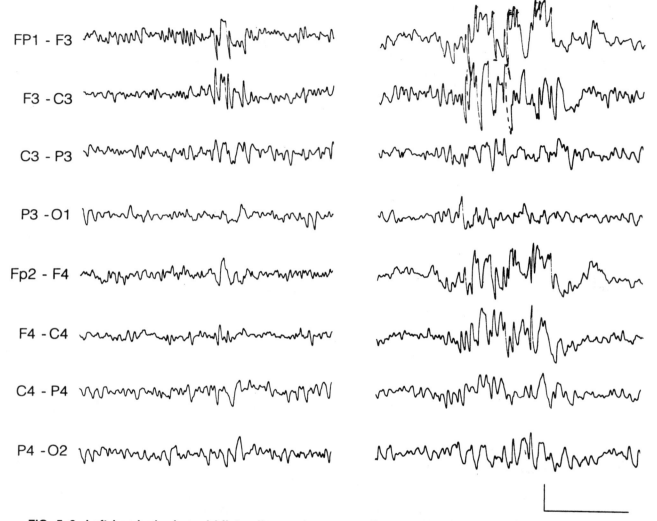

FIG. 5–9. Left hemispheric and bilaterally synchronous spike-waves. 14 years. Careful review of many recordings containing bilaterally synchronous spike-wave or polyspike-wave discharges will reveal some which appear principally or exclusively in one hemisphere. Distinction from focal spikes is made by the similarity of morphology of such regionally accentuated spikes to that of the bilaterally synchronous ones and the lack of any other regional abnormality such as focal delta or theta activity or a reduction of beta (5). Thus, the left frontal (principally F3) spike-waves on the left sample are simply fragments of bilaterally synchronous polyspike-waves in the right sample. Calibration signal 1 sec, 100μV.

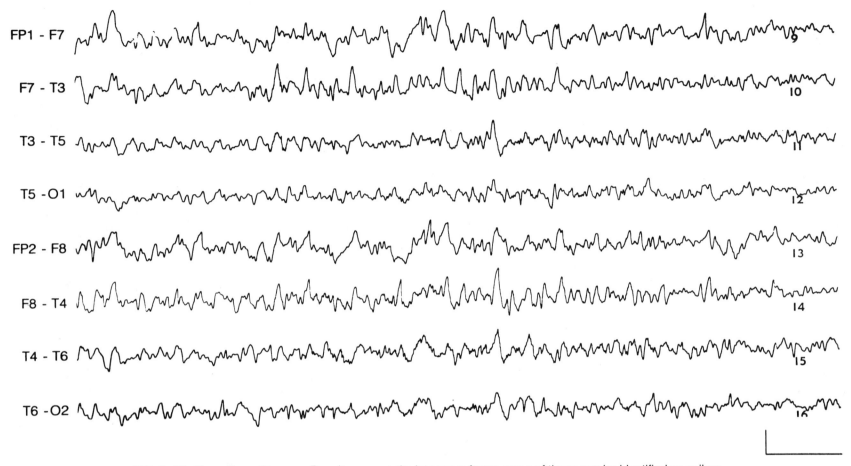

FIG. 5–10. No spikes. 20 years. Despite many apiculate wave forms, none of these can be identified as spikes, because each could be plausibly considered as a product of the rich mixture of wave forms present here. Light sleep tracing. Calibration signal 1 sec, 100μV.

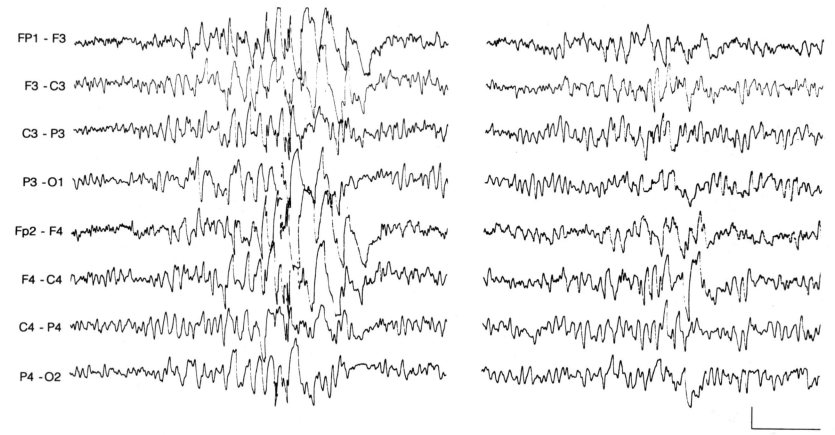

FIG. 5–11. Distorted generalized spike-waves. 24 years. The morphology of diffuse bilaterally synchronous spike-wave discharges can stray considerably from the classical form, either because of superimposition of an irregular background activity containing theta and beta or because of occult secondary bilateral synchrony. The series of spike-wave complexes in the left segment begins as an abrupt augmentation of diffuse, sharply contoured theta for about 1 second before clearly identifiable spikes appear. The center of this burst contains a 6 Hz spikewave. This is followed quickly by spike-wave complexes lasting 300–400 msec. The right sample illustrates even less well defined but clearly present spike-waves, best manifested in the right hemisphere. Calibration signal 1 sec, 70μV.

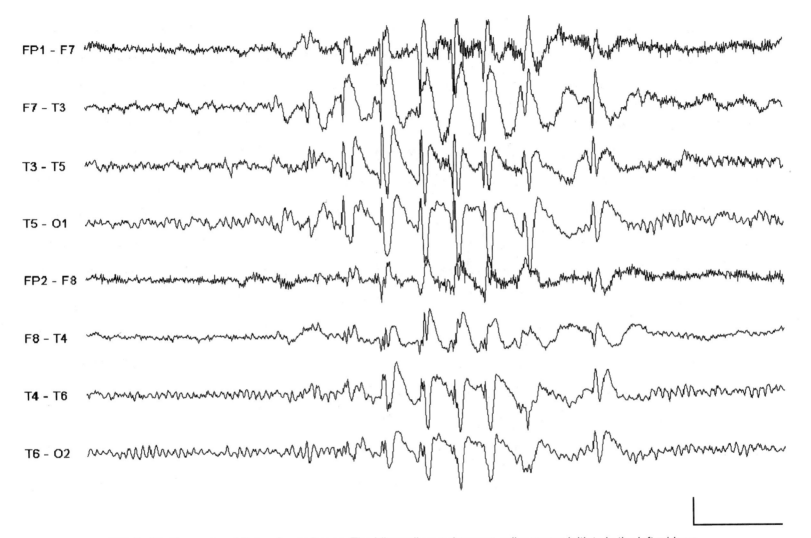

FIG. 5–12. Secondary bilateral synchrony. The bilaterally synchronous spike-waves initiate in the left midposterior temporal region, the site of arrhythmic delta activity which precedes and follows the paroxysm. Calibration signal 1 sec, 100μV.

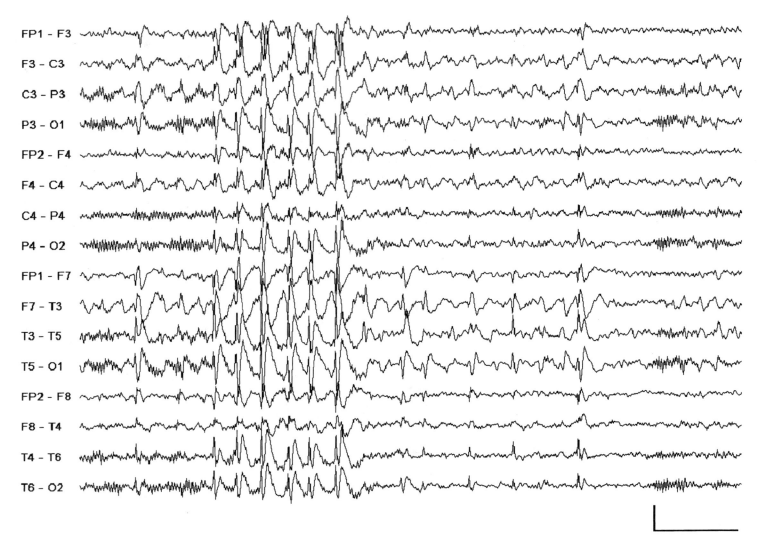

FIG. 5–13. Secondary bilateral synchrony on compressed display. A comprehensive view of this phenomenon can be afforded by viewing at 15 mm/sec. In addition to delta activity involving the left temporal central parietal region (T3, T5, C3, P3), regional left hemisphere spikes precede and follow the more bisynchronous paroxysm in the first third of the illustration. In this example, the field is an expanding and shrinking field, as virtually all spikes have a diffuse and even bilateral distribution. Calibration signal 2 sec, 100μV.

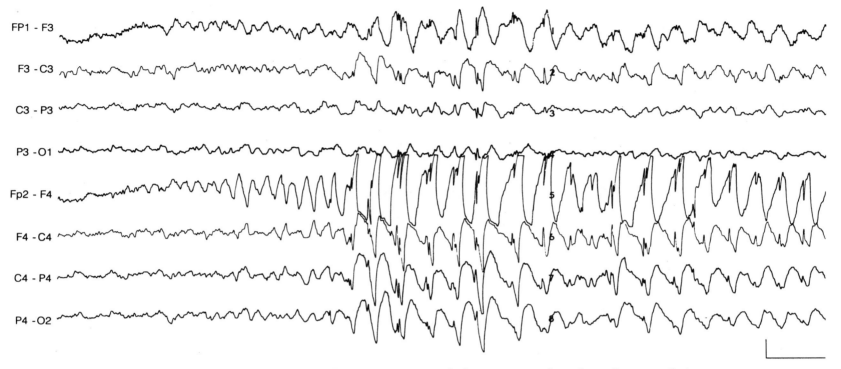

FIG. 5–14. Right hemisphere slow spike-waves. 38 years. A phenomenon such as slow spike-waves that usually appears bilaterally and symmetrically may predominate in one hemisphere. This can result from (a) a focal discharge in one hemisphere, (b) prominent abnormality in the contralateral hemisphere impeding the expression of usually diffuse events there, or (c) simply a hemispheric expression of a usually diffuse phenomenon. The interhemispheric background symmetry of this figure's example excludes the second of these possibilities. The right hemisphere accentuation of 4 Hz rhythmic waves preceding the slow spike-waves raises the first possibility, that is, a regional right frontal onset. In this instance, sagittal leads should be added to seek a possible onset at Fz-F4. Further recording may reveal more symmetrical and diffuse slow spike-waves or even left hemisphere-dominant ones. Calibration signal 1 sec, 50µV.

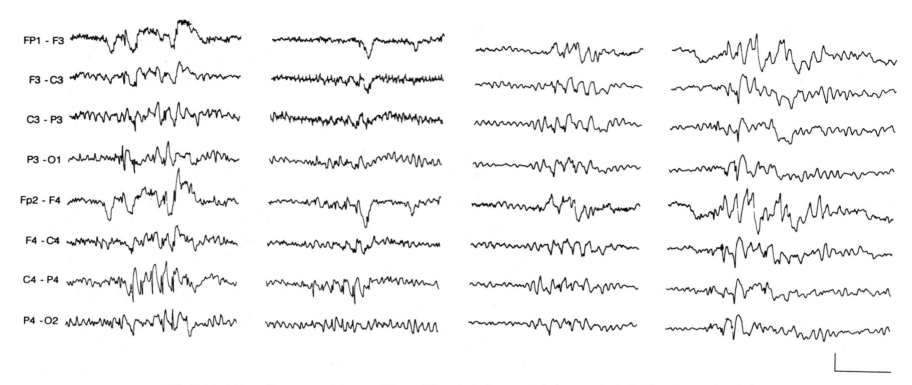

FIG. 5–15. 6 Hz spike-waves. 34 years. These diffuse but often posteriorly accentuated spike-waves repeat at about 6 Hz in these samples. Note the brevity of each spike. The right-sided accentuation of some of these has no clinical significance. Posteriorly accentuated 6 Hz spike-waves are not thought to correlate with a seizure disorder (27, 28). However, the morphology of the more diffuse or anterior-predominant 6 Hz spike-waves may merge with the more clearly epileptogenic 3 Hz spike-waves and therefore correlate more highly with a seizure disorder (28). Such prominent anterior accentuation and merging of morphologies are illustrated in the first and last examples, which may be more epileptogenic than the middle examples. Calibration signal 1 sec, 70μV.

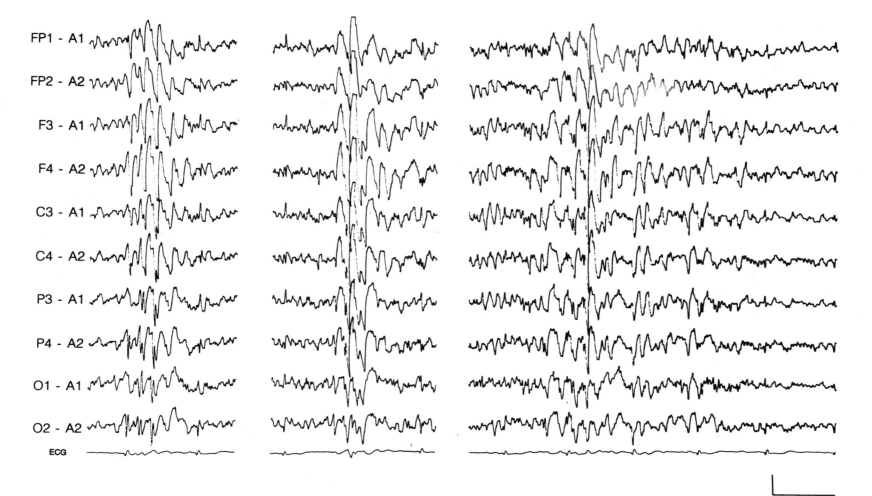

FIG. 5–16. 6 Hz spike and wave on referential montage. 33 years. The full morphology and field distribution of the 6 Hz spike and wave are illustrated in these samples. Note the more restricted field of the spike compared to the wave in the first two samples (from left) in which the spike is accentuated posteriorly; this would be considered nonepileptogenic by most authors (27–29). The initial upward deflection immediately preceding the spike-wave complex on the first (*left*) example resembles a V-wave occurring just before the initial spike of the 6 Hz spike-wave. In contrast, the example on the right merges with the more epileptogenic 3 Hz spike-wave discharge in that its spike distribution is more diffuse and includes the anterior leads, while the repetition rate is slower at about 4–5 Hz. Calibration signal 1 sec, 50μV.

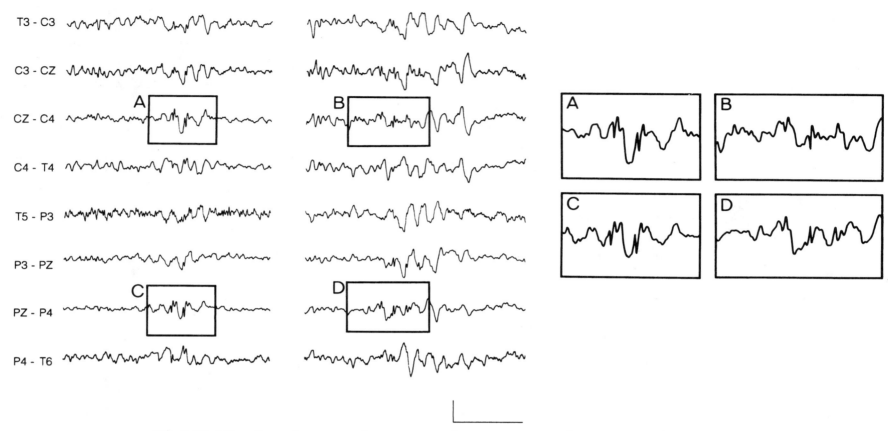

FIG. 5–17. 6 Hz spike and wave complexes on coronal montage. 22 years. Coronal bipolar montages express the 6 Hz spike and wave phenomenon less well than do anterior-posterior bipolar and ear referential montages. However, recognition of their occurrence while using the coronal bipolar montage is important, as shown in these examples. Note how the brief, relatively low-voltage spike component can be somewhat submerged within a theta burst. Calibration signal 1 sec, 50μV.

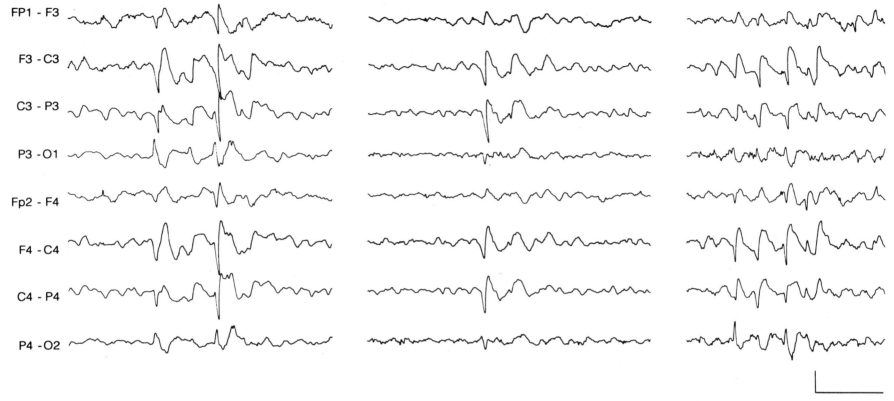

FIG. 5–18. Bisynchronous spikes. 29 years. These bisynchronous apiculate waves resemble V-waves, because their aftercoming slow waves are in opposite phase to that of the spikes. However, the slopes (descending and rising) and consequent peaks of most of these spikes are excessively sharp for V-waves. Moreover, the negative field of these spikes lies in the parietal-occipital region, far more posterior than that of V-waves. Calibration signal 1 sec, 100μV.

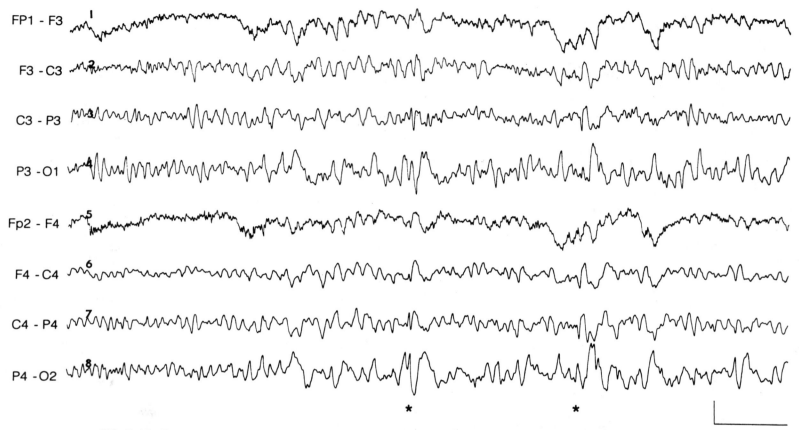

FIG. 5–19. Posterior bisynchronous spike-waves. 18 years. Theta and alpha activity partially obscure the definite posteriorly situated bisynchronous spike-wave complexes (*asterisks*). However, the slopes and peaks of the synchronous spikes differ clearly from those of the background activity. Calibration signal 1 sec, 50μV.

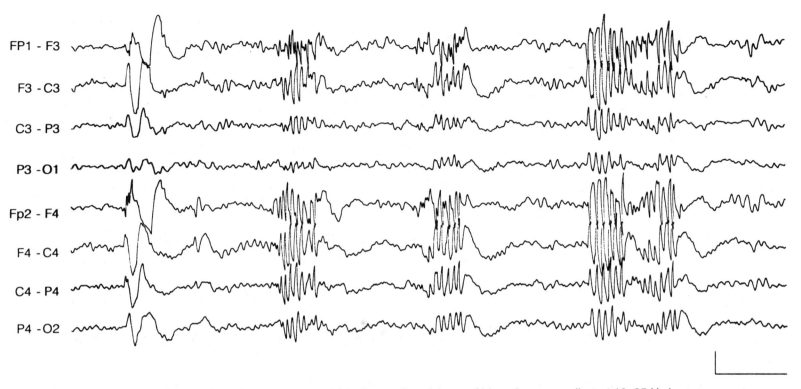

FIG. 5–20. Runs of polyspikes. 21 years. Sleep recording. A burst of bisynchronous spikes at 10–25 Hz is an epileptiform pattern associated with primary generalized epilepsy. Other aspects of the Lennox-Gastaut syndrome may be present (30, 31). This pattern may appear in patients of any age with tonic or absence seizures. Calibration signal 1 sec, 70μV.

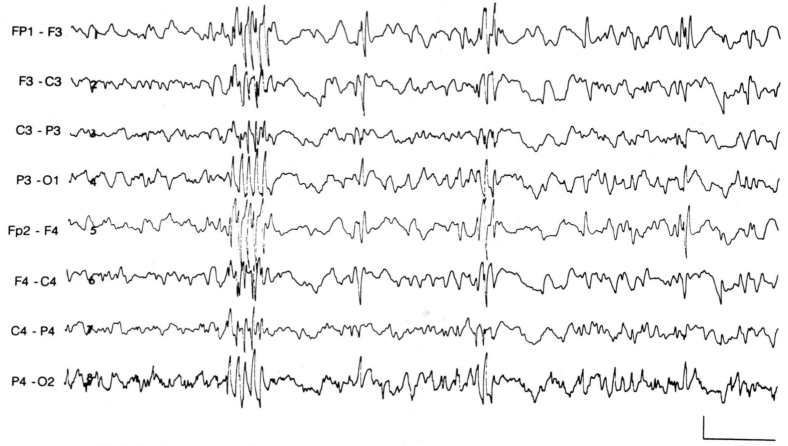

FIG. 5–21. Polyspikes (multiple spikes) among apiculate waves. 25 years. Even though sharply contoured waves characterize some of the background activity here, the four bursts of single spikes and polyspikes can be discerned. The subject's neck flexed tonically in association with the longest burst. Calibration signal 1 sec, 70μV.

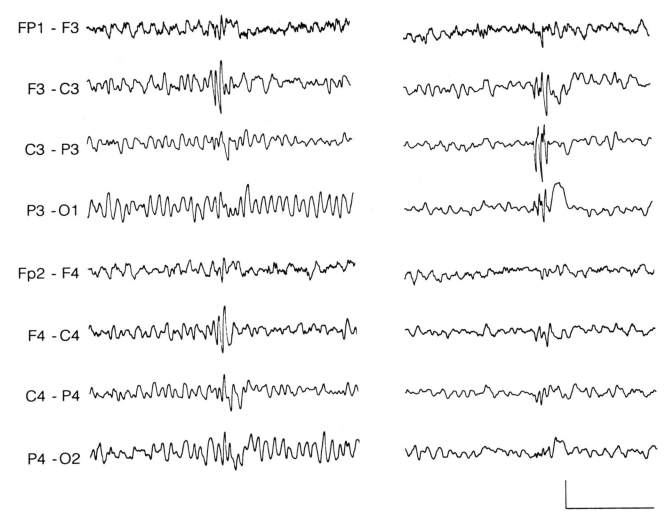

FP1 - F3

F3 - C3

C3 - P3

P3 - O1

Fp2 - F4

F4 - C4

C4 - P4

P4 - O2

FIG. 5–22. Diffuse polyspikes. 24 years. Some bilaterally synchronous epileptiform discharges are not followed by a delta wave. The apiculate morphology of these spikes distinguishes them clearly from the ongoing background activity of these samples. Their identification in a recording containing more beta activity and therefore more sharply contoured waves would be exceedingly difficult. Calibration signal 1 sec, 70μV.

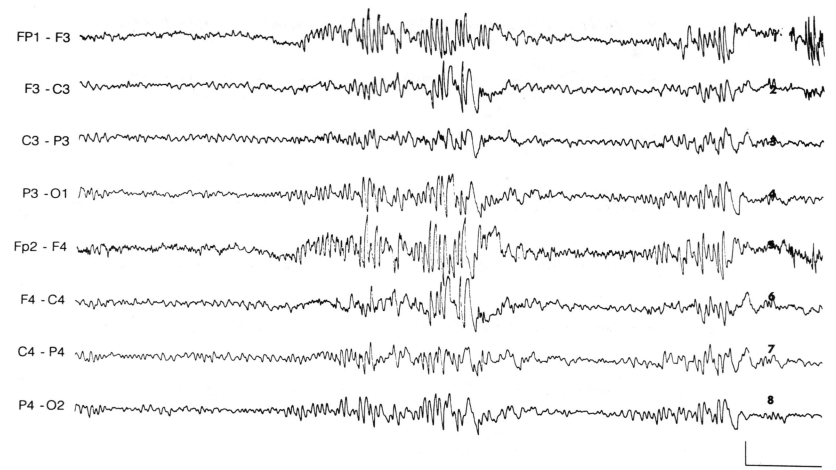

FIG. 5–23. Runs of polyspikes in wakefulness. 26 years. Although some low-amplitude beta activity is present, the abrupt onset of 15 Hz rhythmic waves, becoming spikes, appears diffusely but most prominently in the frontal derivations (Fp1,2-F3,4). Slow waves interrupt the sequential spikes near the end of these spike sequences. Calibration signal 1 sec, 50μV.

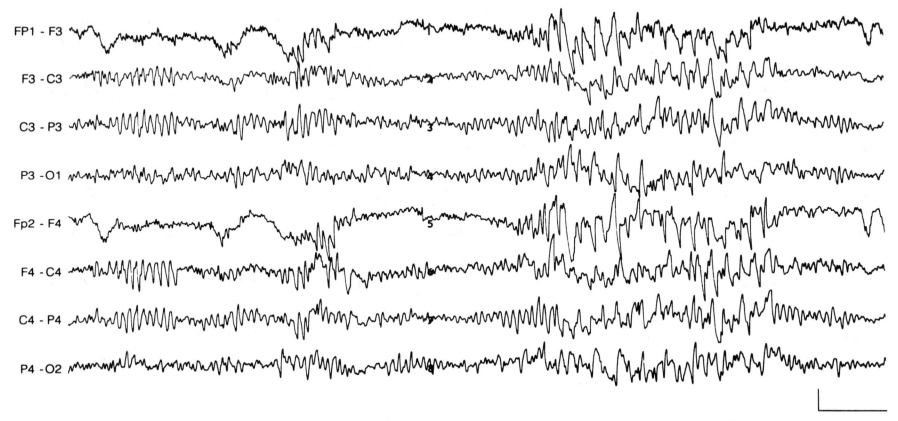

FIG. 5–24. Polyspike-waves in an apiculate background. 20 years. Despite the presence of non-spike apiculate waves as in the first 2 seconds, the morphology of both the diffuse spikes and diffuse waves in the 3½ sec burst of diffuse spike-waves can be clearly distinguished from the background activity. The diffuse 1 sec burst in the 4th second may or may not be a spike-wave burst, because it fails to completely emerge from the background activity. Calibration signal 1 sec, 50µV.

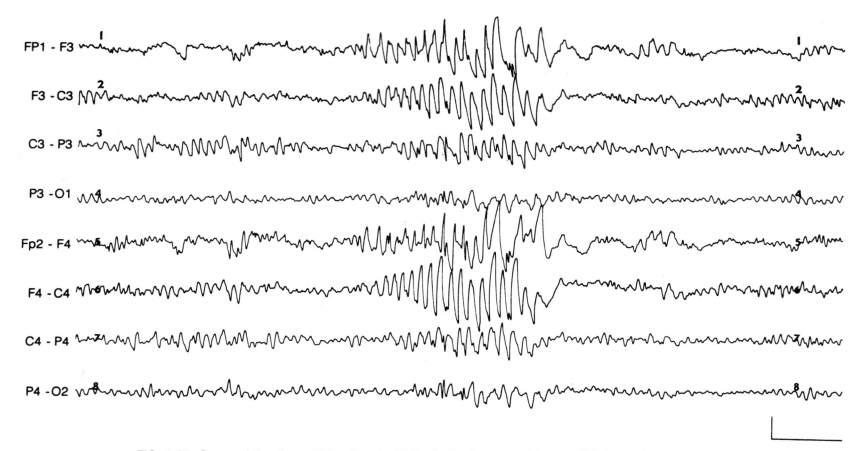

FIG. 5–25. Sequential spikes within a burst of 7 Hz rhythmic waves. 16 years. This burst of 7 Hz waves incompletely hides the bilaterally synchronous spikes which are best expressed in the frontal derivations (Fp1,2-F3,4). Note the gradual slowing in rhythmic wave frequency near the end of the burst. EEG in light drowsiness. Calibration signal 1 sec, 70μV.

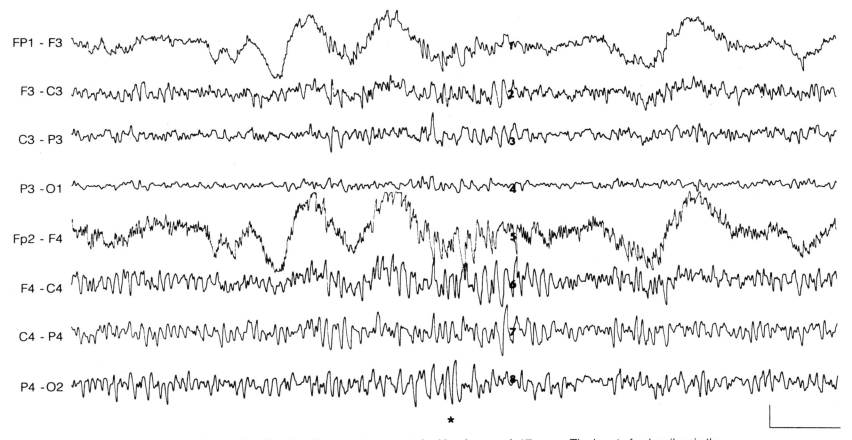

FP1 - F3

F3 - C3

C3 - P3

P3 - O1

Fp2 - F4

F4 - C4

C4 - P4

P4 - O2

*

FIG. 5–26. "Generalized" polyspikes and asymmetrical background. 17 years. The burst of polyspikes in the center of this tracing (*asterisk*) is better expressed in the healthier (right) hemisphere; the diffuse left hemisphere attenuation impedes their expression on that side. Note the prominent eye movement artifacts. Calibration signal 1 sec, 150μV.

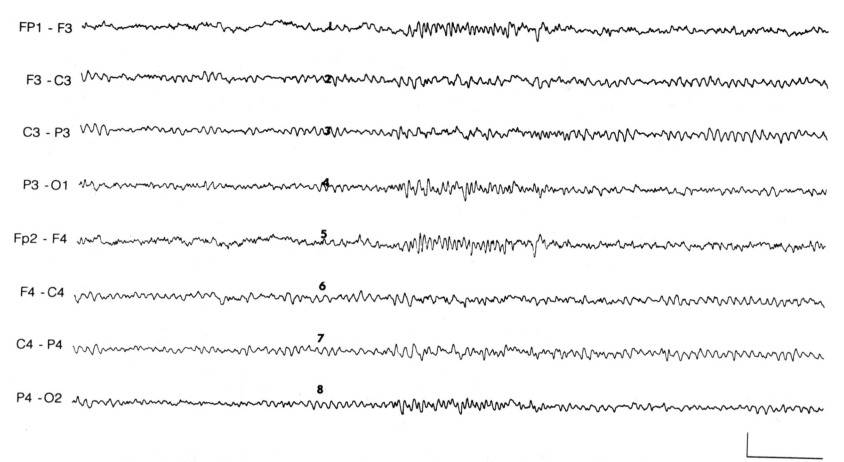

FIG. 5–27. Minimal expression of fast rhythmic waves or polyspikes. 26 years. A considerably lower-voltage version of the polyspikes of Fig. 5–26 appears in the center of this illustration. Runs of polyspikes appear as fast rhythmic waves (5) when they are lower in voltage. Although these resemble beta activity, a burst of beta would not last this long, and such fast rhythmic waves can be easily distinguished from the higher-frequency and lower-voltage beta seen in the frontal polar derivations. Calibration signal 1 sec, 50μV.

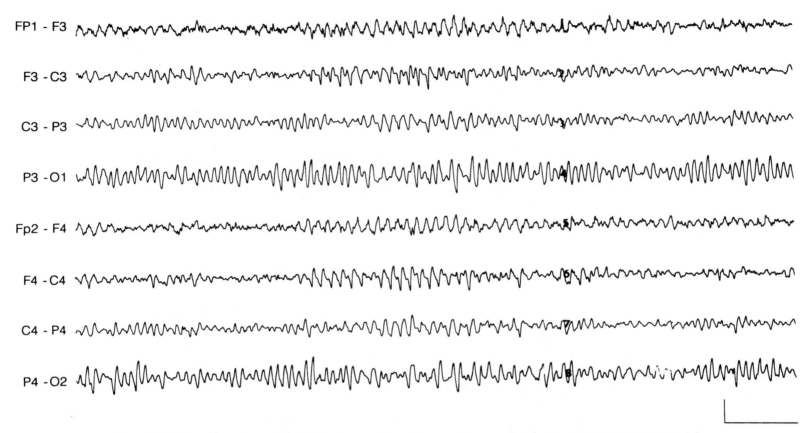

FIG. 5–28. Sharply contoured waves but no spikes. 24 years. The saw-toothed morphology of the potentials seen principally at F3-C3 and F4-C4 indicates their generation as a combination of wave forms (theta and mu) and that they do not represent spikes. As Engel (32) has stated, " . . . anything maintaining an invariably regular frequency is likely to be normal. . ." Calibration signal 1 sec, 70μV.

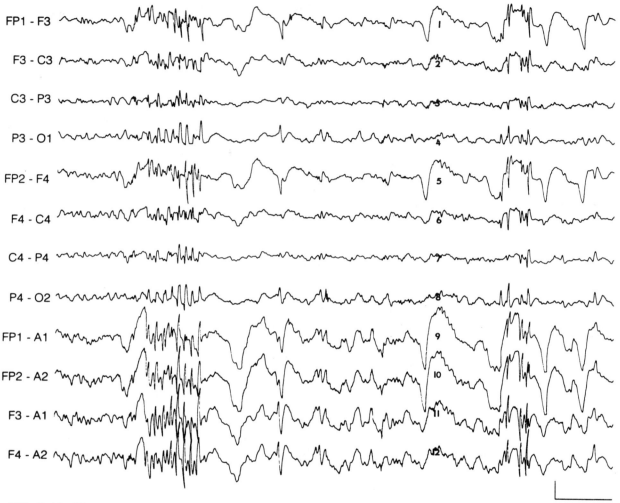

FIG. 5–29. Bisynchronous spikes and polyspikes on bipolar and ear reference montages. 25 years. The referential montage more fully expresses these phenomena than does the bipolar montage, even though each montage records all of these discharges. Speech arrest occurred during the longest polyspike burst. Note the delta activity and attenuation of background rhythms following both the single spikes and polyspikes. Calibration signal 1 sec, 150μV.

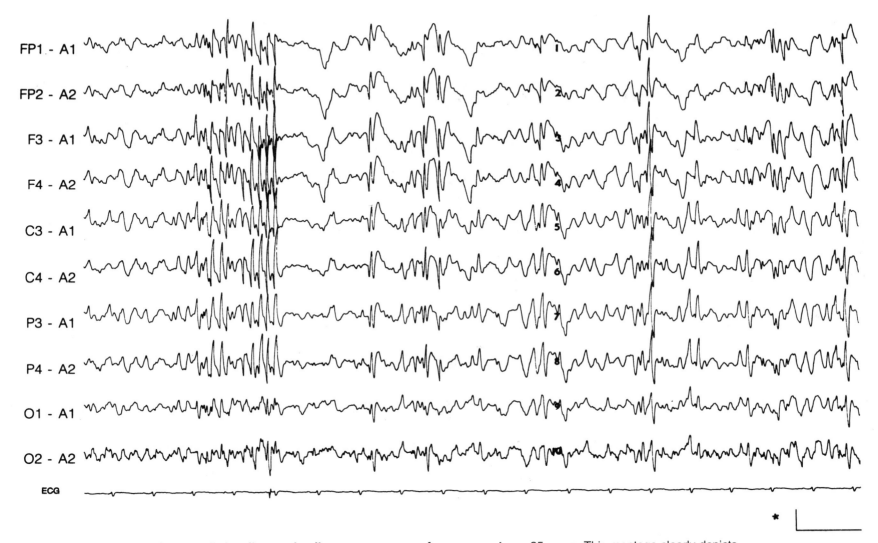

FIG. 5–30. Polyspikes and spike-waves on ear reference montage. 25 years. This montage clearly depicts bisynchronous spikes of several morphologies, including polyspikes, spike-waves, and even subtly appearing bisynchronous spikes (*asterisk*). Low-voltage spikes may require an ECG monitor for distinction from cardiac potentials. Note the transient attenuation of background activity after the 1 sec burst of polyspikes. Light sleep recording. Calibration signal 1 sec, 150μV.

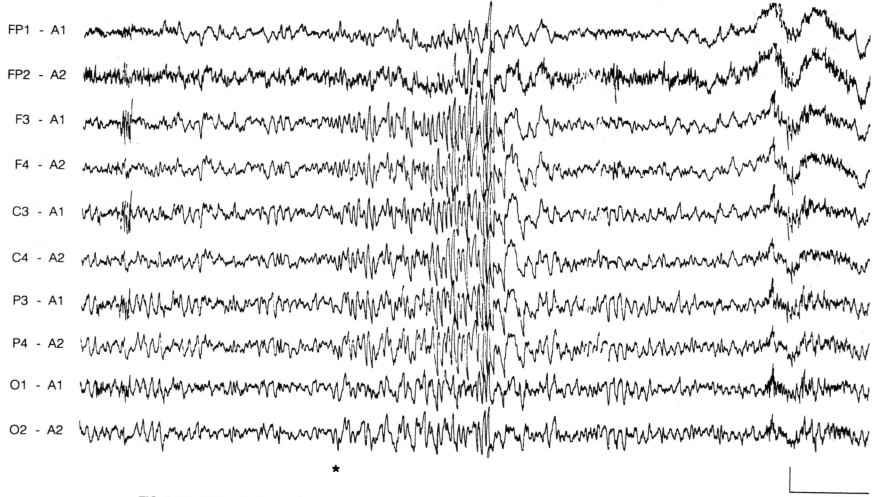

FIG. 5–31. Polyspike bursts in wakefulness. 27 years. Such bursts are more difficult to discern in wakefulness than in sleep because of the greater prominence of background rhythms whose frequencies approach or overlap that of the polyspikes. However, the onset (*asterisk*) can be clearly discerned from the ongoing background activity; the offset is characterized by bisynchronous 200–300 msec waves. Note the brief burst of muscle potentials in the 1st second of this sample and persistent muscle potentials at Fp2. A glossokinetic potential consisting of bisynchronous delta activity with a burst of muscle potentials appears in the last part (*right*) of the sample. Calibration signal 1 sec, 50μV.

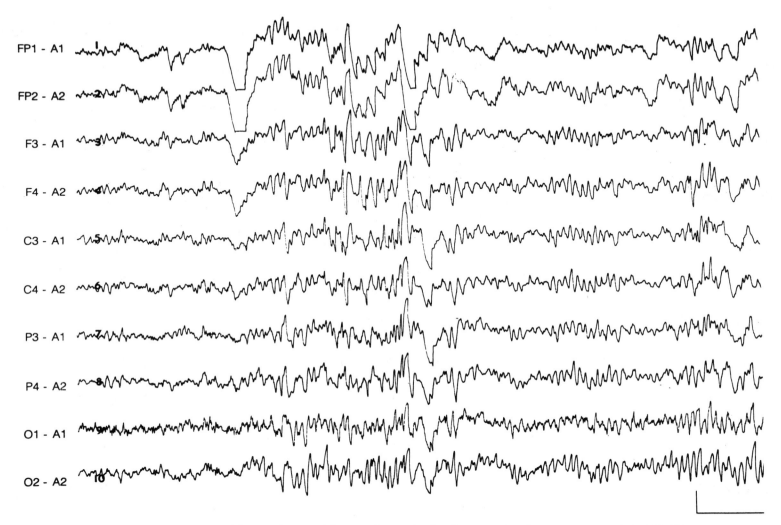

FIG. 5–32. Polyspikes with eye closure. 14 years. Runs of polyspikes or polyspike-waves can occur upon eye closure, as in this sample. Note the clear distinction of this burst, beginning about 200 msec after the eye blink, and the background activities during eyes open (*left*) and eyes closed (*right*). This sample concludes with a brief burst of bilaterally synchronous polyspikes which barely emerges from the background activity. Calibration signal 1 sec, 100μV.

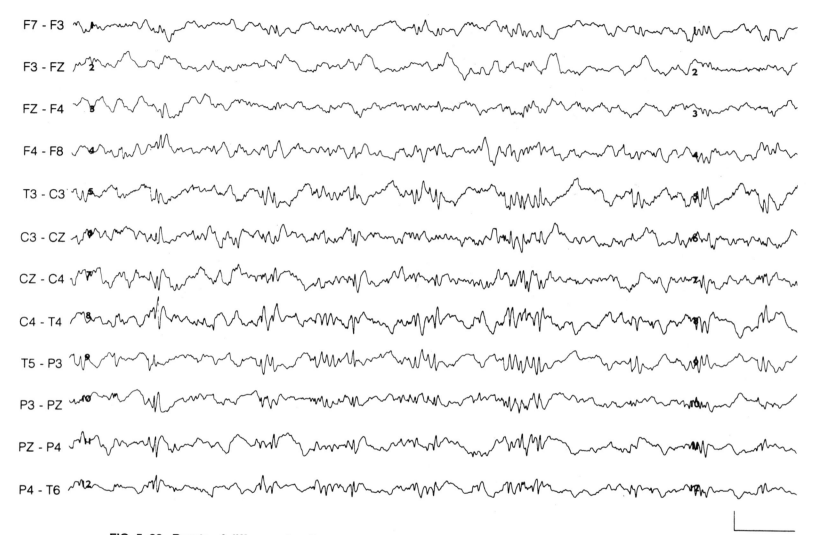

FIG. 5–33. Bursts of diffuse polyspikes. 14 years. The peaks of these spikes contrast sufficiently with the interburst waves for their identification as spikes. Note their diffuse distribution in the central parietal regions and their minimal expression frontally. Recording in non-REM sleep. Calibration signal 1 sec, 100μV.

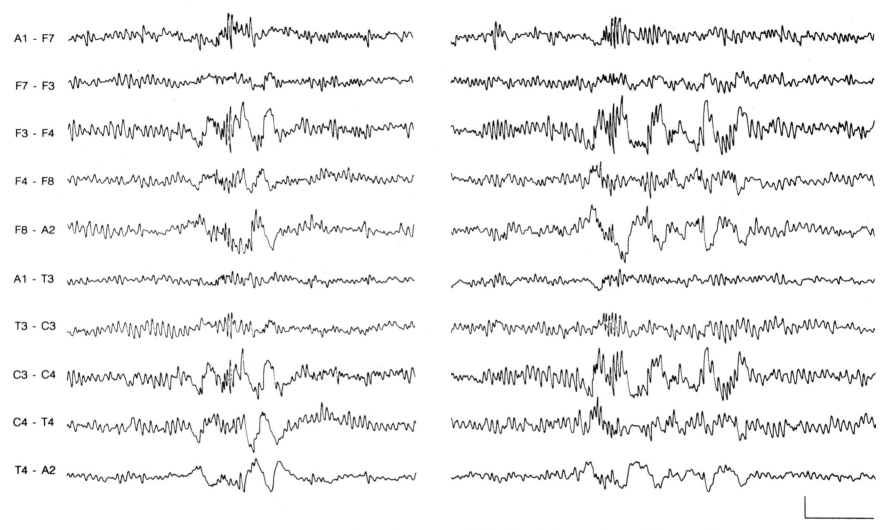

FIG. 5–34. (Almost) unilateral polyspike waves. 20 years. Epileptiform discharges of a morphology usually associated with a bilaterally synchronous distribution may appear unilaterally or even regionally (5, 33). The morphology of these bursts, their widespread distribution throughout the right hemisphere, the moderate expression in the contralateral (left) hemisphere, and the lack of a focal interparoxysmal abnormality all suggest that these spikes do not represent a focal cortical lesion. Nonetheless, recording with parasagittal and sagittal leads during both wakefulness and sleep should be done to seek secondary bilateral synchrony. Note the distinction in frequency between the polyspikes (multiple spikes) and the diffuse background of alpha-beta range. Calibration signal 1 sec, 50μV.

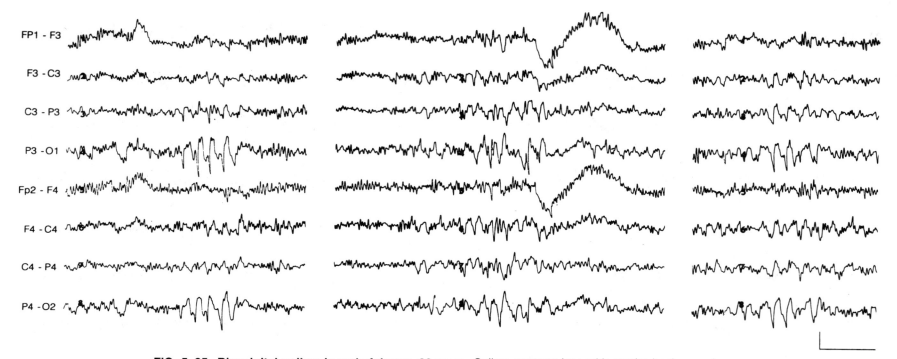

FIG. 5–35. Bioccipital spikes in wakefulness. 38 years. Spikes contrast less with awake background morphology than that of sleep, particularly if beta activity is present. The sharp peaks, accompanying slow-waves, similar morphology in adjacent derivations, and the higher voltage all enable one to identify these bursts as bioccipital spikes. Such patients with bisynchronous posteriorly situated spikes may have a photoparoxysmal response. Calibration signal 1 sec, 50μV.

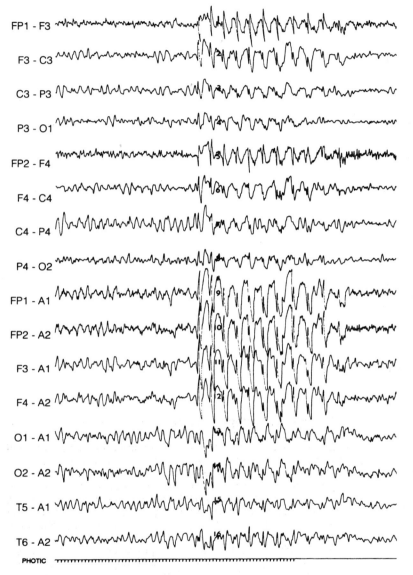

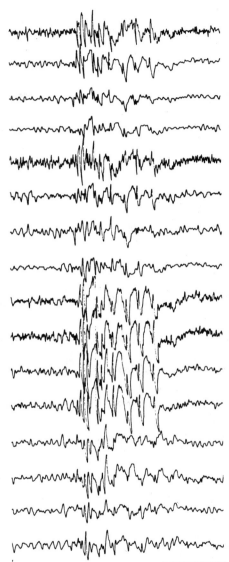

FIG. 5–36. Photoparoxysmal response. 49 years. Stereotypic 3–4 Hz bilaterally synchronous spike-waves at 15 flashes/sec with eyes closed, which is the flash rate with the lowest threshold for production of spike-waves with eyes closed (34). Note the extension of the discharge beyond the cessation of the flash and the lack of any relationship of the spike-wave repetition rate with the flash rate. Spike-waves did not appear until 6 seconds after the onset of the first presentation of 15 flashes/sec (*left*, flash onset not shown) but occurred about 200 msec after the onset of the second presentation (*right*). To prevent convulsive episodes from occurring, technologists should be aware of this gradual lowering of threshold for the photoparoxysmal response with repeated flash stimuli. Calibration signal 1 sec, 100μV.

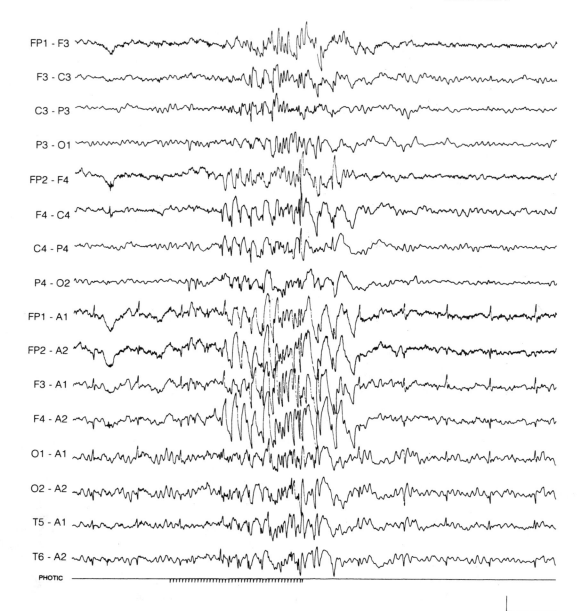

FIG. 5–37. Photoparoxysmal response. 26 years. 15 flashes/sec with the eyes open produced both types of photoparoxysmal response: spike-waves, then polyspikes followed by spike-waves with a lower repetition rate. The frequency of these discharges characteristically varies within the burst and independently of the flash rate; extension beyond the flash sequence occurs commonly. Note the more complete expression of the photoparoxysmal response by the referential portion of the montage compared to the bipolar portion. The initial right hemisphere expression of the spike-waves illustrates again that phenomena whose mechanism and appearance are that of generalized discharges may appear unilaterally. The out-of-phase sequential potentials in the referential portion of the recording are ECG artifact. Calibration signal 1 sec, 70μV.

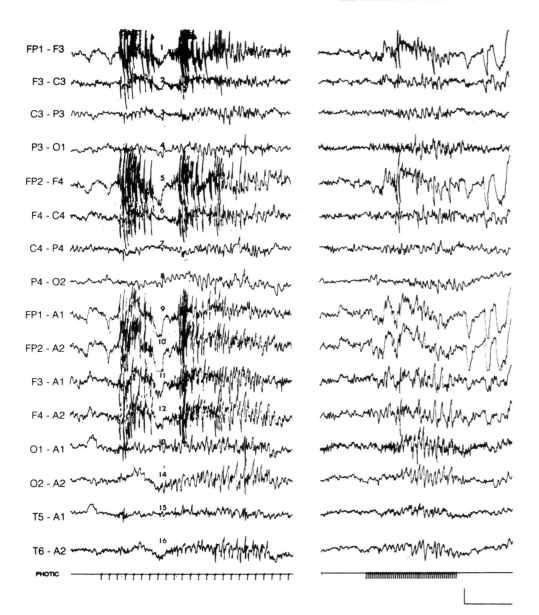

FIG. 5–38. Photomyogenic response and photoparoxysmal response. 24 years, 22 years. Repetitive frontal muscle spikes constitute the photomyogenic response, which may occur in association with the photoparoxysmal response (35). In each instance, the very brief-duration muscle spikes are gradually replaced by slightly longer-duration cerebrally originating spikes as the 6 and 25 flashes/sec with eyes open proceed. Calibration signal 1 sec, 70μV.

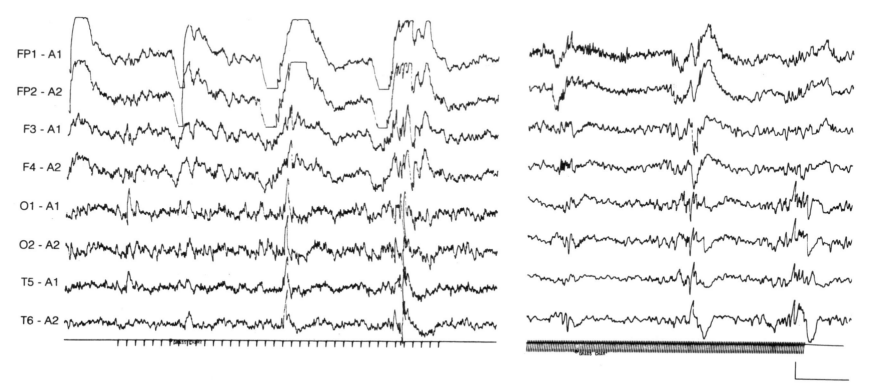

FIG. 5–39. Photoparoxysmal response with eye closure. 29 years. In most patients, the threshold for eliciting the photoparoxysmal response is lowest with eye closure as opposed to eyes closed or eyes open. The eye blinks occurring during the presentation of 6 Hz and 30 Hz flashes are evident as large-amplitude positive-negative deflections maximally in the Fp1,2 leads. These are associated with bilaterally synchronous and transient spikes and polyspikes. Onset of 30 Hz flash not shown. Calibration signal 1 sec, 70μV.

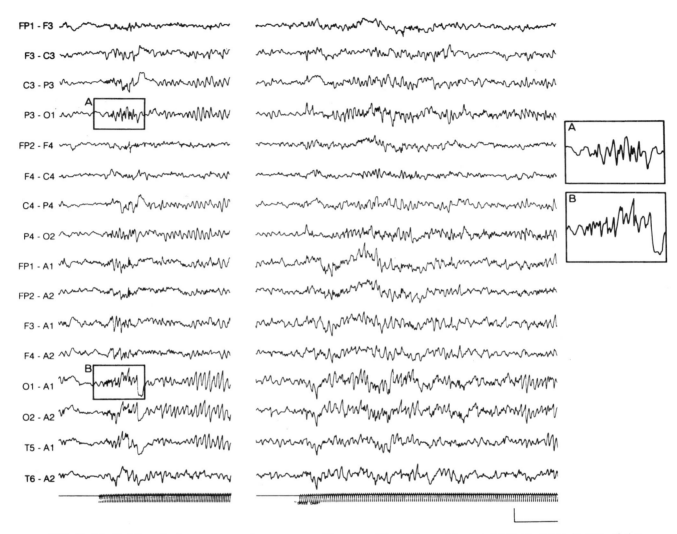

FIG. 5–40. Subtle photoparoxysmal response. 16 years. The enlarged boxes (*A,B*) illustrate in two of the derivations (P3-O1, O1-A1) the generalized sequential spikes elicited by photic stimulation. Note the delayed appearance of photically-induced polyspikes in the right segment. Calibration signal 1 sec, 70μV.

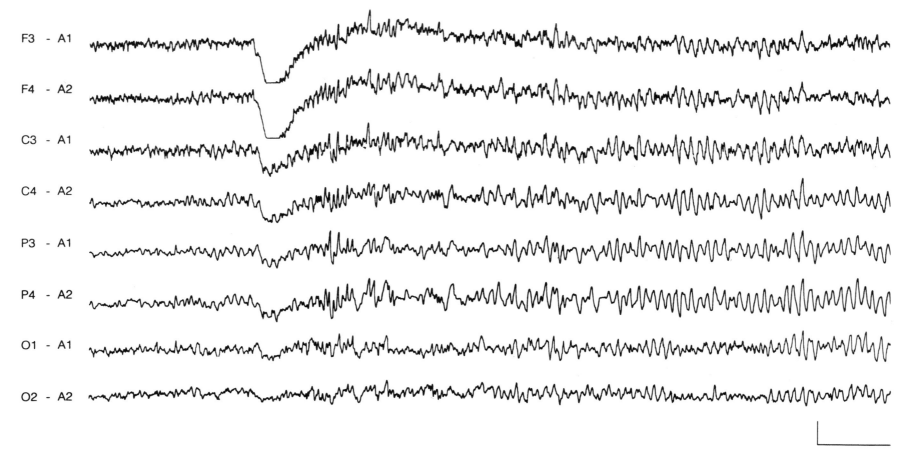

FIG. 5–41. Polyspikes on eye closure. 39 years. Because they merge somewhat with background activity, these diffuse or posteriorly accentuated discharges occurring on eye closure may be overlooked. Compare background activity with eyes open (first 2 seconds), and that of eyes closed (last 4 seconds) with that of the 1st second after eye closure, which contains widely synchronous sequential 15 Hz spikes. Calibration signal 1 sec, 70μV.

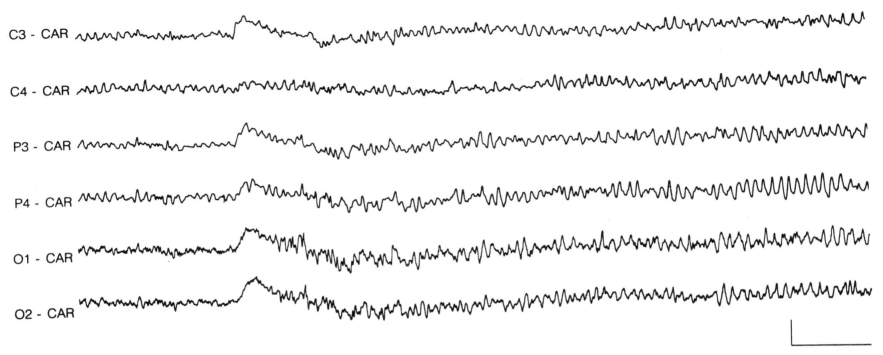

FIG. 5–42. Minimal expression of polyspikes on eye closure. 39 years. Scrutiny of occipital (O1, O2) derivations will reveal the low-amplitude, briefly-occurring sequence of 20 Hz spikes occurring on eye closure. Calibration signal 1 sec, 70μV.

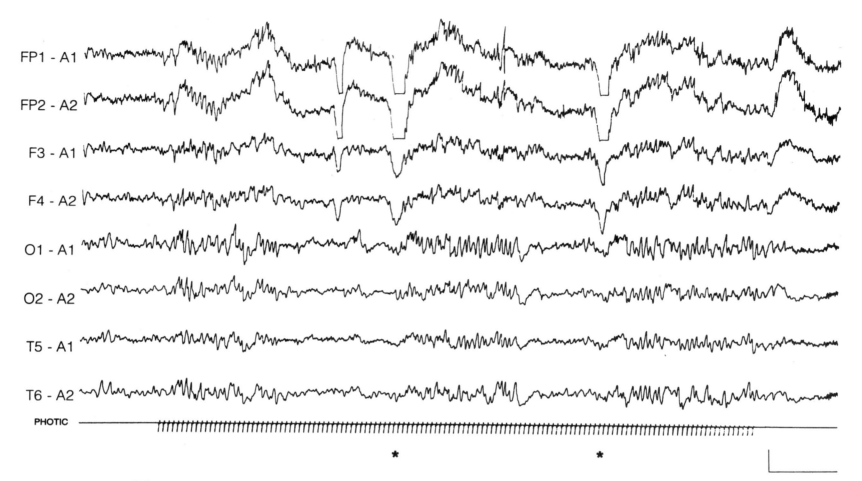

FIG. 5–43. Photic stimulation with eyes closed and with eye closure elicits spikes. 39 years. Same patient as in Figs. 5–41 and 5–42. High-frequency (15 Hz) photic stimulation with eyes closed (beginning of photic stimulation) and with eye closure (*asterisks*) (*center* and last part of photic stimulation) elicits polyspikes. Flash stimuli usually elicit polyspikes when eye closure on the resting record does so. Calibration signal 1 sec, 70μV.

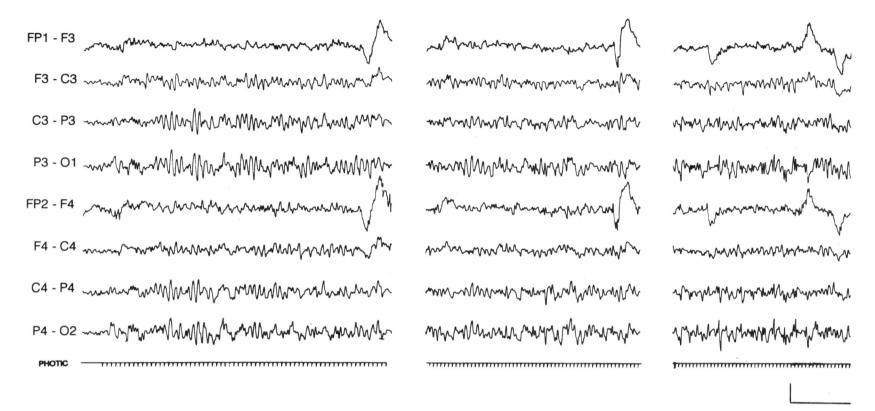

FIG. 5–44. Variations in prominence of photoparoxysmal response with frequency. 21 years. At 14 flashes/sec (*left*), the photoparoxysmal response appears only subtly but becomes progressively more evident in the posterior head regions at 16 and 17 flashes/sec (*center and right*)—all with eyes closed. Calibration signal 1 sec, 50μV.

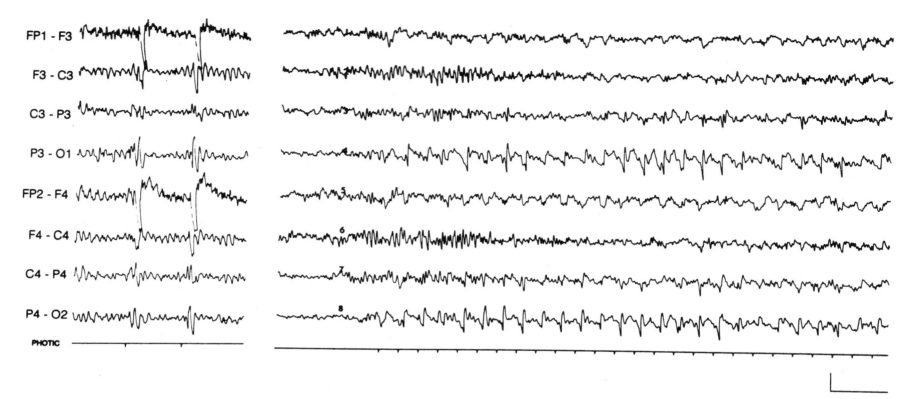

FIG. 5–45. Bisynchronous spikes elicited by low flash rates. 43 years (*left*), and 23 years (*right*). Rarely, low flash rates will elicit prominent single spikes or polyspikes. In the left tracing, they appear just before the eye blinks in response to single flashes. In the right tracing, these spikes are time-locked to the 3 Hz flash rate; in this instance, they might be considered an exaggerated following response. This type of response has been reported in children with neuronal ceroid lipofuscinosis (36). Responses to flash stimuli are usually of higher voltage while the eyes are closed than when open (4). Certain metabolic conditions or other diffuse encephalopathies may produce such high-amplitude discharges (4, 35). Left calibration signal 1 sec, 70μV. Right calibration signal 1 sec, 50μV.

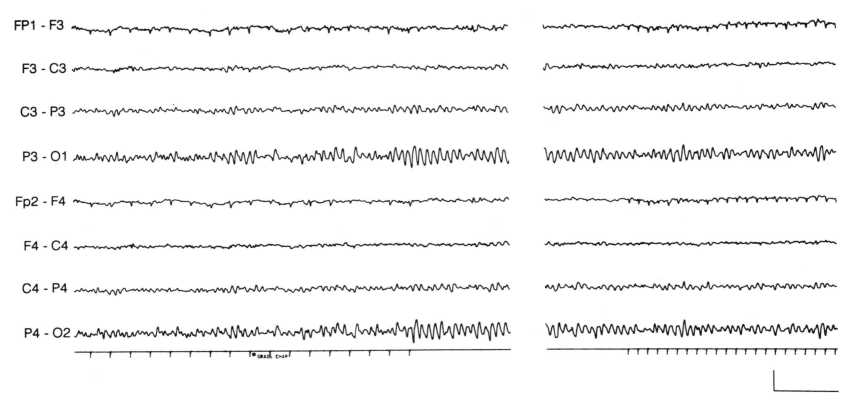

FIG. 5–46. Photomyoclonic response to low-frequency flash with eyes closed. 46 years. These synchronous spike-like potentials recorded in the frontal polar (Fp1,2) leads occur about 50 msec after each flash and represent contractions of the orbicularis oculi and other facial muscles. Electrostatic artifact, representing a photochemical response occurring with high electrode impedance, would not have this delay. Calibration signal 1 sec, 50μV.

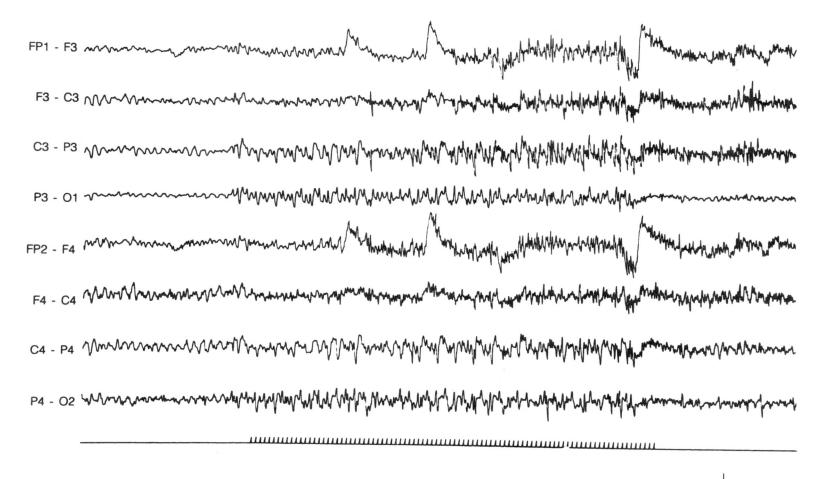

FIG. 5–47. Photomyogenic response. 76 years. Repetitive muscle spikes appear and gradually augment during photic stimulation at 15 flashes/sec and subside promptly with the flash, leaving some muscle artifact. Extending posteriorly, the muscle spikes intermingle with photic driving to resemble a photoparoxysmal response. The simultaneous termination of the muscle potentials with flash is more suggestive of a photomyogenic response. Calibration signal 1 sec, 50μV.

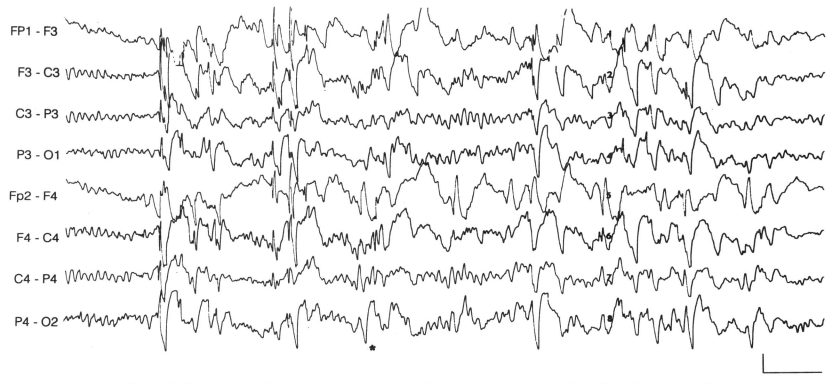

FIG. 5–48. Toranomaki. 29 years. Roughly translated, this Japanese term means "revealing all in a nutshell." Thus, this single prolonged burst demonstrates 3 Hz spike-waves, slow spike-waves, and bisynchronous polyspikes (*asterisk*). Note the subtle shifting of the maximum field of spikes between the right and left hemispheres. Calibration signal 1 sec, 50µV.

Chapter 6

Epileptiform Abnormalities: Seizures

Focal Seizures (Figs. 1–29)
- Focal seizures produce sequential new EEG phenomena in one region whose morphology progressively evolves and may spread to adjacent regions or contralaterally.
- Postictally focal abnormalities usually appear in the region of maximum seizure intensity which is usually the area of onset. Such abnormalities may include: attenuation, delta, and increased interictal spike activity.

Generalized Seizures (Figs. 30–40)
- Generalized seizures consist of bilaterally synchronous sequential spike-waves, spikes, or rhythmic waves.
- Higher frequency phenomena (fast rhythmic waves, polyspikes) usually appear earlier in the seizure than lower frequency ones (spike-waves, rhythmic delta).
- Usually an abrupt non-focal onset and offset.

Periodic Lateralized Epileptiform Discharges (PLEDs) (Figs. 41–45, 47–50)
- Diphasic or polyphasic spike.

- Usually electronegative.
- Slow wave follows spike.
- Duration of each complex about 200–500 msec.
- Hemispheric or regional; not confined to single electrode position.
- Recur every 0.5 to 2 seconds.
- Abnormal background in area of PLEDs.
- Acute or subacute cerebral process.
- Synchronous contralateral myoclonic jerks in minority.

PLEDs Plus (Fig. 46)
- Low amplitude rhythmic, high frequency discharge superimposed upon conventional PLEDs, usually the second slope.
- Partial seizure within 30 minutes is more likely than with conventional PLEDs alone.

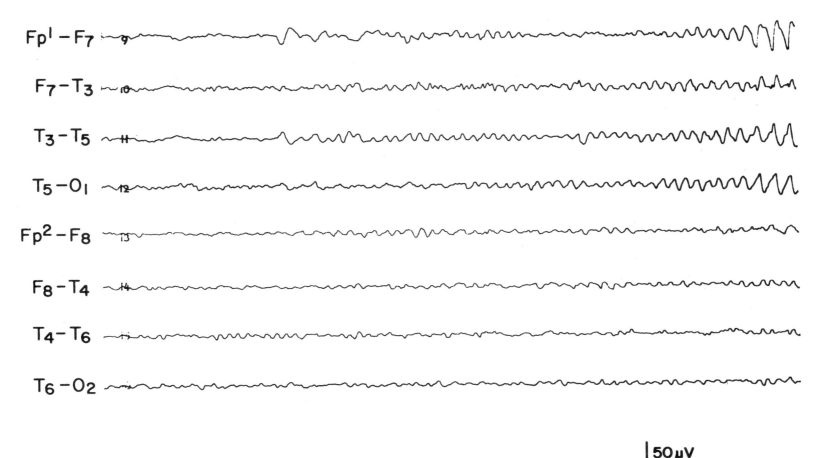

FIG. 6–1. Left temporal seizure: onset. This and following tracings illustrate features which characterize focal epileptic seizures: a progressive evolution of both morphology, repetition rate and location of sequential epileptiform discharges. The seizure begins as a single diphasic wave followed by rhythmic 5 Hz sequential waves in the left anterior-mid temporal (F7-T3) region which increase in voltage and become more apiculate near the end of this segment.

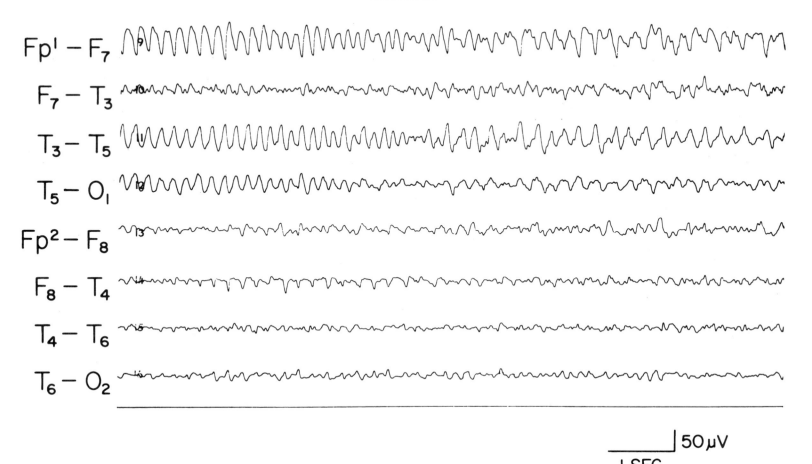

FIG. 6–2. Left temporal seizure: continuation. The 5 Hz higher voltage rhythmic waves continue for an additional 4–5 seconds and change abruptly to sequential blunted 4–5 Hz apiculate waves at F7-T3 which continue for most of the seizure.

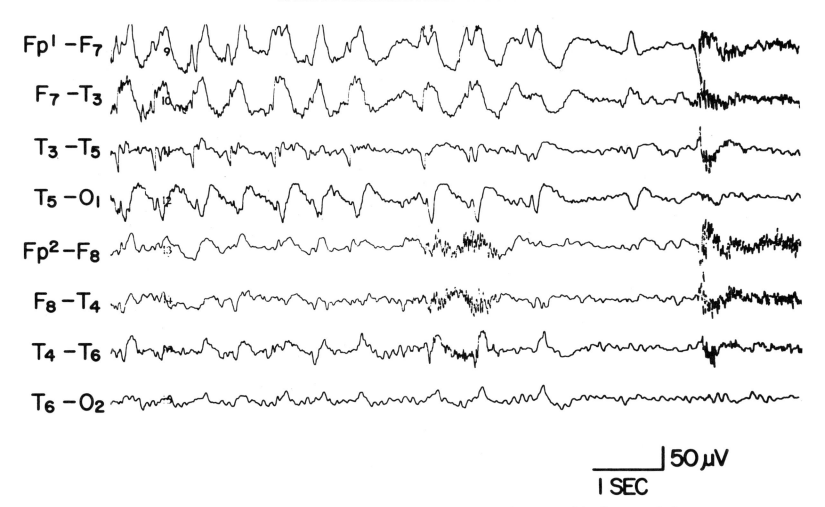

FIG. 6–3. Seizure termination. The previous phenomena have converted to sequential spike-wave discharges and have propagated to the posterior temporal region (T5). Note the chewing artifact at seizure termination.

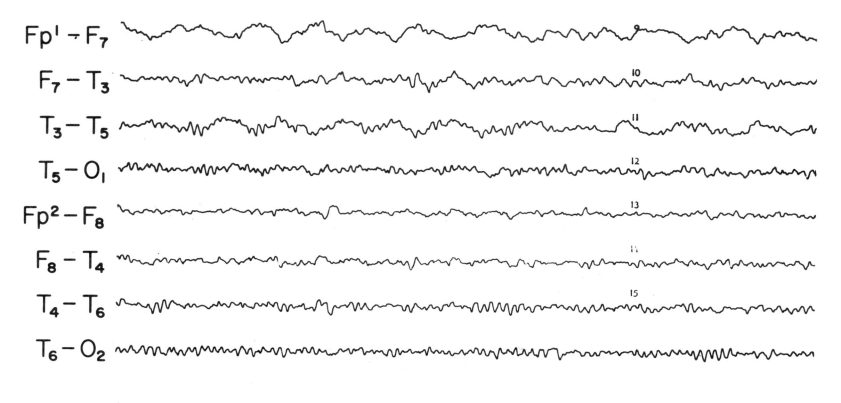

FIG. 6–4. Left temporal seizure: postictal phase. Focal arrhythmic persistent but gradually declining delta activity postictally correlates very well with side of seizure onset (37).

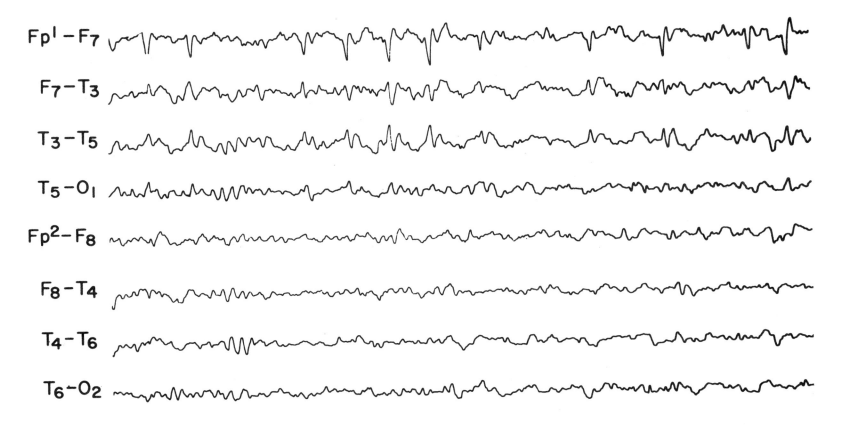

FIG. 6–5. Left temporal epileptogenesis: interictal recording. Abundant left anterior temporal (F7-T3) spikes, if consistent over multiple recordings, give strong evidence for seizure localization (38).

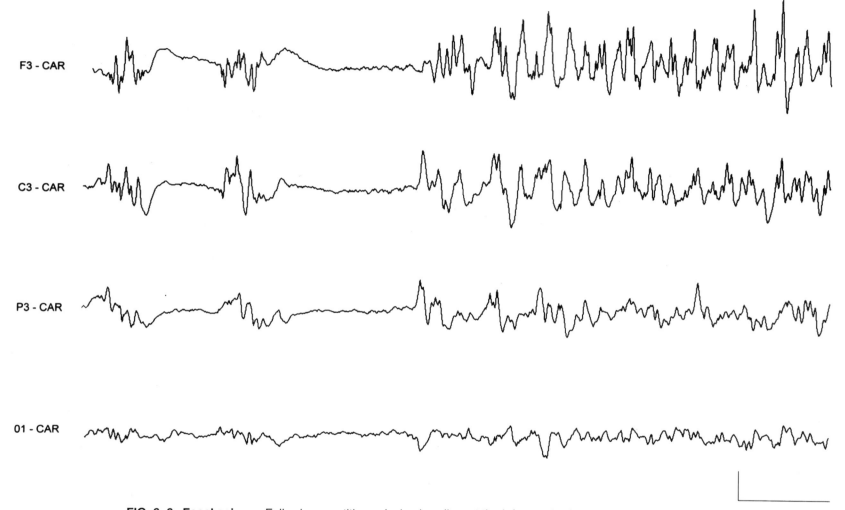

FIG. 6–6. Focal seizure. Following repetitive polyphasic spikes at the left superior frontal central (F3, C3) positions, the seizure begins as sequential spikes at F3, C3 with minimal left parietal involvement. Calibration signal 1 sec, 70μV.

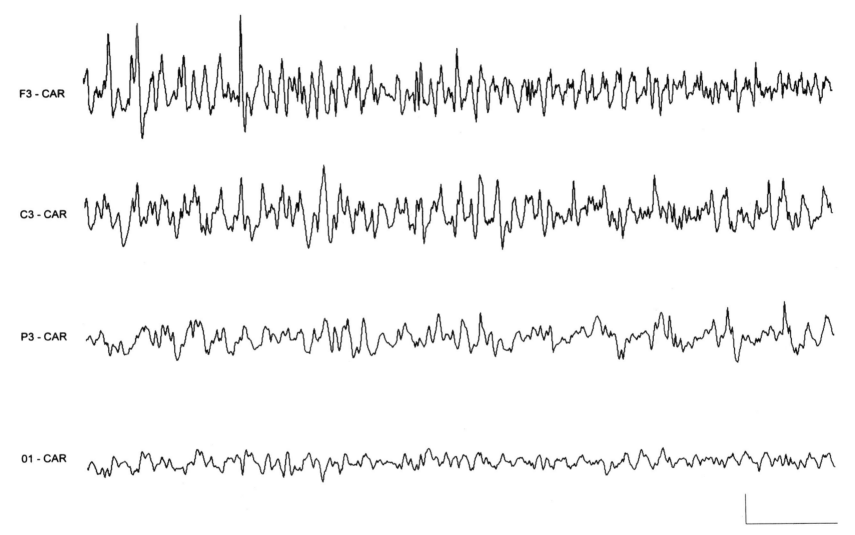

FIG. 6–7. Focal seizure, continued. About 15 seconds later, the seizure has spread more prominently to the left parietal (P3) region and the frequency of the sequential spikes has increased. Diffuse theta also appears. Progressive evolution of multiple morphologies characterizes and defines focally originating seizures. Calibration signal 1 sec, 70μV.

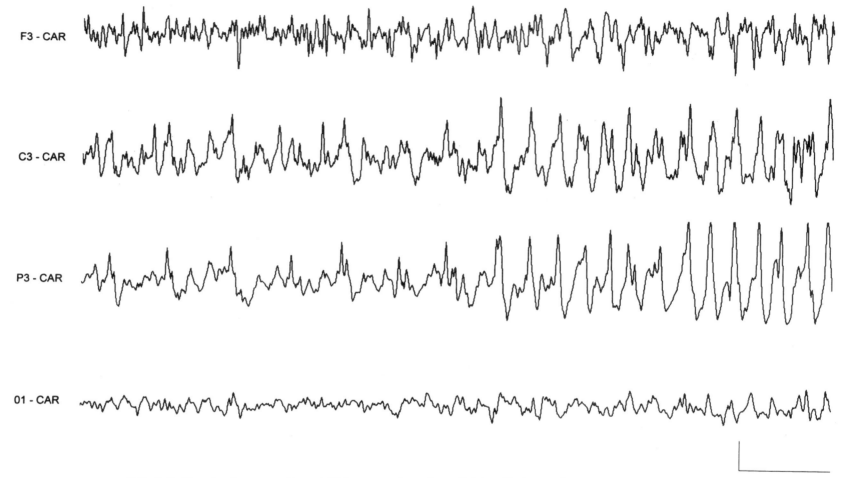

FIG. 6–8. Focal seizure, continued. This segment overlaps slightly with the previous one and shows the slowing and then increase in sequential spike rate, principally in the left central parietal (C3, P3) regions with some spread to the left superior frontal region (F3). Calibration signal 1 sec, 70 μV.

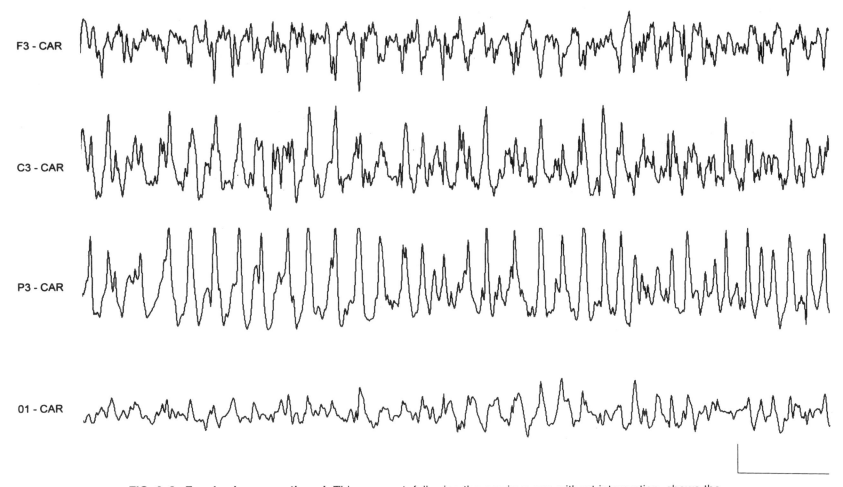

FIG. 6–9. Focal seizure, continued. This segment, following the previous one without interruption, shows the continued focal spikes, in-phase at C3, P3 and principally out-of-phase at F3 indicating an electrical dipole between F3 on the one hand and C3, P3. Calibration signal 1 sec, 70µV.

F3 - CAR

C3 - CAR

P3 - CAR

01 - CAR

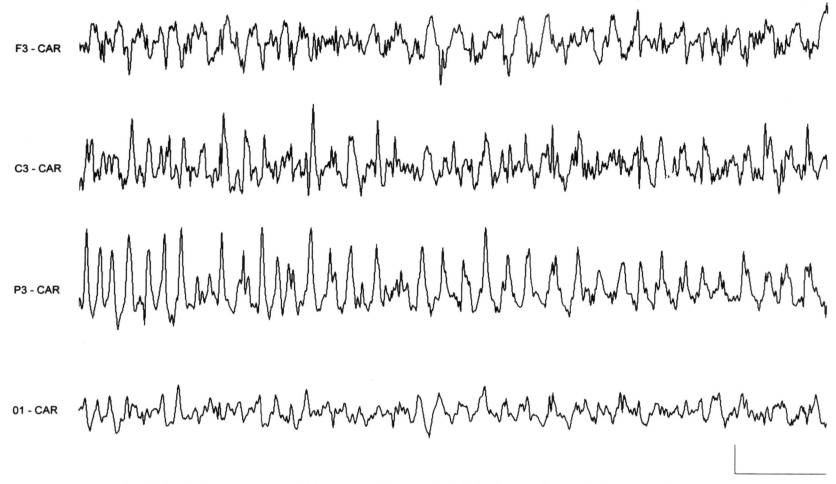

FIG. 6–10. Seizure, continued. This segment shows gradual diminution in spike amplitude as the seizure proceeds. Calibration signal 1 sec, 70μV.

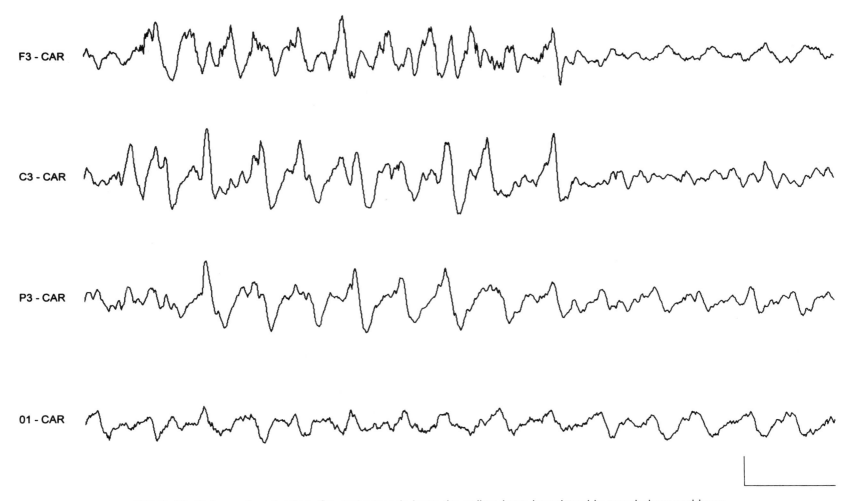

FIG. 6–11. Seizure, termination. Several seconds later, the spikes have broadened in morphology and have slowed in rate and then cease suddenly. Calibration signal 1 sec, 70μV.

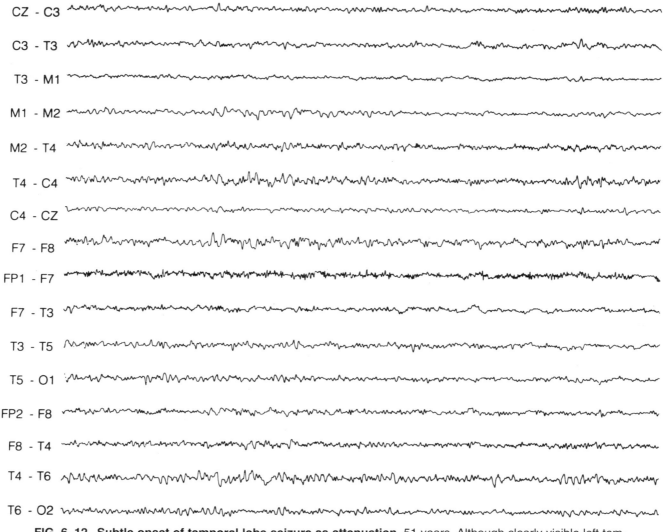

FIG. 6–12. Subtle onset of temporal lobe seizure as attenuation. 51 years. Although clearly visible left temporal (T3-M1-F7) seizure activity appears in the right-hand segment, the initial manifestation appears subtly in this segment as left temporal attenuation as depicted in the F7-T3, T3-T5, T5-O1 derivations; compare these to the unchanged right temporal derivations. Unfortunately, the presumed attenuation in the Fp1-F7 derivation is obscured by muscle artifact. About 11% of partial seizures begin with such attenuation (39). In the right segment, the left temporal attenuation changes abruptly to 4–5 Hz rhythmic waves in the left inferior anterior midtemporal region (M1-T3-F7). Calibration signal 1 sec, 70μV.

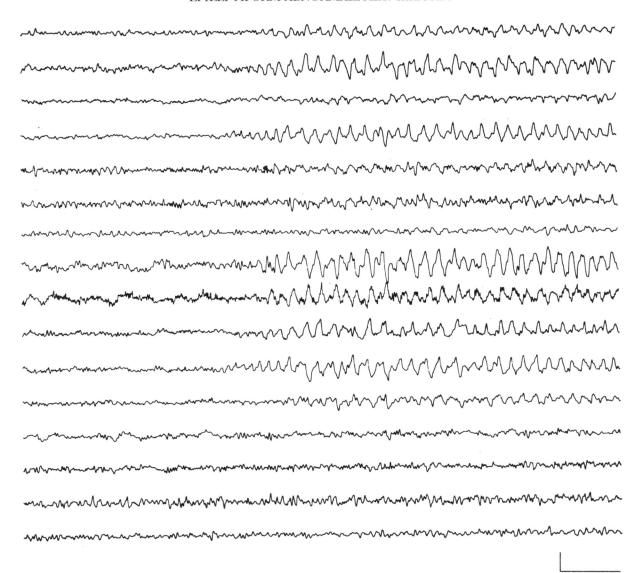

FIG. 6–12. *Continued.*

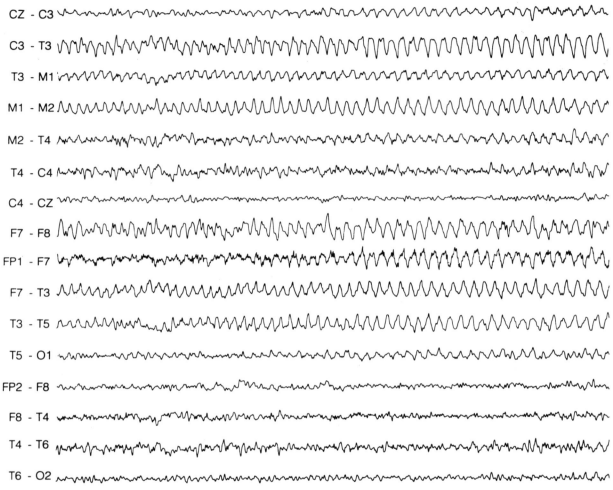

FIG. 6–13. Same seizure, termination. The apiculate 4–5 Hz rhythmic waves change gradually to 3 Hz spikes near seizure termination. No independently occurring right-sided involvement appeared. Calibration signal 1 sec, 70μV.

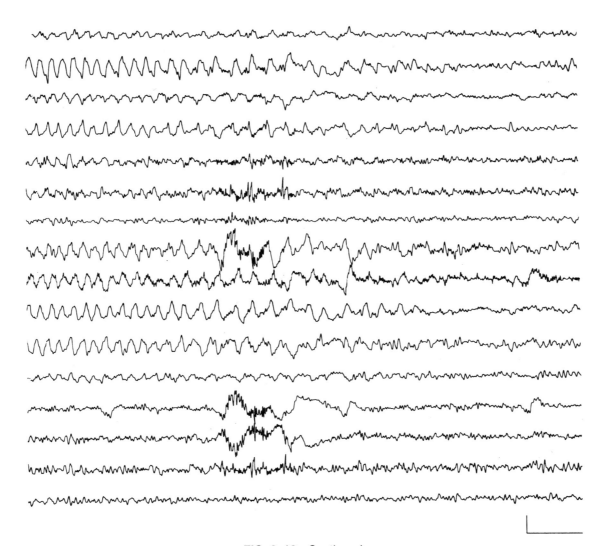

FIG. 6–13. *Continued.*

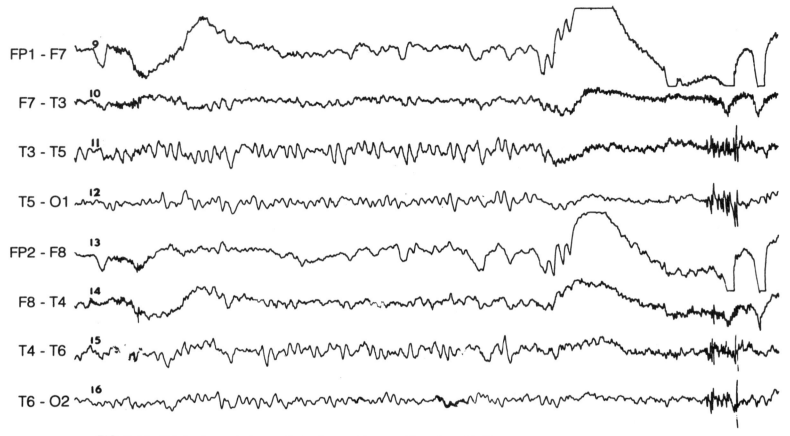

FP1 - F7

F7 - T3

T3 - T5

T5 - O1

FP2 - F8

F8 - T4

T4 - T6

T6 - O2

FIG. 6–14. Gradual onset of a partial seizure. 16 years. Together with Figs. 6–12 and 6–13, this illustrates the very gradual evolutionary nature of some partial seizures and their probable incomplete expression on a less-than-optimum montage. The left segment, preictal, shows bilateral theta and delta, slightly more on right. To the right, sequential low voltage right anterior temporal (F8-T4) spikes mark the onset of the attack. Eye opening attenuates background activity. Calibration signal 1 sec, 100μV.

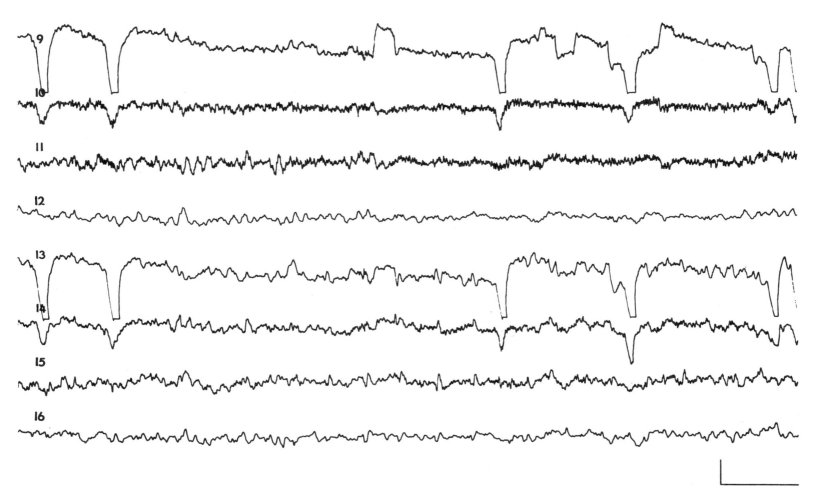

FIG. 6–14. *Continued.*

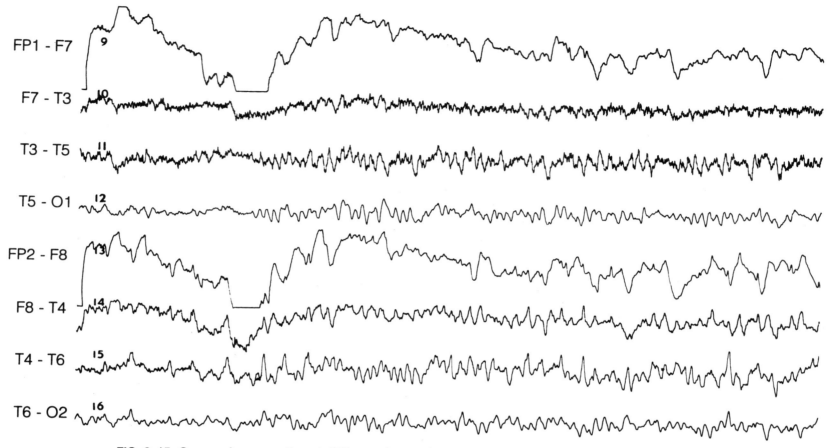

FIG. 6–15. Same seizure, continued. With eye closure, the reappearance of background activity partially obscures the sequential right temporal spikes. The right hand segment shows further evolution as 4–5 Hz rhythmic waves and 2–3 Hz delta activity appear in the right temporal region (compare with left). Profuse eye blinks partially obscure the right temporal phenomena. Calibration signal 1 sec, 100μV.

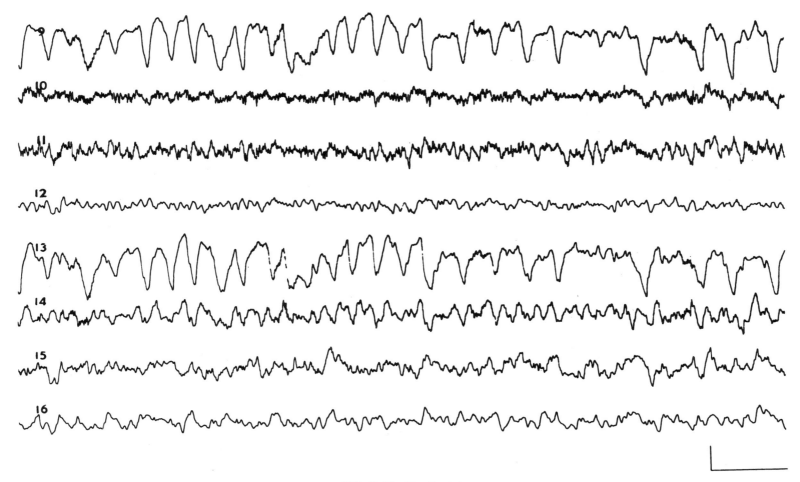

FIG. 6–15. *Continued.*

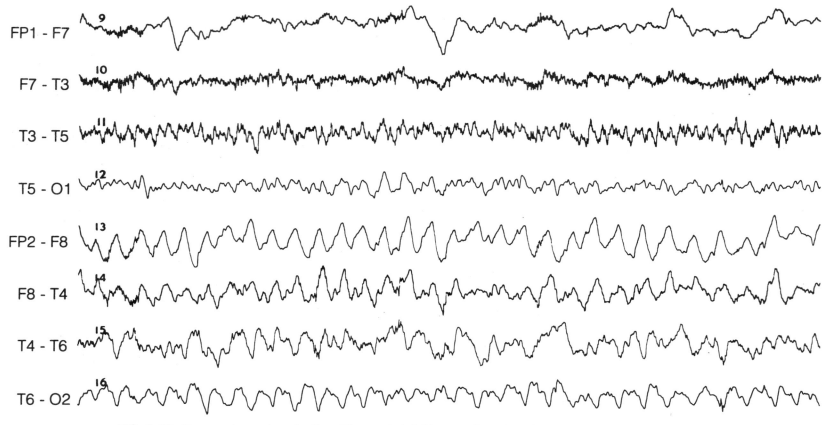

FIG. 6–16. Same seizure, termination. The most definitive manifestation of this seizure is 3–4 Hz rhythmic waves at T4-F8 with spread to T6. Note the slowing of wave repetition rate and loss of its rhythmicity as the attack gradually terminates. Nausea was the only symptom. Calibration signal 1 sec, 100μV.

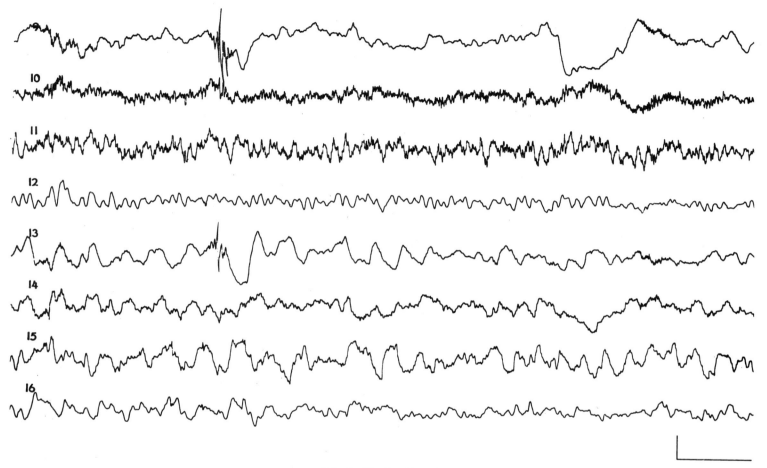

FIG. 6–16. *Continued.*

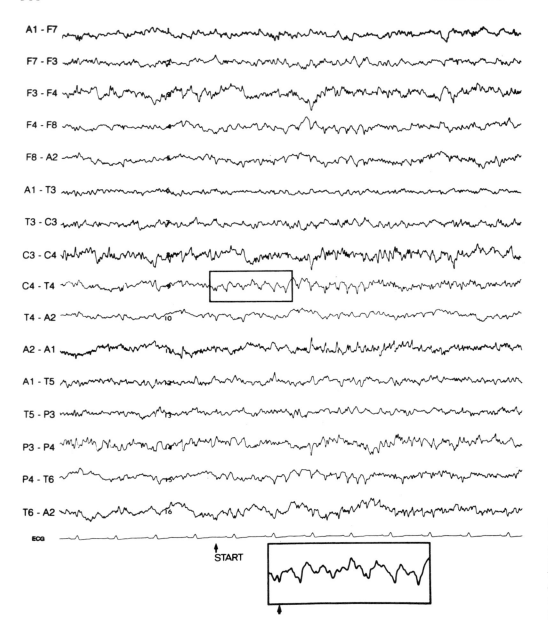

FIG. 6–17. Subtle and gradual seizure onset. 69 years. This and Fig. 6-16 illustrate the "start-stop-start" of seizure onset (40), and the gradual evolution of a partial seizure. Only minimal evidence of the impending seizure appears in the left side of this figure, as a 3–4 second train of 5 Hz sequential spikes in the right temporal region (A2-T4-T6) constituting the "start" and the "stop" of the start-stop-start phenomenon. Ten seconds later *(right)*, 5 Hz right temporal spikes reappear. Calibration signal 1 sec, 50μV.

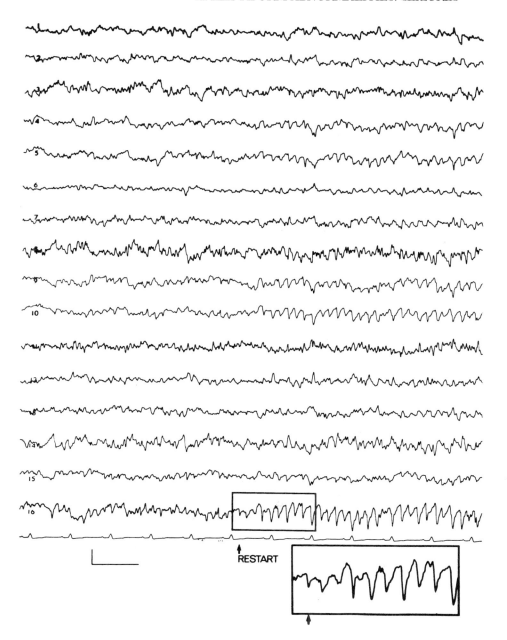

FIG. 6–17. *Continued.*

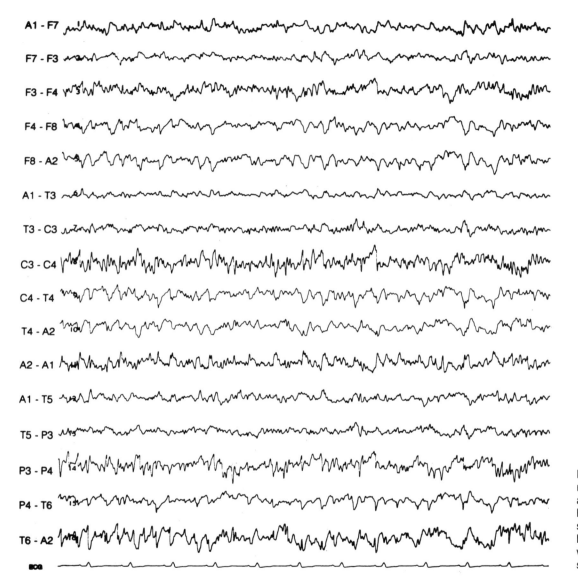

FIG. 6–18. Same seizure, continued. No time lapse. The spike rate slows to about 4 Hz; the spikes involve T6, P4, T4, A2, C4, and F8 but are somewhat buried in 4 Hz theta *(left)*. Whether the higher frequency (15 Hz) waves constitute part of the seizure itself or represent an alerting phenomenon is unclear. 20 seconds later *(right)*, the seizure consists of right temporal-parietal spikes with metronomic repetition. These continued an additional 12 seconds (not shown). Calibration signal 1 sec, 50μV.

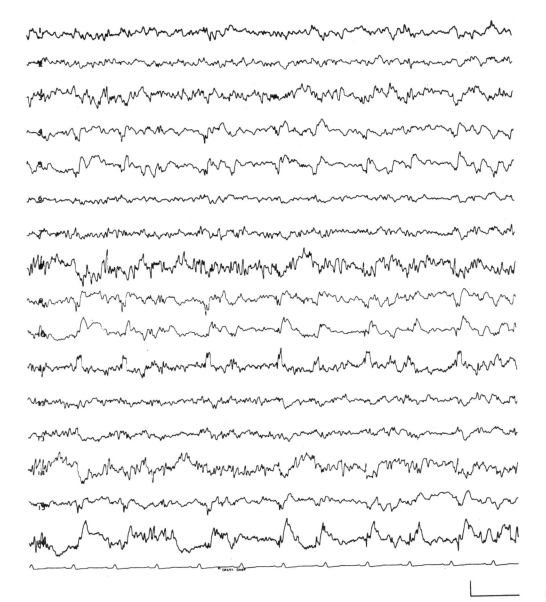

FIG. 6–18. *Continued.*

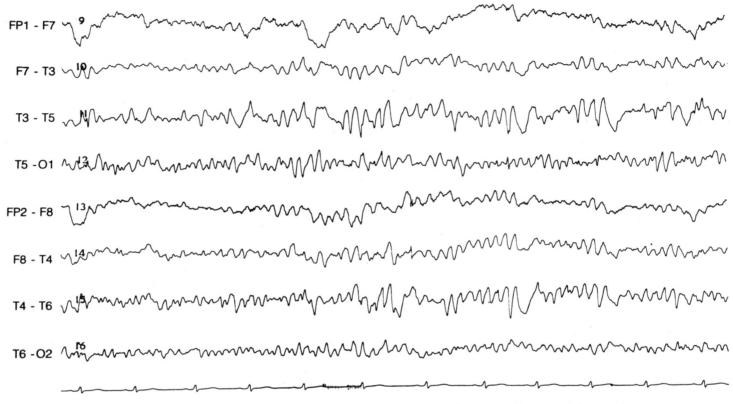

FIG. 6–19. Subclinical attack at delta focus. 37 years. Preictal. The left segment illustrates left posterior temporal-occipital delta with intermingled low amplitude electronegative spikes in the same region; both phenomena appear in minimal form contralaterally. In the right segment, note the abrupt appearance of about 12 Hz sequential spikes in the left posterior temporal region (T5) with some spread (as partial cancellation) to the left occipital area (O1) and with slight homologous spread. After 3 1/2 seconds of continuous spikes, they become intermittent as this subclinical seizure abates. Calibration signal 1 sec, 70μV.

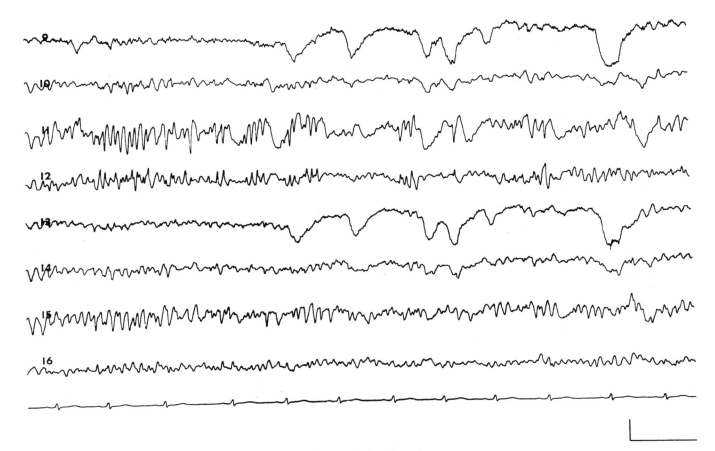

FIG. 6–19. *Continued.*

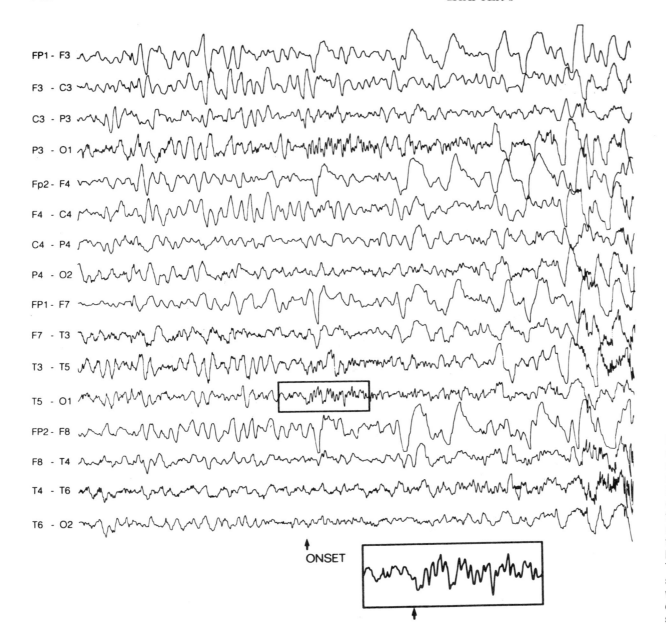

FIG. 6–20. **Left occipital and secondarily generalized seizure.** 14 years. Diffuse theta and delta may obscure the focal onset of this ultimately generalized seizure. Note the 15 Hz rhythmic waves in the left occipital (O1) region extending to the left posterior temporal area (T5) for about 3 seconds changing to diffuse 3–4 Hz rhythmic waves with intermingled spikes in the following two segments. The spikes gradually become more prominent as the attack proceeds. The patient had a "funny feeling" in her eyes then stared straight, fell backwards tonically, and then walked about in a confused manner with multifocal intermittent myoclonus. Calibration signal 1 sec, 70μV.

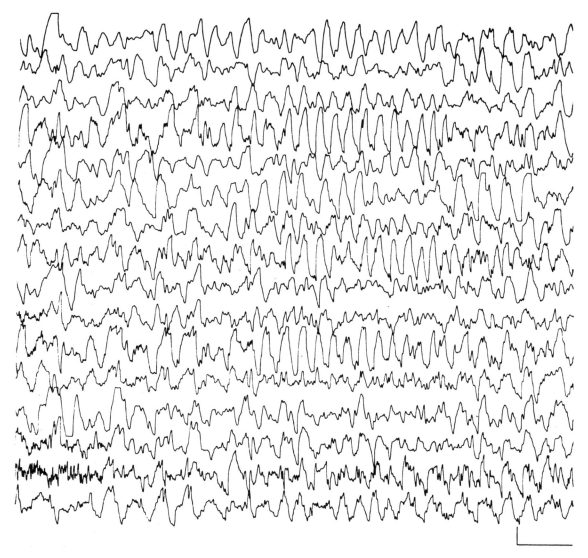

FIG. 6–20. *Continued.*

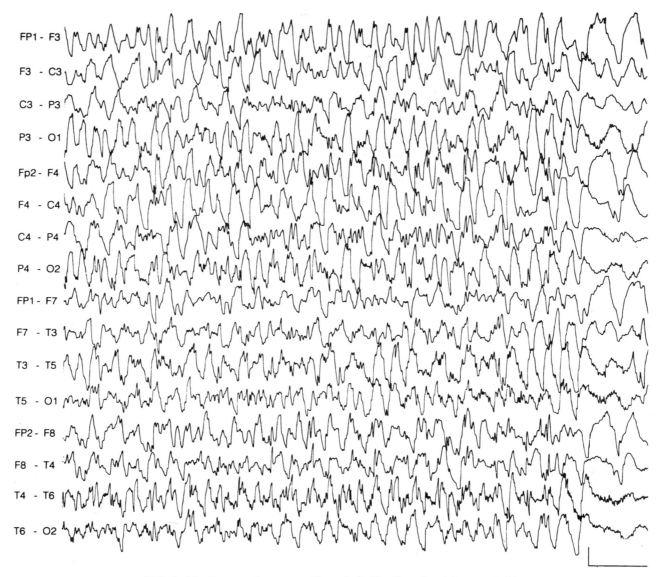

FIG. 6–21. Same seizure, continued. Calibration signal 1 sec, 70μV.

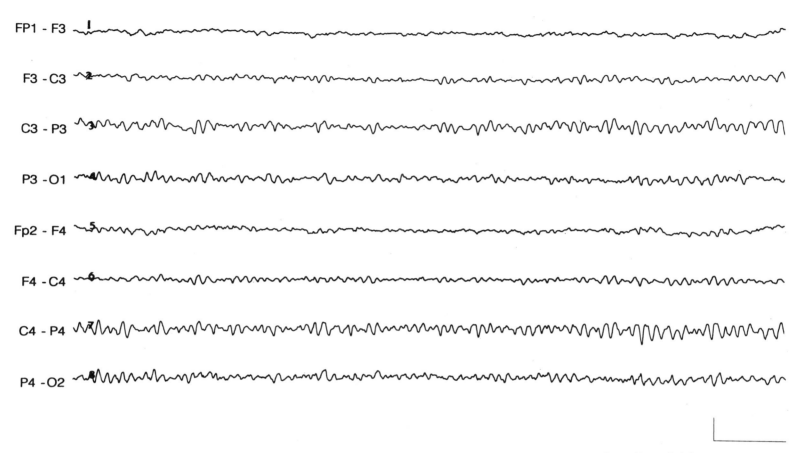

FIG. 6–22. Gradual onset of left frontal-central (F3-C3) seizure. 77 years. Preictal recording with a slightly greater quantity of theta in the left parasagittal region as compared to the right. Calibration signal 1 sec, 70μV.

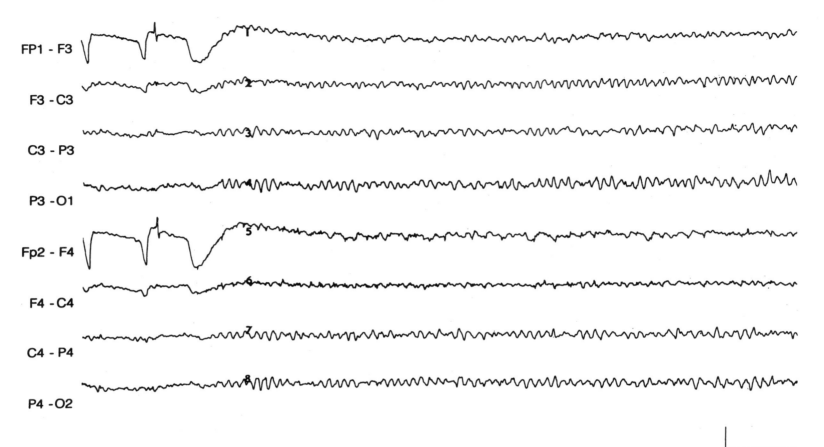

FIG. 6–23. Same seizure, continued. Early Ictal. Although the 9–10 Hz sustained rhythm seen principally at the F3-C3 derivation resembles alpha, it contrasts clearly with the preictal recording and with the contralateral (F4-C4) derivation. Note the slight spread to the Fp1-F3 derivation indicating F3 involvement; involvement of C3 is more difficult to assess because of the alpha field. 10 seconds later *(right)*; a relative pause. 10 Hz rhythm at F3-C3 and Fp1-F3 slows to about 6–8 Hz and is interrupted by sporadic apiculate waves in the F3-C3 derivation. Calibration signal 1 sec, 70μV.

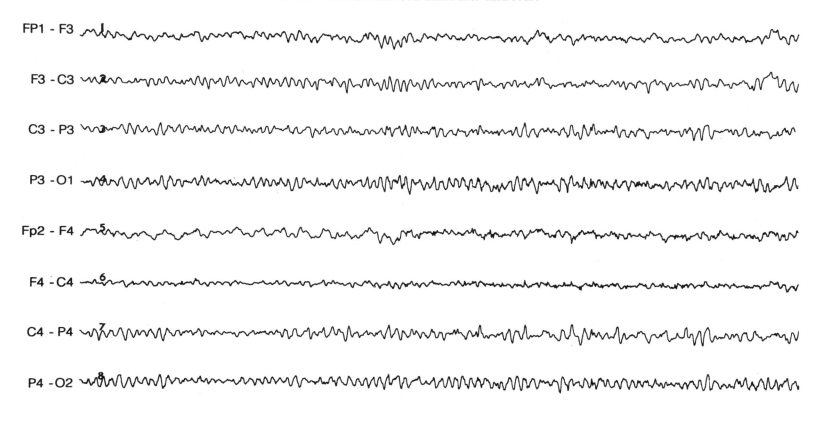

FIG. 6–23. *Continued.*

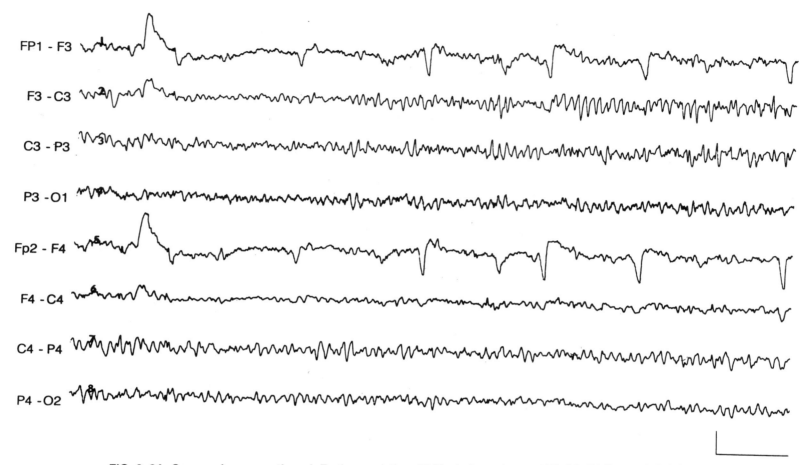

FIG. 6–24. Same seizure, continued. Further evolution. 10 Hz rhythm returns at F3-C3, C3-P3, and slightly at Fp1-F3 derivations, indicating F3-C3 involvement; accompanied by spikes *(left)*. Jerking of the right arm began. Right segment shows a complex intermixture of about 9 Hz and about 20 Hz waves principally at C3. Patient stated "Ah, ah"; right arm adducted at shoulder, rotated inwardly and flexed at elbow. Calibration signal 1 sec, 70μV.

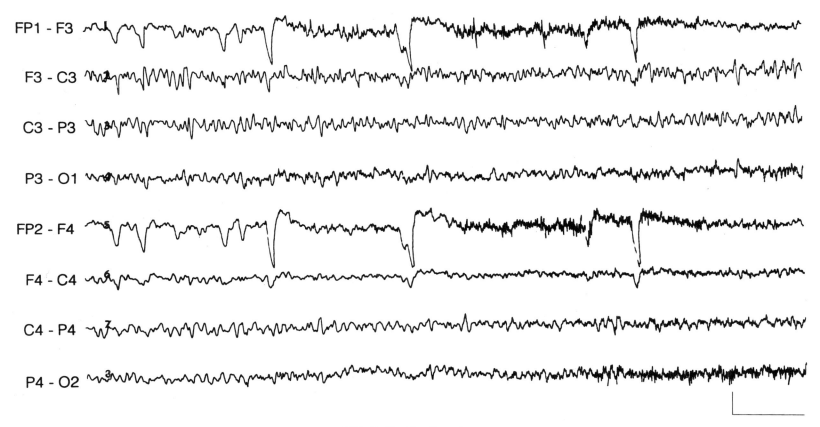

FIG. 6–24. *Continued.*

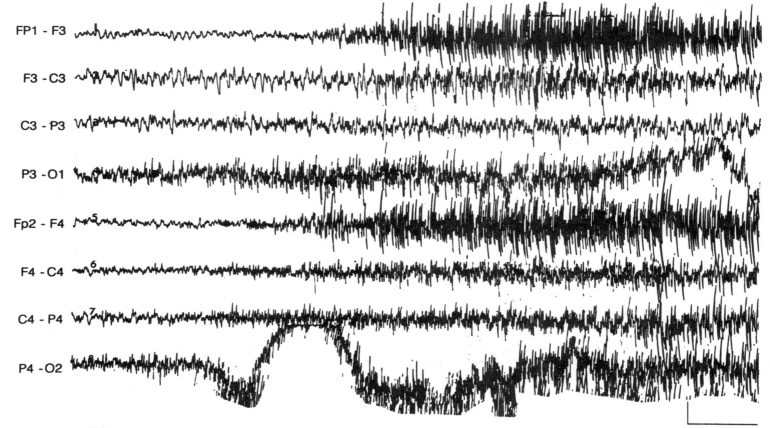

FIG. 6–25. Same seizure, continued. Seizure proceeded to generalized tonic-clonic seizure. 8 Hz apiculate waves principally at C3 become submerged in diffuse tonic muscle artifact *(left)*. Termination of grand mal component *(right)*. The seizure has slowed to synchronous polyspike-waves repeating at every 800–1000 msec, which then terminate slightly earlier in the originating left hemisphere. Calibration signal 1 sec, 70μV.

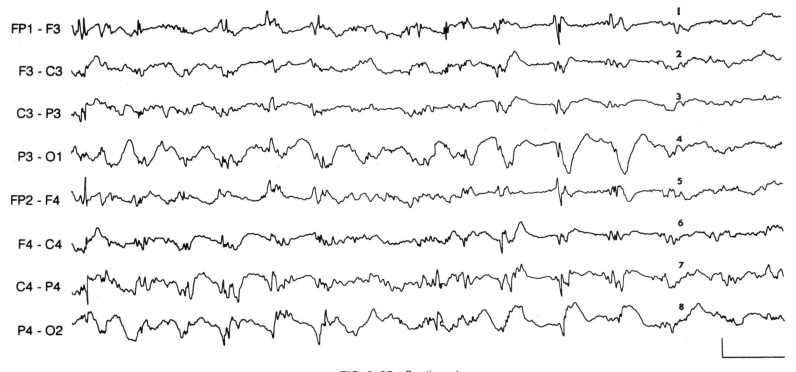

FIG. 6–25. *Continued.*

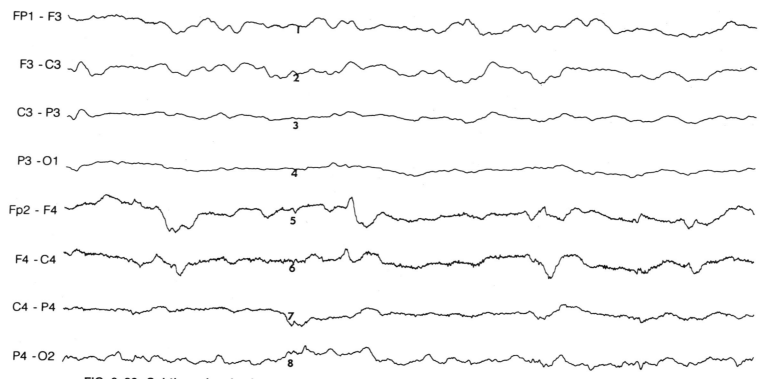

FIG. 6–26. Subtle regional seizure onset in a comatose patient. 79 years. In a patient whose encephalopathy is sufficiently severe to reduce the quantity of cerebral activity diffusely, a seizure may begin in the less affected of the two hemispheres, the right in this case. Thus, the better-developed background activity appears in the right occipital (O2) region in the preictal recording *(left)*. Two to three Hz rhythmic waves with intermittent low voltage right frontal central (F4-C4) spikes gradually appear *(right)*. Calibration signal 1 sec, 70μV.

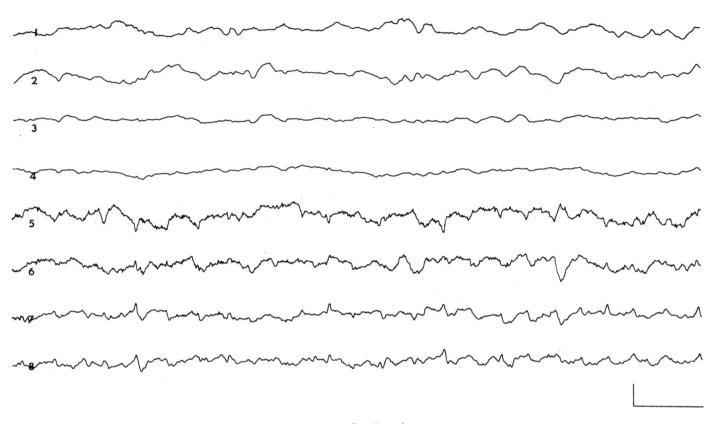

FIG. 6–26. *Continued.*

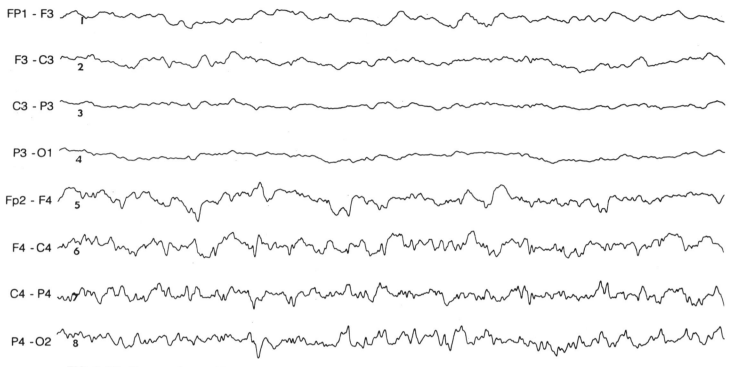

FIG. 6–27. Same seizure, 80 seconds later. The right hemisphere seizure continues as a mixture of intermittent low voltage spikes, delta, and theta activity *(left)*. Such activity can only be identified as a seizure by assessing the preictal background activity in the same area. The morphological development of this attack, although slow, conforms to the criteria of a partial seizure as a progressive modification of the background rhythms (39). Calibration signal 1 sec, 70μV.

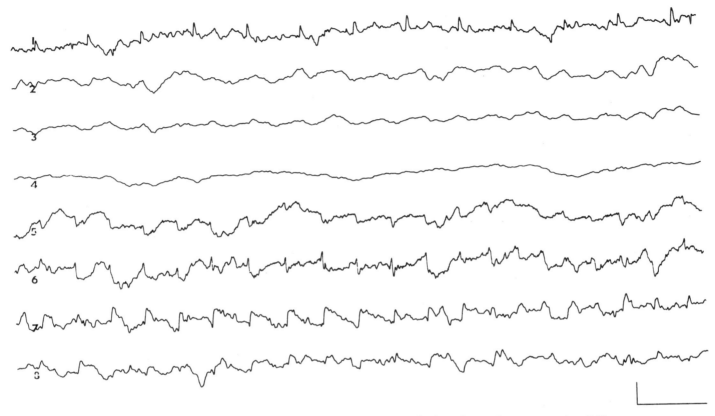

FIG. 6–28. Same seizure. Ten seconds after the last segment, a further change has occurred as 2 Hz sequential electropositive spikes in the right central (C4) region followed by apiculate delta *(right)*. Note the independently occurring left frontal polar (Fp1) seizure. Seizures in severely encephalopathic adults share several characteristics of neonatal attacks: gradual evolution, slow topological spread or confinement to one area, coexistence of two seizures of independent morphology and evolution, and emergence of such patterns from an attenuated (suppressed) background (41). Calibration signal 1 sec, 70μV.

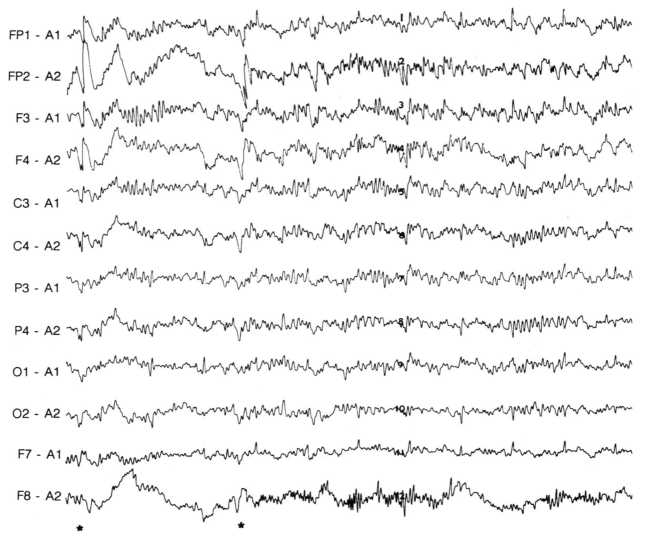

FIG. 6–29. Right frontal seizure partially obscured by spindles; the "start-stop-start" phenomenon. 39 years. After two irregular-appearing right frontal spikes *(asterisks)*, 25–30 Hz, low to medium voltage waves appear at F8 and spread slightly to Fp2, F4 within 1 second. The amplitude of such ictal potentials partially abates over the last 3 seconds of this segment. This constitutes the "start-stop" of the "start-stop-start" phenomenon (40). Ongoing spindles partially occlude expression of such high frequency rhythmic waves. 25 Hz medium voltage rhythmic waves augment again at F8, Fp2 and slightly at F4 completing the "start-stop-start" phenomenon *(right)*. This term describes the manner in which some clinical and subclinical partial seizures begin, i.e., a partial seizure either ceases or decreases in amplitude of expression for a few seconds before recommencing; the second start is usually in the same region as the first. Calibration signal 1 sec, 50μV.

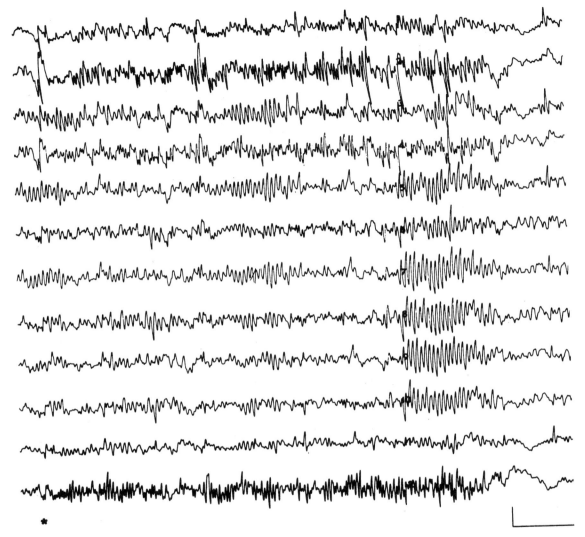

FIG. 6–29. Continued.

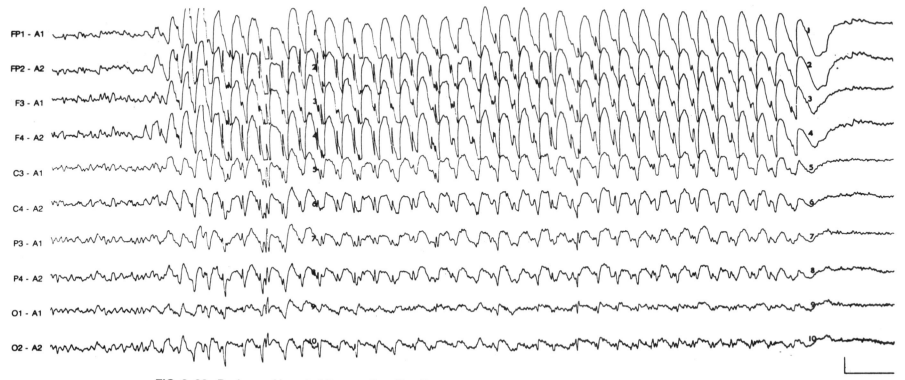

FIG. 6–30. Prolonged burst of "generalized" spike-waves. 20 years. Befitting their bilaterally synchronous nature, these spike-waves begin and end suddenly and simultaneously in all regions. At onset, the slightly more prominent 150–200 msec waves on the right and the usually slightly higher spikes on the right do not necessarily indicate occult secondary bisynchrony. Scrutiny of many bisynchronous spike-waves will reveal such minor asymmetries. As is usual, the spike-waves are slightly higher in voltage at F4,3 than Fp2,1. Compared to baseline, note the prominent electropositive trough between the spike and the wave, a feature particularly prominent on field plots (26). As commonly occurs, the spike-wave repetition rate is slightly faster at burst onset. "Generalized" spike-waves rarely engulf all electrode positions. Only a minimal impairment of consciousness occurred during this prominent burst and the patient recalled a number given during its 5th second. Calibration signal 1 sec, 200μV.

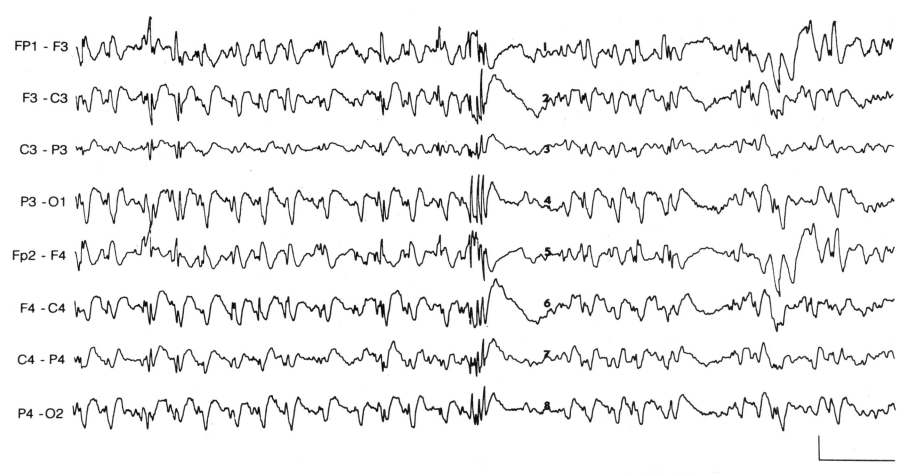

FIG. 6–31. Absence status epilepticus with electrodecremental events. 46 years. 2–3 Hz, bilaterally synchronous spike-waves and polyspike-waves become interrupted by sudden diffuse attenuation of potentials, known as electrodecremental events. These are occasionally preceded by widely synchronous polyspikes (42). Calibration signal 1 sec, 100μV.

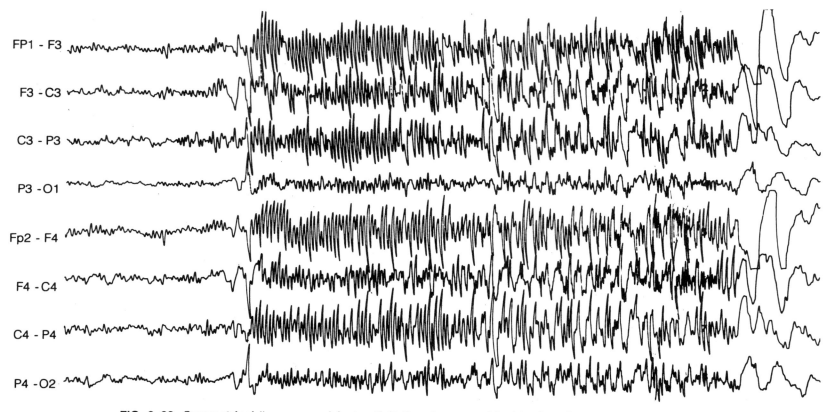

FP1 - F3

F3 - C3

C3 - P3

P3 - O1

Fp2 - F4

F4 - C4

C4 - P4

P4 - O2

FIG. 6–32. Symmetrical "paroxysmal fast activity" and asymmetrical tonic seizure. 32 years. From light sleep and a background of low voltage beta activity, sequential polyspikes suddenly appear, initially associated with a diffuse V-wave *(left)*. This phenomenon is also termed "generalized paroxysmal fast activity" (31) and "runs of rapid spikes" (43). Although such polyspikes appear symmetrical in onset, maximum expression, and offset, the clinical association contained many asymmetries: right arm elevation with elbow flexion, leftward cephalic deviation, and left arm flaccidity. Calibration signal 1 sec, 70μV.

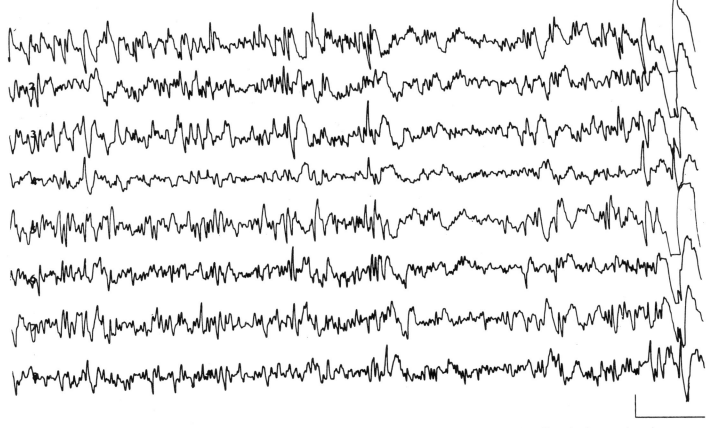

FIG. 6–32. Same seizure, continued. Twenty seconds later *(right)*, such diffuse polyspikes had waxed and waned in the interval and now appear interrupted by diffuse irregular 200–400 msec waves creating bisynchronous polyspike-waves. Despite the diffuseness of the spikes, the principal clinical sign was multiple single elevations and flexions of the right arm only. Calibration signal 1 sec, 70μV.

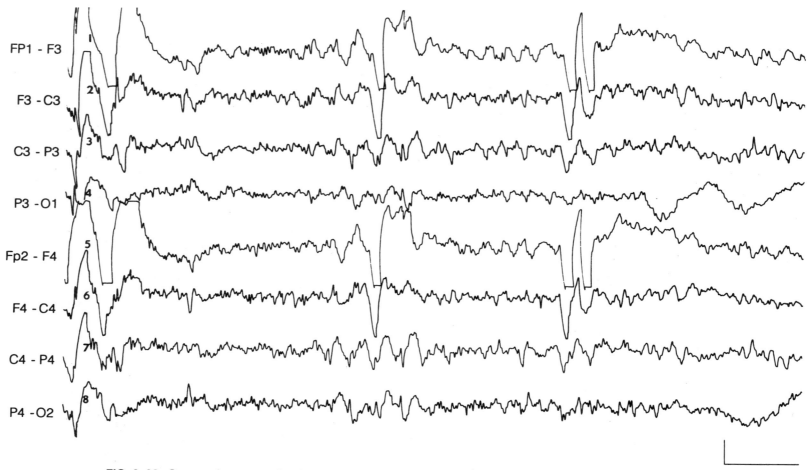

FIG. 6–33. Same seizure, termination. This diffuse seizure ends gradually as intermittent 300–400 msec theta with intermingled bisynchronous spikes. Bilateral myoclonus of arms accompany this phase. Calibration signal 1 sec, 70μV.

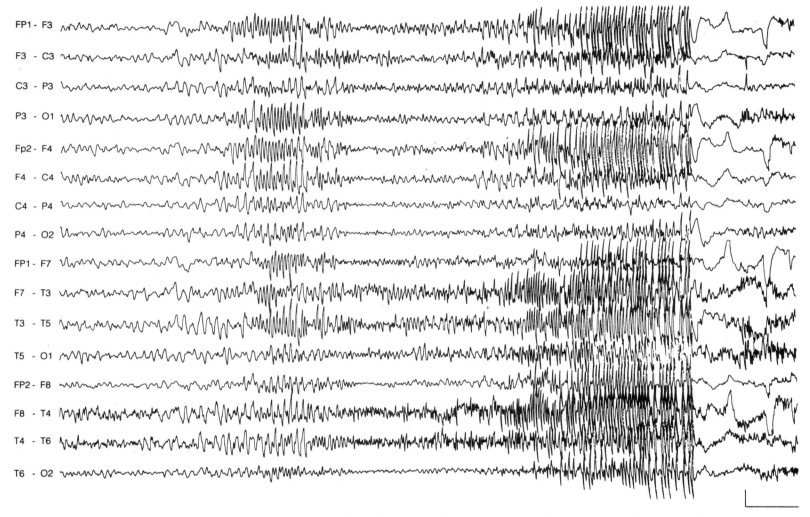

FIG. 6–34. Generalized seizure as polyspikes. 32 years. Following a non-specific burst of 6–7 Hz theta for 1 second, 15 Hz sequential polyspikes (multiple spikes) with intermixed 7 Hz waves appear diffusely for 3 seconds then abate for an additional 2 seconds only to recur in more vigorous fashion. Diffuse, sequential spikes are usually accompanied by a brief generalized tonic seizure which may be restricted to the trunk and proximal extremities, as in this instance. As the morphology of these discharges merges with that of the epileptic recruiting rhythm (33), this morphology may also be associated with atypical absence attacks with or without minor tonic features. Calibration signal 1 sec, 50µV.

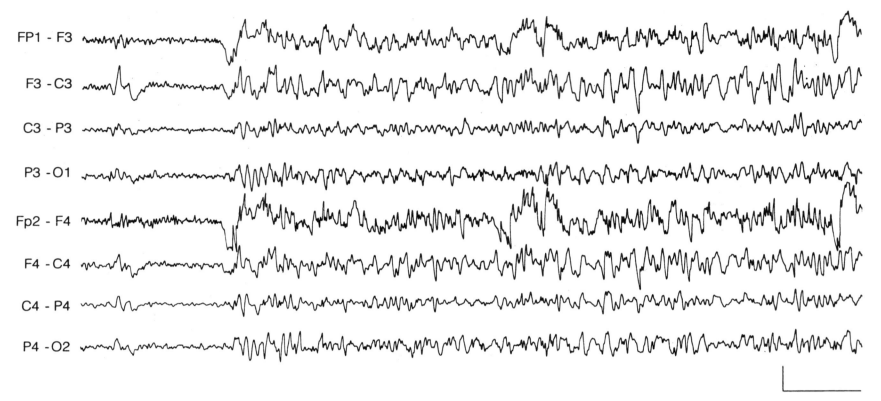

FIG. 6–35. Seizure as generalized paroxysmal fast activity (generalized polyspikes) and theta. 43 years. After a non-specific theta burst, sustained 15 Hz diffuse waves appear, maximum anteriorly, with intermingled 5 Hz semi-rhythmic waves *(left)*. As consciousness was only partially lost during this attack, the patient experienced light headedness in association with this discharge. Other, often bizarre, symptoms may accompany such diffusely appearing epileptic discharges (44). Calibration signal 1 sec, 100μV. Seven seconds later, the absence attack continues *(right)*. The 15 Hz rhythmic waves with intermingled 3–4 Hz waves and spike-waves continue, then end abruptly and synchronously. This discharge is identical to the epileptic recruiting rhythm of Gastaut (33). Calibration signal 1 sec, 100μV.

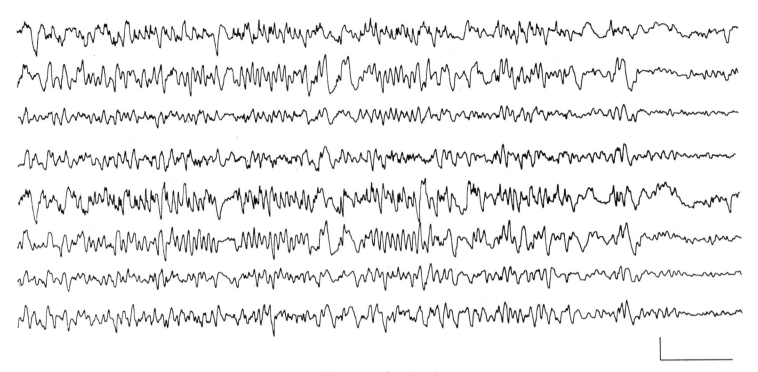

FIG. 6–35. *Continued.*

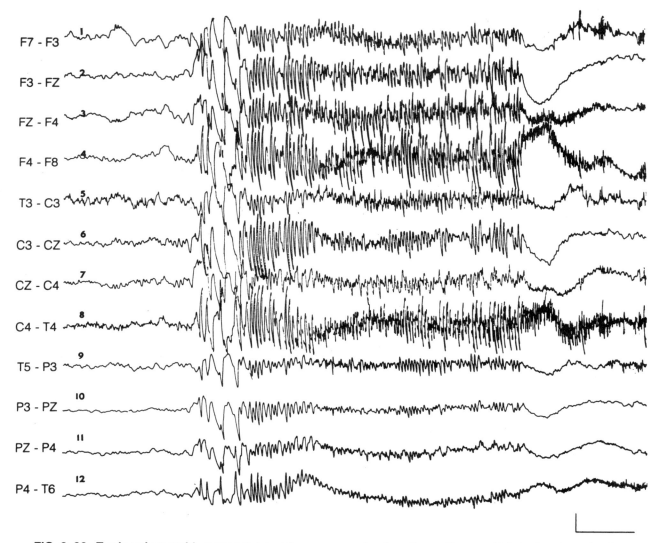

FIG. 6–36. Tonic seizure with generalized spike-waves and polyspikes. 46 years. This tonic seizure begins diffusely as 4–7 Hz spike-waves followed by 15 Hz generalized polyspikes, also termed "generalized paroxysmal fast activity" (31). During this attack the patient's eyes deviated rightward, the trunk flexed, both arms stiffened symmetrically, and the right leg stiffened. Lateralizing features of tonic seizures occur commonly, even when the epileptic discharge is diffuse and symmetrical as in this instance. The tonic muscle artifact extends beyond the end of the EEG-recorded seizure. Calibration signal 1 sec, 70μV.

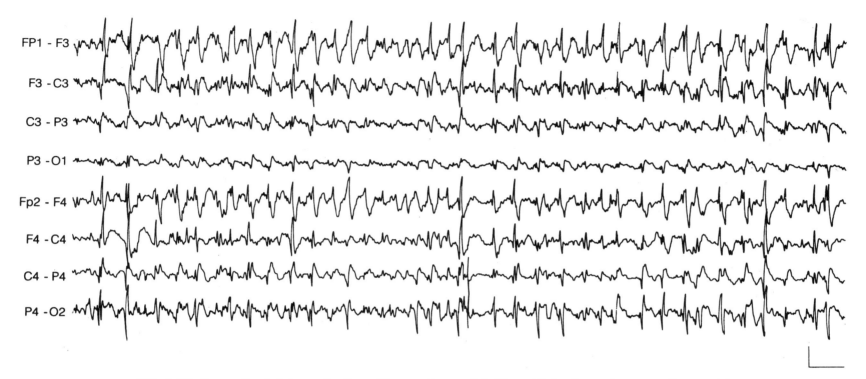

FIG. 6–37. Generalized status epilepticus. 29 years. Sequential, diffuse, bilaterally synchronous spikes persist in this patient in whom the peripheral manifestations of this status epilepticus were abolished by curare and light anaesthesia. Note slow paper speed. Calibration signal 1 sec, 50μV.

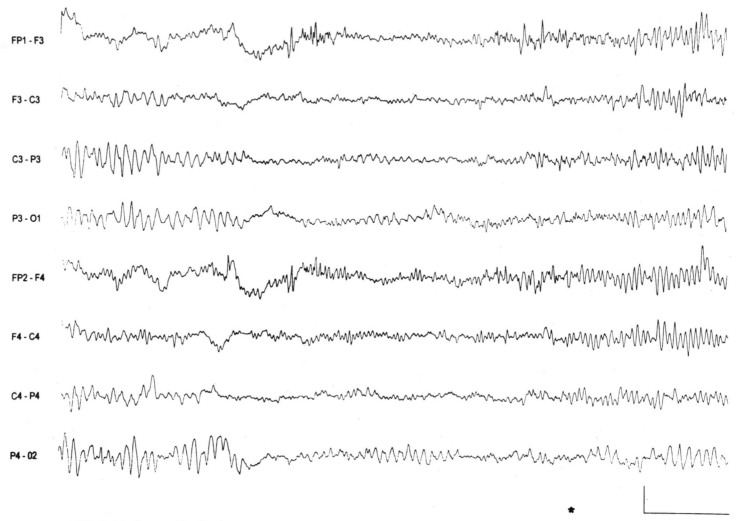

FIG. 6–38. Generalized seizure with possible regional onset. 14 years. The first 2 seconds depict the interictal recording with generally symmetrical 9 Hz background activity. The 15–20 Hz beta activity is higher in the right frontal region as compared to the left. The first clear modification is a diffuse attenuation in the 3rd second with slightly more prominent right frontal-predominant beta activity which has quickened slightly to about 22 Hz. Whether this is sufficiently distinct from the ongoing beta activity to constitute a regional onset of a diffuse seizure is unclear. Four seconds later *(asterisk)*, 15 Hz epileptic recruiting rhythm appears diffusely but more on the right frontal central region than elsewhere for 1 second before becoming diffuse and occasionally maximum in the left hemisphere *(right)*. The "epileptic recruiting rhythm" continues for 4 seconds in this segment, being more prominent in the left hemisphere as compared to the right. This activity is partially replaced by 9–12 Hz semi-rhythmic waves diffusely for about 2 seconds. Sequential spike-waves and myoclonic muscle artifact dominate the remainder of this segment. Calibration signal 1 sec, 100μV.

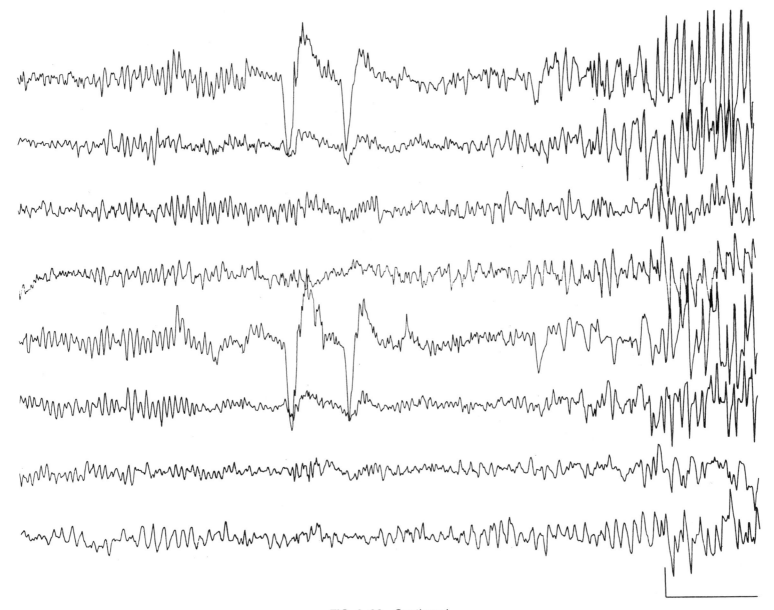

FIG. 6–38. *Continued.*

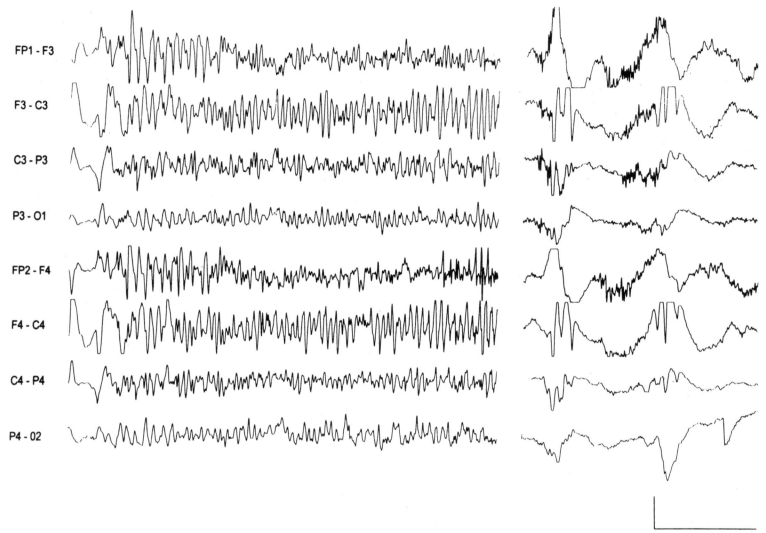

FIG. 6–39. Generalized tonic-clonic seizure with diffuse polyspikes (epileptic recruiting rhythm). 30 years. From sleep, 1–2 V-waves occur followed by diffuse, bilaterally synchronous, 20–30 Hz sequential spikes constituting the "epileptic recruiting rhythm" lasting 5–6 seconds before becoming interrupted by delta activity. Generalized tonic seizure accompanied the sequential polyspikes, followed by synchronous clonus during the polyspike-wave phase (not fully shown). Calibration signal 1 sec, 100μV.

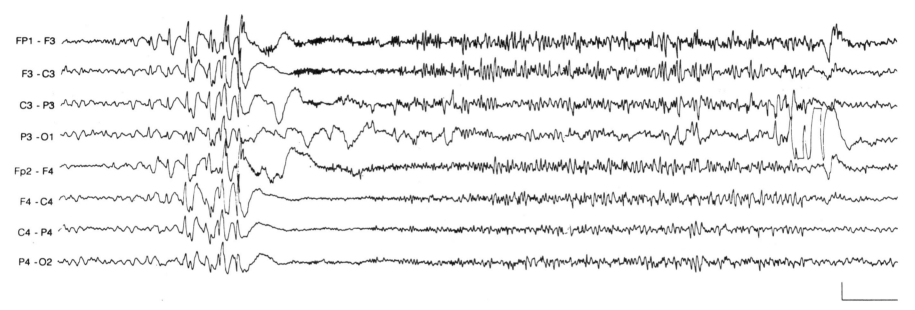

FIG. 6–40. Diffuse, principally left hemisphere seizure of multiple morphologies. 29 years. Diffuse epileptiform potentials in the form of polyspike-waves, then attenuation, and then paroxysmal fast activity dominate this picture. Note artifacts at 01, P3. Calibration signal 1 sec, 70μV.

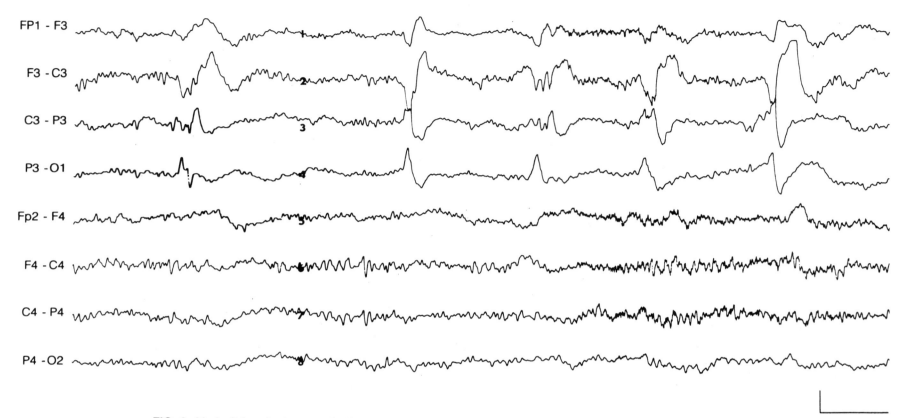

FIG. 6–41. Left hemisphere periodic lateralized epileptiform discharges (PLEDs). 40 years. These repetitive left central parietal (C3, P3) broad spikes recur with only mild variations in interburst interval and arise from an attenuated background with delta. Discharges of PLEDs may be biphasic (as occurs here), triphasic, or even polyphasic. Evidence, even minimal, of focal motor status epilepticus (epilepsia partialis continua) should be sought in limbs contralateral to such prominent PLEDs. The contralateral (right) delta activity is likely propagated from the left as the background is minimally disrupted. Recording situations of patients with PLEDs are often fraught with movement-related or sweat-related artifact. Calibration signal 1 sec, 70μV.

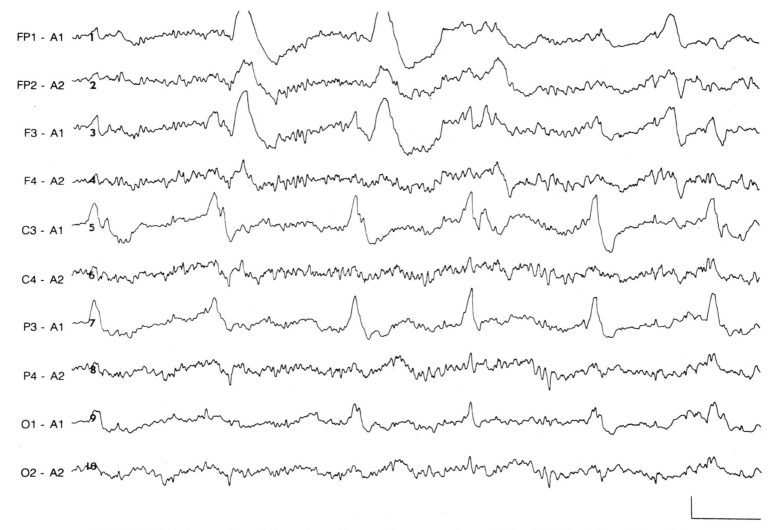

FIG. 6–42. PLEDs on referential montage. 40 years. Same recording as in Fig. 6-41. The left central-parietal (C3, P3) PLEDs together with left hemisphere background attenuation and delta are again evident. That the reference (A1) is not significantly involved by these periodic discharges is seen by their considerably lower voltage at O1-A1 and their virtual absence at Fp1-A1. The sporadically appearing bifrontal (Fp1, F3, Fp2) delta waves are "projected" activity and not PLEDs. Acute processes underlie each of these phenomena more commonly than chronic ones, but exceptions occur (22). Calibration signal 1 sec, 70μV.

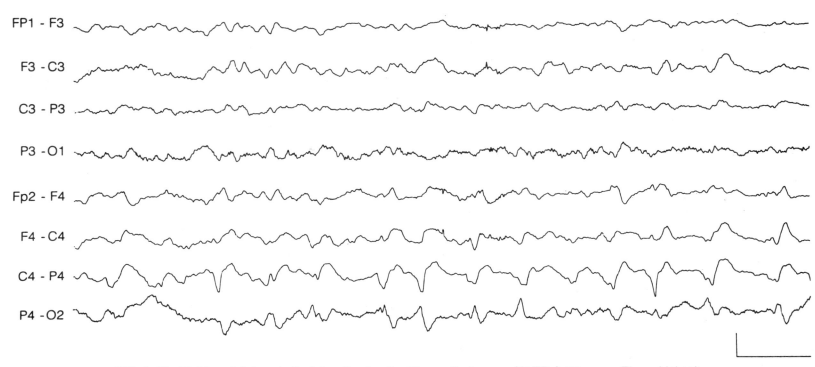

FIG. 6–43. Right parietal periodic lateralized epileptiform discharges (PLEDs). 75 years. These biphasic, principally negative right parietal (P4) spikes spread moderately to the right occipital (O2) region. The diffuse delta activity is accentuated in the right hemisphere while the more sustained and higher frequency background activity appears principally in the left hemisphere. Calibration signal 1 sec, 70μV.

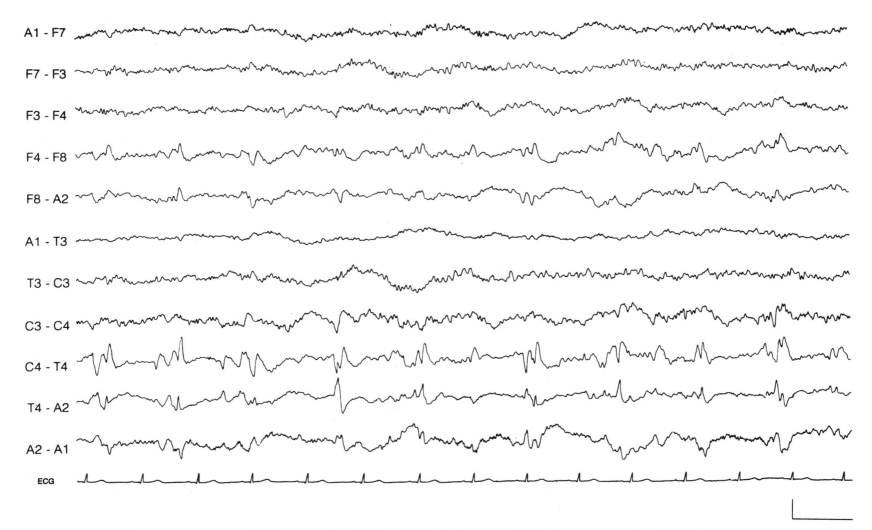

FIG. 6–44. Right temporal PLEDs. 81 years. These polyphasic PLEDs are clearly depicted by this coronal montage along with the right hemisphere delta activity. Both the periodicity and the delta activity represent a physiologically evolving process such as a postictal condition, a cerebral viral infection or a recent stroke. Calibration signal 1 sec, 70μV.

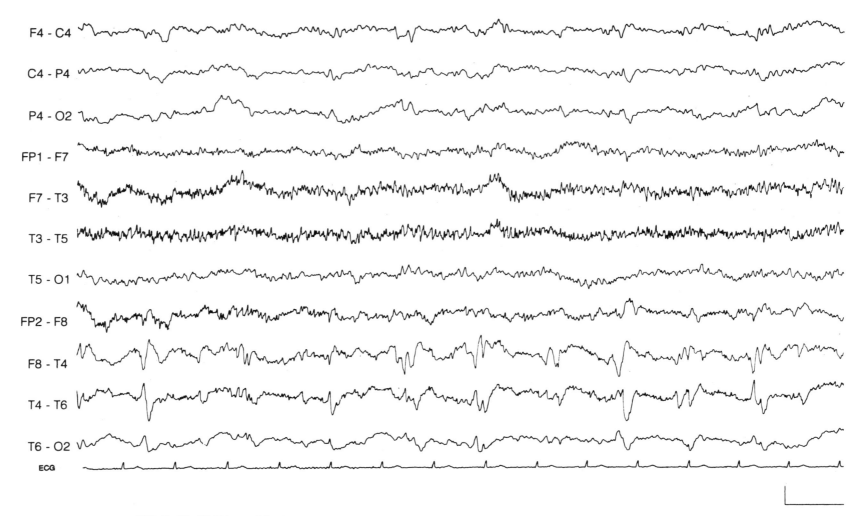

FIG. 6–45. PLEDs on bipolar anterior-posterior montage. 81 years. Same recording as in Fig. 6–44. Polyphasic PLEDs in the right midtemporal (T4) region with some posterior and suprasylvian spread. Right hemisphere delta activity is low frequency and persistent. The left temporal delta may be artefactual in this acutely ill patient. Calibration signal 1 sec, 50μV.

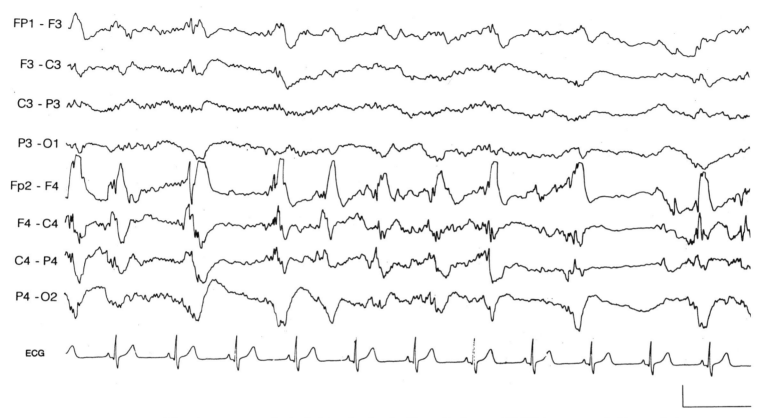

FIG. 6–46. PLEDs plus. 76 years. Periodic lateralized epileptiform discharges (PLEDs) accompanied (preceded or followed) by low voltage high frequency rhythms constitute "PLEDs plus" which is associated with a high likelihood of a seizure occurring within the next 15–30 minutes of recording (45). This activity is accompanied by diffuse delta, more prominent in the right hemisphere, the side of the "PLEDS plus". Note the diffuse right hemisphere electrodecremental events. Calibration signal 1 sec, 50μV.

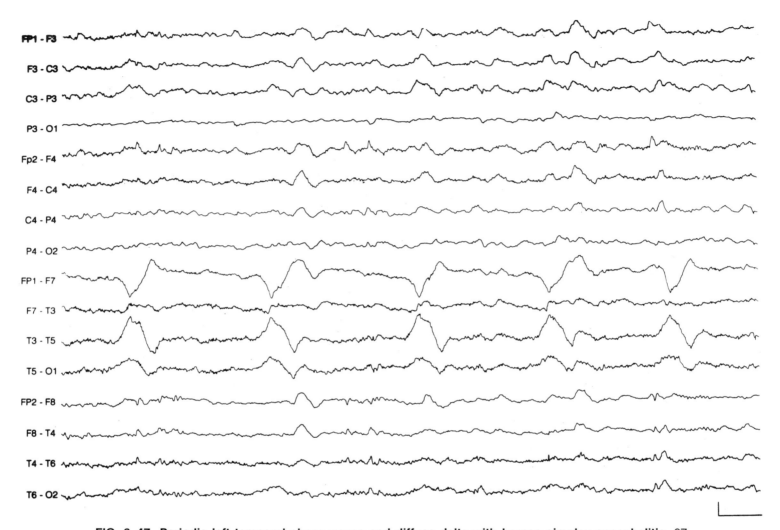

FIG. 6–47. Periodic left temporal sharp waves and diffuse delta with herpes simplex encephalitis. 67 years. Regularly repetitive sharply contoured diphasic delta waves appear over the left anterior-midtemporal (F7, T3) area in association with left temporally accentuated diffuse continuous delta. This combination of EEG features, in association with an encephalitic-like clinical picture, suggests herpes simplex as its cause—as was the case here. Note the sporadically appearing low voltage right temporal (F8, T4) spikes. Calibration signal 1 sec, 50μV.

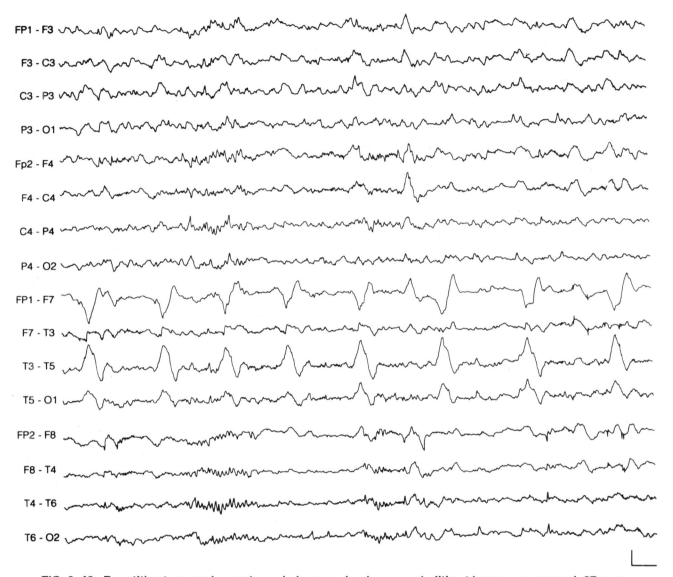

FIG. 6–48. Repetitive temporal complexes in herpes simplex encephalitis at lower paper speed. 67 years. The regular repetition of these stereotyped left anterior-midtemporal (F7-T3) diphasic sharply contoured delta waves is even more evident at 15 mm/sec paper speed. Diffuse delta activity is accentuated in the left temporal region and left hemisphere. Bursts of spindle-like alphoid activity are lower in the left hemisphere as compared to right. EEG abnormalities with herpes encephalitis eventually become bilateral in most cases, in our experience. Calibration signal 1 sec, 50μV.

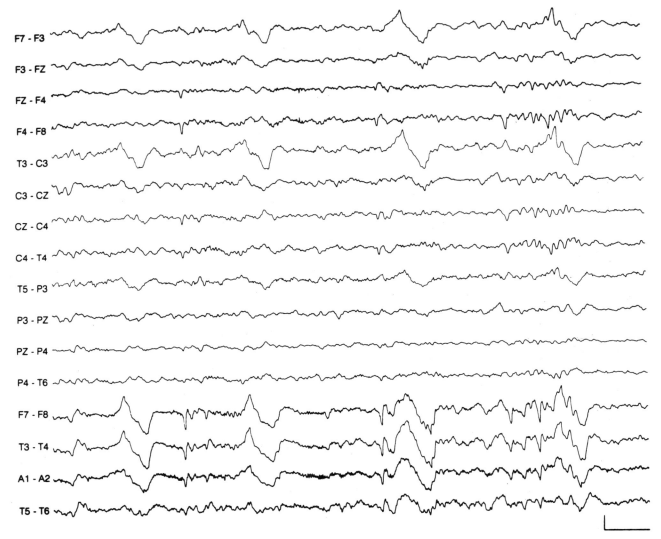

FIG. 6–49. Periodic complexes in herpes simplex encephalitis on a coronal montage. 67 years. The temporal location (F7, T3) of these repetitive discharges is clear on this coronal montage. Note the slightly variable morphology. The essential features are the sharply contoured delta waves, their regular repetition rate, and the diffuse delta activity which is accentuated in the hemisphere of the repetitive complexes. Note the right temporal (F8, T4, A2) spikes, evidence that the process is bitemporal. Calibration signal 1 sec, 50 μV.

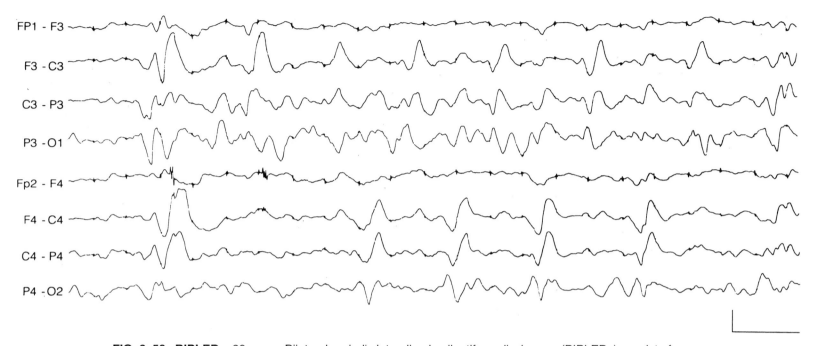

FIG. 6–50. BIPLEDs. 66 years. Bilateral periodic lateralized epileptiform discharges (BIPLEDs) consist of asynchronously and independently occurring complexes in each hemisphere which differ in morphology, rate, and site of maximal involvement. BIPLEDs may be produced by anoxic encephalopathy or encephalitis and are commonly associated with coma (46;47). Note the faster repetition rate in the left hemisphere which also has the higher voltage and more sustained background activity. This tracing would therefore indicate severe bihemispheric abnormalities, principally right. Transformer artifact at Fp1,2. Calibration signal 1 sec, 50μV.

Chapter 7

Nonepileptiform Abnormalities

Abnormal Alpha Symmetry (Figs. 1–4, 6–8)
- Lower side < 50% higher side.
- Persistent throughout recording.
- Assessed on ipsilateral ear or common average referential montages.
- Scrutinize for frequency asymmetry—lower is abnormal side.
- Scrutinize for reactivity asymmetry—less reactive is abnormal side.

Mu and Beta Asymmetries (Figs. 5, 9–12)
- Mu asymmetry indicates dysfunction of the lower side, if: no skull defect, persistent, and associated beta reduction.
- Persistent beta asymmetry *usually* indicates dysfunction of lower side.

Regional Attenuation (Figs. 13–22, 25–28)
- Overlies the center of dysfunction or lesion.
- Better localizing feature than associated delta.
- Represents more severe dysfunction than regional delta.
- Often inapparent on scalp EEG.
- More difficult to assess in areas whose normal rhythms are low-voltage, i.e., frontally.

Asymmetrical Sleep Spindles (Figs. 23, 24)
- Distinguish persistent (abnormal) from shifting (normal) asymmetry.
- < 50% lower indicates ipsilateral dysfunction of thalamocortical pathway.

Skull Defect Effects: Breach Rhythm (Figs. 29–36)
- Accentuates beta and theta rhythms in central, parietal, and frontal regions.
- Central rhythms attenuate to extremity movement, like mu.
- Steeply sloped field, thus accentuated on bipolar montages.
- Apiculate negative phases of waves.
- Alpha amplitude enhanced if defect posterior.

Regional Delta Activity (Figs. 20, 32, 36–40, 42–61, 63–76, 78–81, 83–85, 93, 94)
- Arrhythmic 0.5 to 3 Hz waves.
- Near lesion slowest, least reactive, no superimposed faster frequency.
- Variable persistence, greater with acute lesion.
- Posterior delta more attenuated with eye opening than anterior delta.
- Almost always with abnormal background rhythms in same region—attenuation or excess theta. If not, suspect artifact.
- Posterior delta disrupts alpha more so than does anterior delta.
- May appear only in drowsiness, light sleep, or with hyperventilation.

Bi-occipital Delta (Fig. 52)
- Postictal effect of generalized tonic-clonic seizure.
- Alpha preserved or minimally slowed.

Intermittent Rhythmic Delta Activity (IRDA) (Figs. 28, 59, 77–79, 81–85)
- Rhythmic 1–3 Hz delta.
- Bursts or brief runs.
- Widely distributed.
- Usually anterior maximum.
- Appears with diffuse encephalopathies, including postictal states.
- Not localizing but more common with anterior lesions than posterior ones.
- Regional or focal delta may coexist.

Focal and Regional Theta (Figs. 33, 39, 40, 41, 47, 72, 86–95)
- Persistently lateralized to one hemisphere or localized to one region to indicate regional dysfunction.
- Disrupts background less than regional delta.
- May not react to eye opening or alerting.
- May appear only in repose and drowsiness.

Slow Background and Diffuse Theta (Figs. 96–98)

- Exclude drowsiness as cause.
- 7–8 Hz posterior rhythm.
- Diffuse theta increases.
- Slight accentuation of theta in left temporal region occurs commonly with diffuse increase; does not imply focal lesion.
- Medication, metabolic abnormality most common causes.
- Often with diffuse excess beta-medication effect.

Medication Effect (Beta) (Figs. 99–101)

- Benzodiazepines and barbiturates.
- Combines with background to produce apiculate forms.

Diffuse and Bilateral Arrhythmic Delta (Figs. 102–112, 114)

- Continuous arrhythmic 0.5–3 Hz diffuse waves.
- Theta replaces alpha as highest-frequency background rhythm.
- Severity inversely proportional to: delta frequency, reactivity to afferent stimuli, and background frequency.
- Severity and/or acuteness directly proportional to persistence.

Triphasic Waves and Diffuse Delta (Fig. 106)

- Metabolic encephalopathy.
- Dementia.

Dementia (Figs. 107–114)

- Diffuse delta.
- Spikes: multifocal, bisynchronous, periodic or aperiodic.
- Triphasic waves.
- Rapidity of cognitive decline correlates with prominence of EEG abnormalities.

FIG. 7–1. Abnormal asymmetry of background potentials. 76 years. A left thalamic infarct has almost abolished the left-side 9 Hz alpha activity, creating an asymmetry which clearly exceeds the usual 50% rule: an asymmetry in which the lower-side voltage is < 50% of the higher-side voltage indicates an abnormality on one side, usually the lower. Note that the alpha activity as recorded at P3-O1 and P4-O2 derivations is nearly symmetrical in certain portions of this tracing, but that the more anterior expression of the alpha rhythm is always lower on the left. This finding suggests that the degree of asymmetry may vary within the alpha field and that reasonable stretches of the recording should be examined in assessing asymmetry. The near symmetry of alpha activity at derivations T5-O1 and T6-O2 may be produced by a lack of alpha on the left and a cancellation of potentials within the alpha field on the right. A referential recording (Fig. 7–2) examines this further. Calibration signal 1 sec, 50μV.

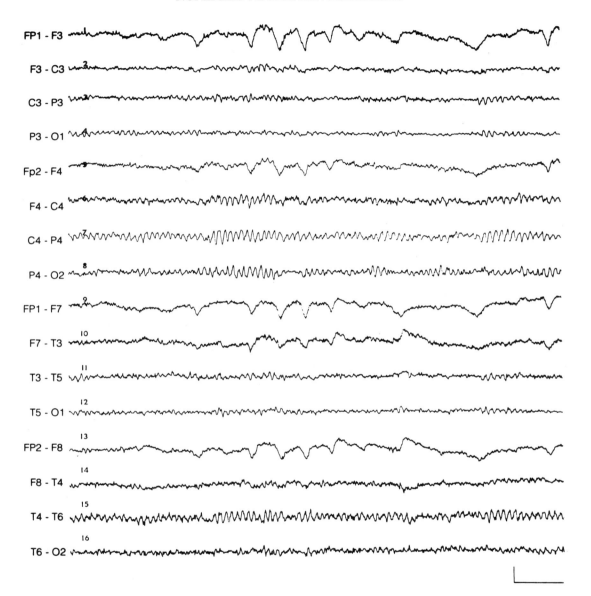

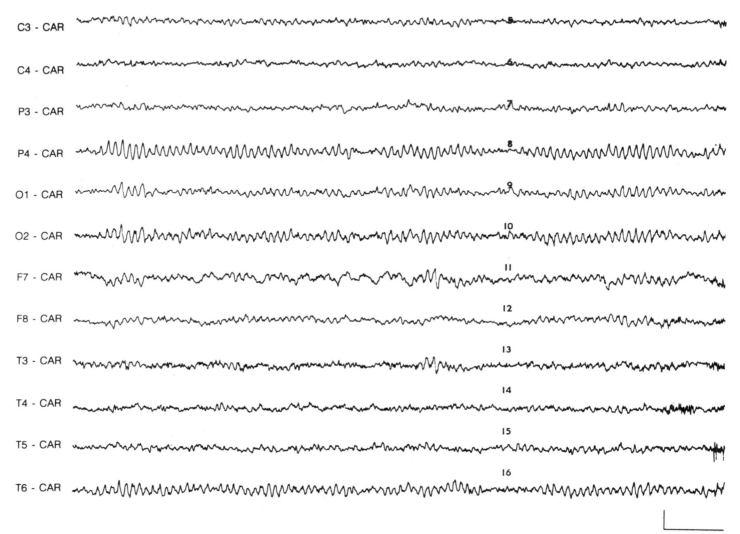

FIG. 7–2. Common average reference depicts asymmetry of alpha field. 76 years. Although the slightly lower alpha at O1, compared to O2, is within normal limits, there is marked alpha reduction in the left parietal (P3) and left posterior temporal (T5) regions compared to the right (P4, T6). Left thalamic infarct. Left inferior frontal (F7) delta also appears. Calibration signal 1 sec, 50μV.

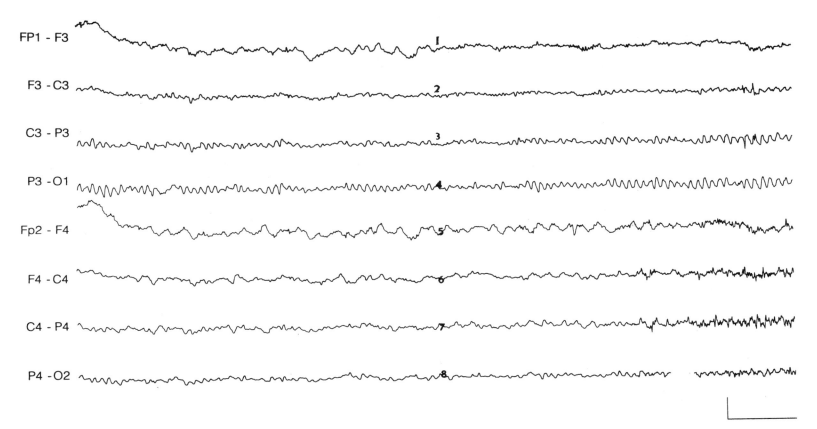

FIG. 7–3. Reduction of alpha activity in right hemisphere. 34 years. The first clue to other abnormalities in a hemisphere may be a reduction of its alpha activity, reflecting occipital lobe or thalamic dysfunction. In addition to the loss of alpha activity, note the 5 Hz theta activity in the right frontal-central regions. Time constant 0.12 seconds. Calibration signal 1 sec, 50µV.

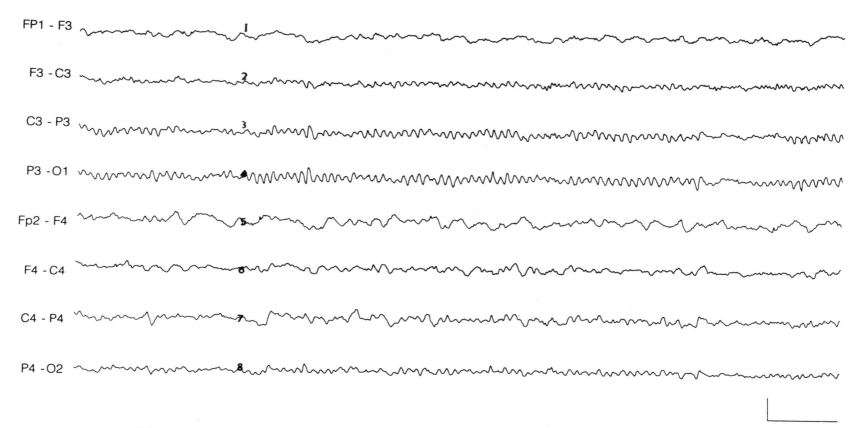

FIG. 7–4. Reduction of alpha activity in right hemisphere; effect of time constant on anterior abnormalities. 34 years. Same recording as in Fig. 7–3 at a longer (0.4 seconds) time constant. Right frontal-central delta activity becomes apparent. Calibration signal 1 sec, 50μV.

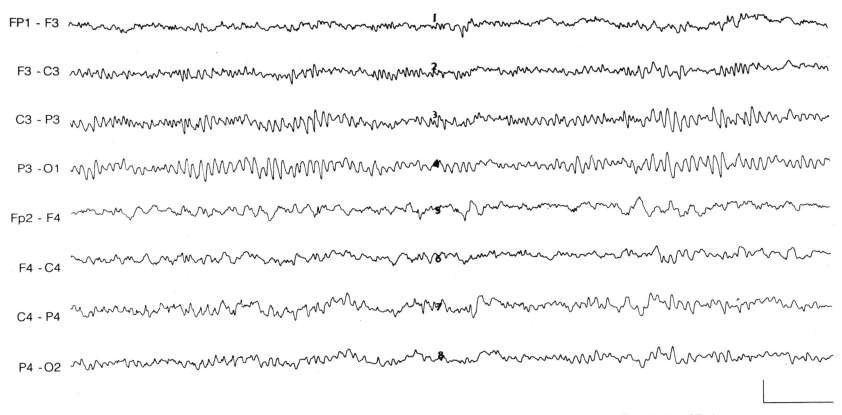

FIG. 7–5. Increasing sensitivity reveals beta asymmetry. 34 years. Same recording as in Figs. 7–3 and 7–4. Increasing the sensitivity to 30 μV/10mm more prominently displays the alpha asymmetry and also reveals a small beta asymmetry (minimally evident in Figs. 7–3 and 7–4). These findings indicate a widespread right hemisphere abnormality: alpha reduction representing posterior or thalamic dysfunction and beta reduction with excess delta and theta activity representing central and anterior dysfunction. Calibration signal 1 sec, 30μV.

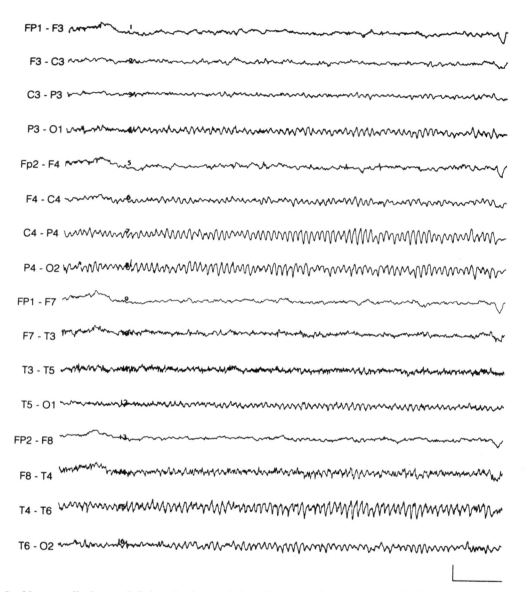

FIG. 7–6. Abnormally lower left hemisphere alpha. 18 years. Acknowledging that alpha activity is usually higher in the right hemisphere in most normal subjects, this left hemisphere alpha is abnormally low; its amplitude rarely attains 50% of the rightside activity. However, a closer side-to-side approximation appears between derivations involving the occipital leads (P3-O1 vs. P4-O2 and T5-O1 vs. T6-O2) because the widespread right alpha field causes partial cancellation of alpha among the right posterior temporal, parietal, and occipital regions on this bipolar montage. Note the considerably less anterior spread of the alpha field in the left hemisphere compared to the right hemisphere. Calibration signal 1 sec, 50μV.

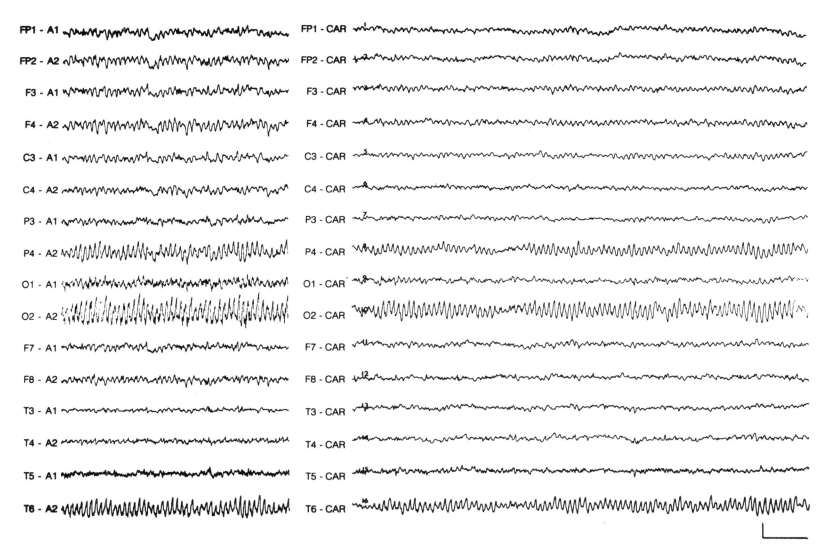

FIG. 7–7. Referential recordings depict asymmetry of alpha field. 18 years. Same patient as in Fig. 7–6. The ear reference montage (*left*) illustrates the prominent reduction of alpha at O1, P3, and T5 compared to homologous positions on the right. The slightly lower potentials in the derivations including frontal leads (channels 1–4, 11, 12) likely reflect greater recording of the alpha field by the right ear (A2) than the left ear (A1) reference. Common average reference (CAR) (*right*) reliably demonstrates the marked reduction in leftside alpha. The symmetrical alpha range potentials in the channels containing anterior leads reflect slight CAR involvement by alpha. Calibration signal 1 sec, 50μV.

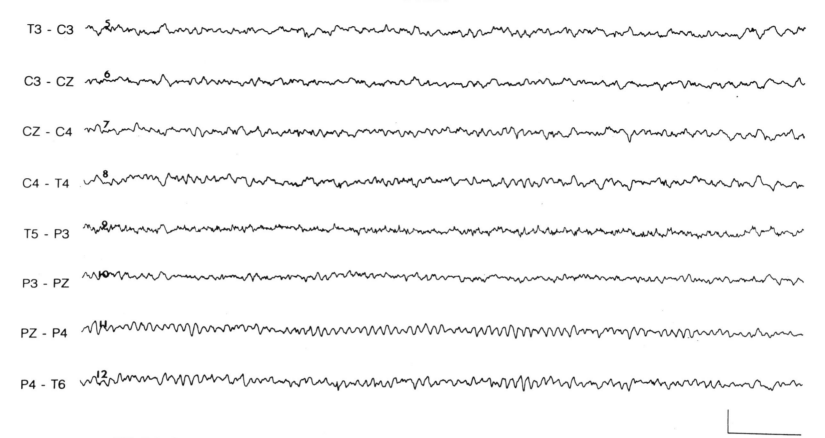

FIG. 7–8. Alpha asymmetry with a coronal montage. 18 years. Coronal montages usually depict background asymmetries less well than do anterior-posterior bipolar and referential montages. However, the confinement of the asymmetry to the posterior head regions is shown here and in Fig. 7–9. Note the reduction of alpha activity in the left posterior temporal parietal derivations (T5-P3, P3-Pz) compared to those on the right, whereas only a minimal background asymmetry for higher frequencies, reduced left, appears in the central leads. Involvement of both P4 and T6 by the alpha field causes some cancellation in this (P4-T6) derivation. Calibration signal 1 sec, 50μV.

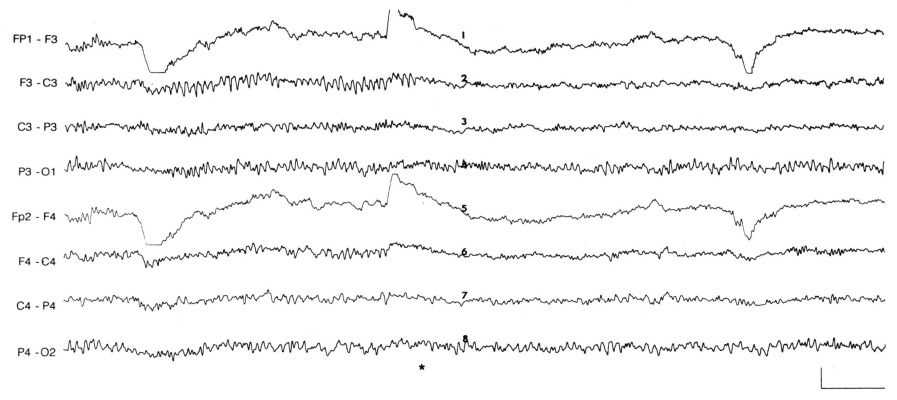

FIG. 7–9. Asymmetrical mu rhythm. 11 years. Mu rhythm, an arciform phenomenon close to alpha in frequency, may shift in prominence from side to side. In some instances, the asymmetry may be consistent without suggesting underlying dysfunction on either side. Wiggling the right thumb (*asterisk*) attenuated the asymmetrical mu rhythm (higher left) bilaterally, leaving a virtually symmetrical central rhythm, suggesting that the mu asymmetry does not reflect a central abnormality. Calibration signal 1 sec, 70μV.

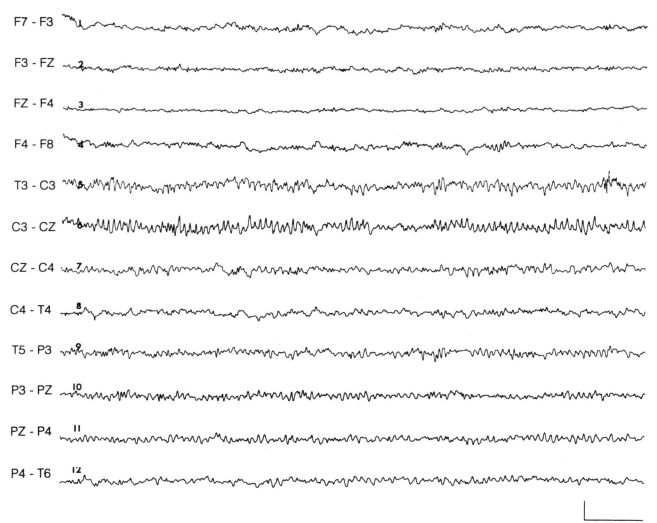

FIG. 7–10. Abnormal mu asymmetry on coronal montage. 11 years. Compare this tracing to those depicting alpha asymmetry on a coronal montage. The asymmetry in this instance appears principally in central derivations (*lower right*), although it appears minimally in the parietal portion of this montage. Because of within-field cancellation effects on bipolar montages (for example, Fz-F4), a referential montage (*next illustration*) more reliably assesses an asymmetry. Calibration signal 1 sec, 70μV.

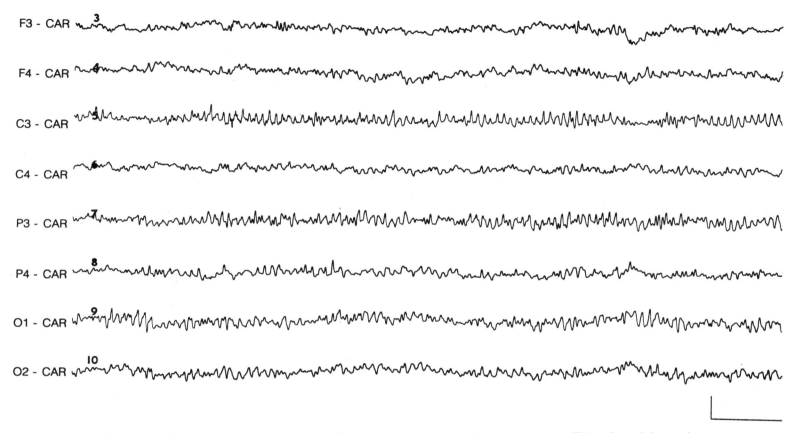

FIG. 7–11. Abnormal mu asymmetry and the common average reference. 11 years. This referential recording illustrates the marked reduction in mu rhythm in the right central-parietal (C4, P4) leads compared to left. The associated beta reduction suggests that the mu asymmetry reflects right central dysfunction, but these asymmetries would have to persist throughout the awake recording to establish significance. Calibration signal 1 sec, 70μV.

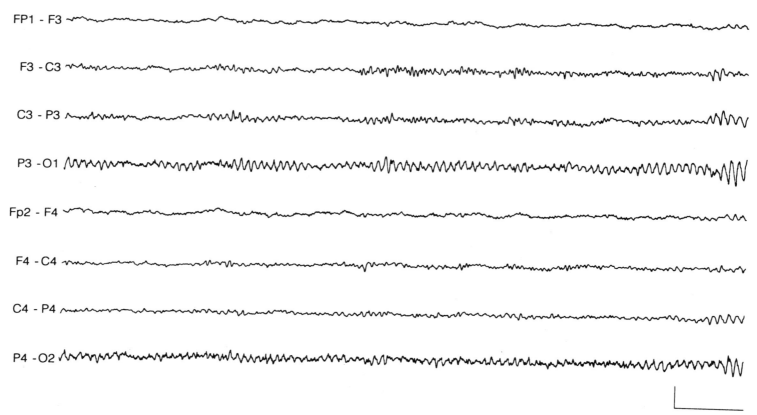

FP1 - F3

F3 - C3

C3 - P3

P3 - O1

Fp2 - F4

F4 - C4

C4 - P4

P4 - O2

FIG. 7–12. Beta asymmetry. 71 years. In addition to a mild alpha asymmetry (*lower right*), the beta activity is moderately less abundant on the right compared to left. The assessment should include an ear reference montage to exclude cancellation effects. As beta may be up to 35% lower on one side in normal subjects (48), a beta asymmetry should be at least moderate and persistent before it is given clinical significance. This patient had a previous right hemisphere stroke. Calibration signal 1 sec, 50μV.

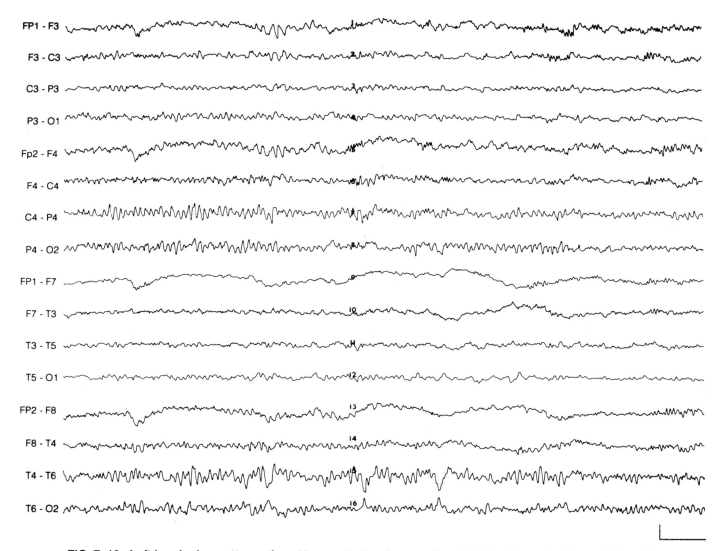

FIG. 7–13. Left hemisphere attenuation. 18 years. In the absence of a skull defect (none in this case), the side of lower alpha activity is usually the abnormal one. In youth, such alpha attenuation will also include posterior slow of youth, which could give a falsely lateralizing impression of a right posterior slow wave abnormality. Note that the beta activity and frontal theta activity are the least attenuated of the left hemisphere components. Therefore, the attenuation involves principally the left occipital, parietal, and temporal regions. Calibration signal 1 sec, 40 μV.

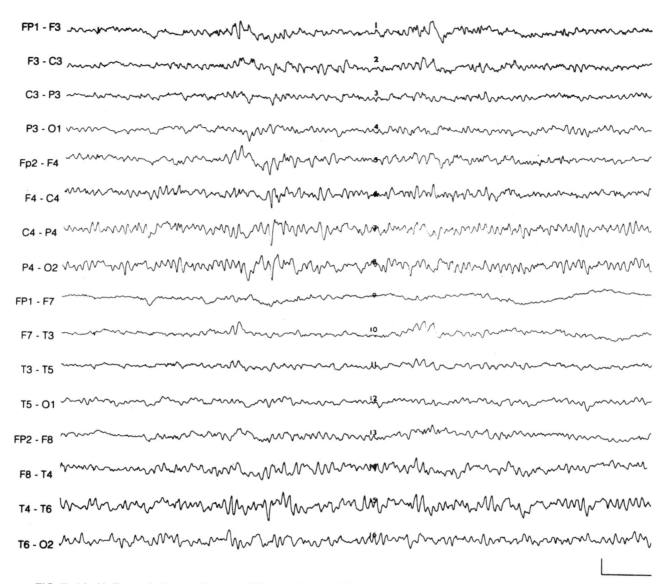

FIG. 7–14. Unilateral attenuation and diffuse abnormalities. 19 years. Same patient as in Fig. 7–13, one year later. Attenuation of alpha and other wave forms on the left indicate that the principal abnormality resides on that side. Any process such as metabolic derangements which normally would have produced bilaterally symmetrical and diffuse abnormalities will also be attenuated on the abnormal (left) side and therefore appear principally in the healthier (right) hemisphere. Thus, posterior delta and diffuse theta appear principally over the healthier right hemisphere, and bilateral abnormalities, principally left, are depicted. Calibration signal 1 sec, 70μV.

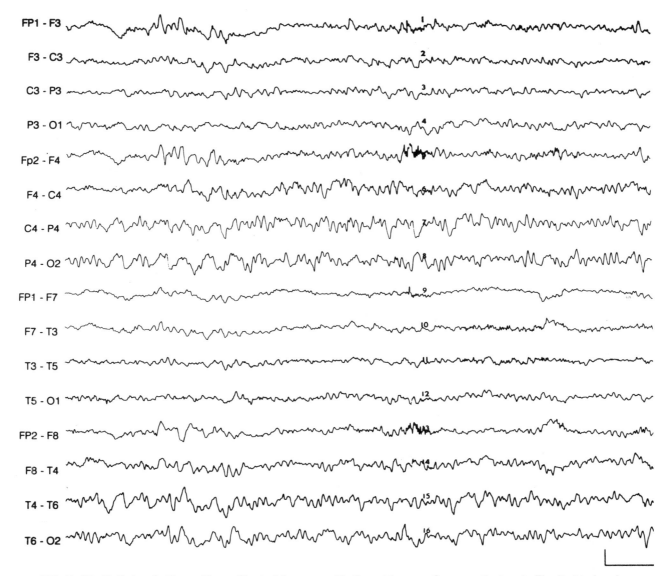

FIG. 7–15. Unilateral attenuation: effect of hyperventilation. 19 years. Same patient as in Fig. 7–14 showing that the hyperventilation "build-up" will also appear principally in the healthier (right) hemisphere: delta and theta augment on right. Calibration signal 1 sec, 70μV.

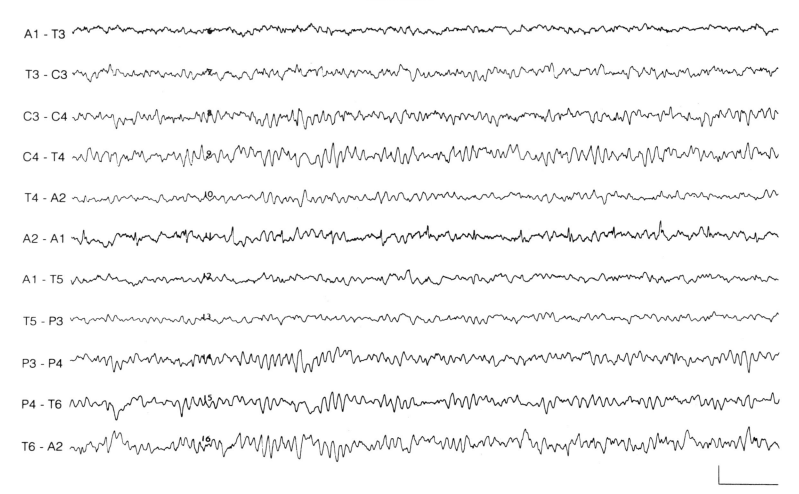

FIG. 7–16. Attenuation on a coronal montage. 19 years. Same patient as in Figs. 7–14 and 7–15. Coronal montages can occasionally demonstrate the anterior-posterior extent of attenuation, particularly when the side of abnormality has been determined by other montages. Note the greater attenuation at positions A1, T5, P3, and T3, with less attenuation at C3. In assessing the distribution of attenuation, compare homologous bipolar derivations. Any derivation with lower activity indicates that both positions of the derivation are attenuated; for example, both P3 and T5 are attenuated. Cancellation effects will have been largely excluded by anterior-posterior bipolar and referential montages. Evidence of anterior attenuation is often less than that posteriorly because of the relative paucity of activity anteriorly (not shown). Note the low amplitude 1–2 Hz activity which is normally present in healthy hemispheres and is seen therefore more on the right side compared to left. ECG artifact in A2-A1 derivation. Calibration signal 1 sec, 50μV.

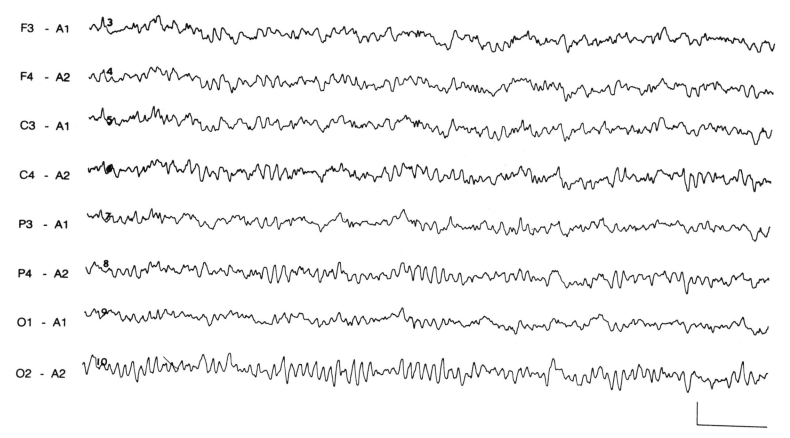

FIG. 7–17. Attenuation on referential montage. 19 years. Same patient as in Figs. 7–14 to 7–16. An ear referential montage may clearly depict attenuation, providing that the quantity of activity at each ear reference (A1, A2) is approximately the same. In this instance, one sees a more prominent attenuation at P3 and O1 than elsewhere. Note again the small amount of delta activity, which normally appears in both hemispheres in youth and is slightly more evident on referential montages. Delta on the left posteriorly appears more prominent but it may have been revealed by the lack of ongoing alpha and other background activity. Calibration signal 1 sec, 70μV.

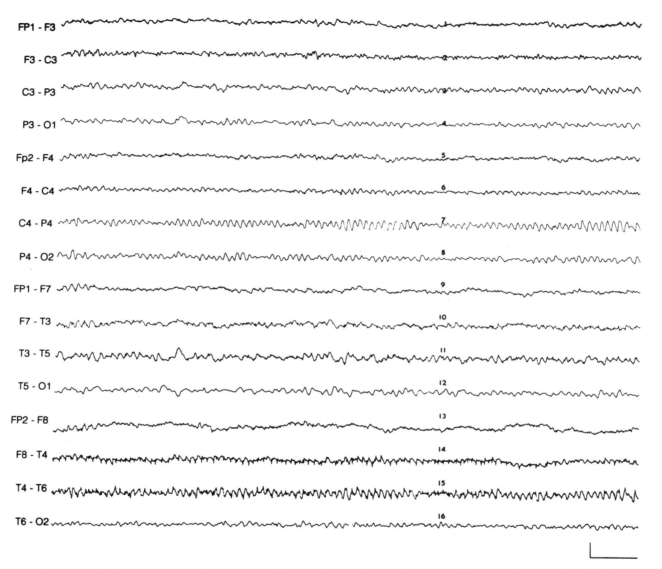

FIG. 7–18. Mild focal abnormality. 49 years. The 4–7 Hz semirhythmic theta activity is easily appreciated in the left posterior temporal region with moderate involvement of the left occipital region, using the T3-T5 and T5-O1 derivations. As with other posteriorly situated abnormalities, the 7 Hz background activity is markedly diminished in the left hemisphere. When an easily recognizable abnormality appears in one portion of a tracing, seek its minimal presence elsewhere to sharpen your detection ability. Therefore, the teaching value of this tracing lies principally in the C3-P3 and P3-O1 derivations; compare these with the homologous ones of the right. Calibration signal 1 sec, 50μV.

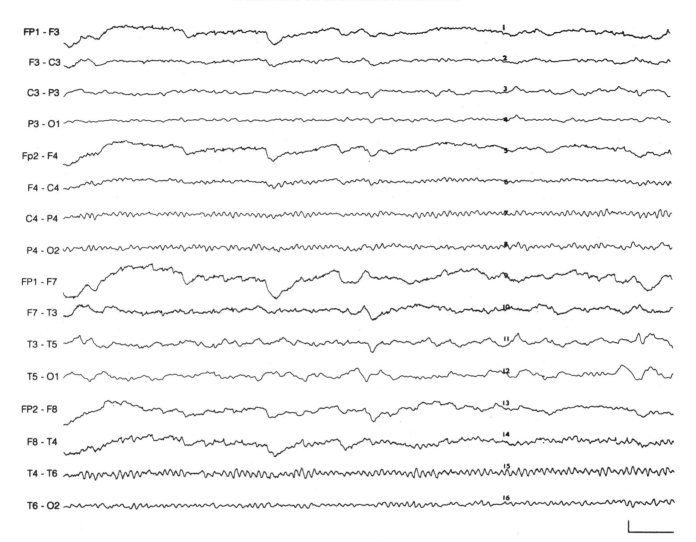

FIG. 7–19. Left hemisphere attenuation and delta. 48 years. Even though the left temporal delta activity is the most prominent abnormality, the diffuse attenuation of higher-frequency background rhythms in the left hemisphere is the more significant one and indicates the widespread nature of the left hemisphere dysfunction, extending beyond the left temporal area. The very-low-amplitude apiculate frontal polar (Fp1, Fp2) potentials likely emanate from periocular muscles, but bifrontal spikes rarely have the same morphology. This possibility should be sought by use of an anterior coronal montage, greater sensitivity, and a shorter time constant. Calibration signal 1 sec, 50μV.

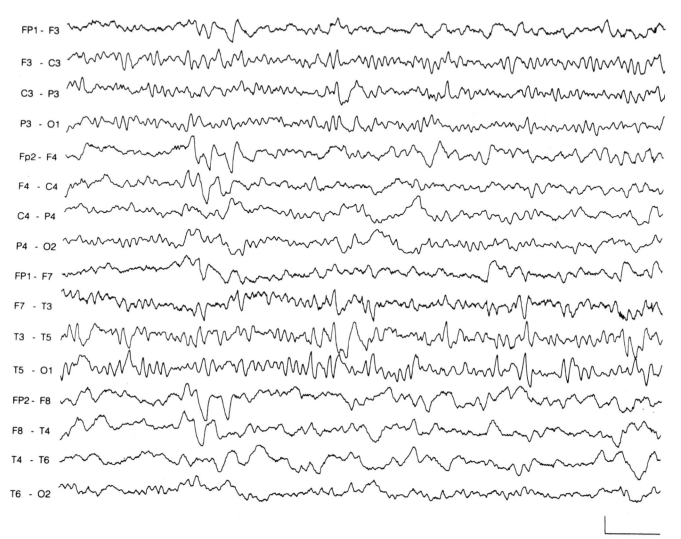

FIG. 7–20. Unilateral attenuation and delta. 17 years. Although there is clear evidence of right hemisphere delta activity, the major finding is an attenuation of occipital and central rhythms on the right compared to left. However, frontal rhythms (compare Fp1-F3 derivation with Fp2-F4) are symmetrical, and the single intermittent rhythmic delta activity (IRDA) burst appears principally in the right and anteriorly. Calibration signal 1 sec, 70μV.

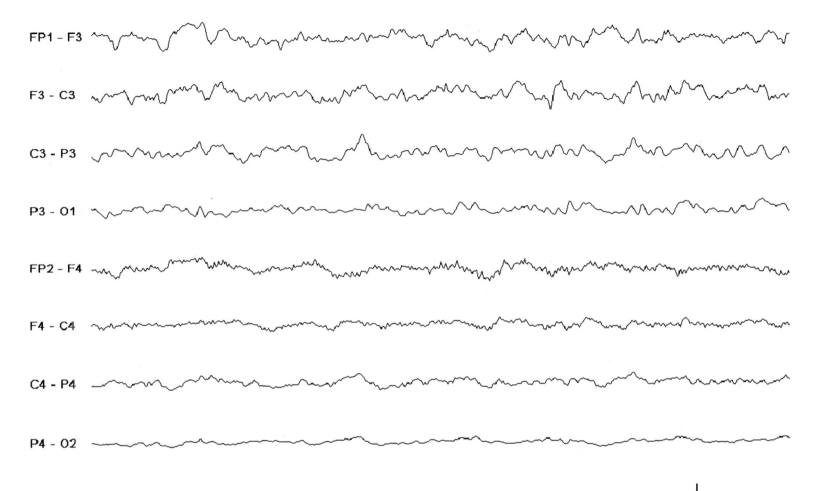

FIG. 7–21. More delta in healthier hemisphere. The principal abnormality is a reduction in potentials in the right hemisphere which "allows" an abnormal delta activity to be better expressed on the healthier left. Calibration signal 1 sec, 50μV.

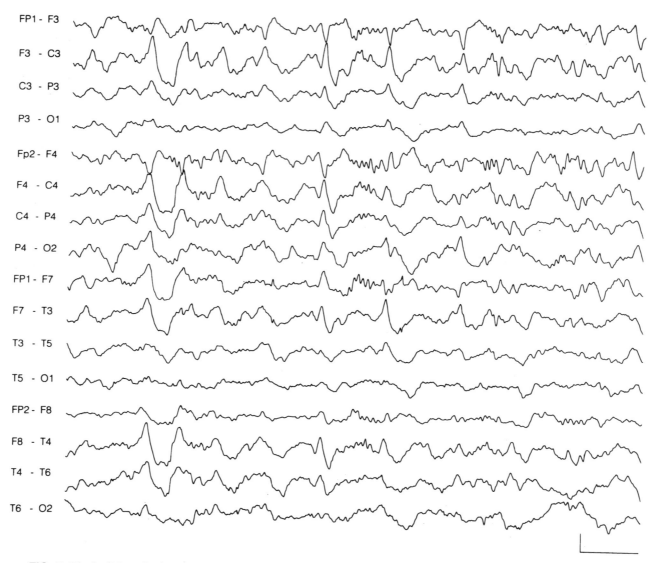

FIG. 7–22. Left hemisphere attenuation in sleep. 20 years. The principal attenuation appears in the left occipital (O1) and left parietal (P3) regions with moderate attenuation in the left posterior-midtemporal regions (T3,T5). In assessing the distribution of attenuation remember that, unlike localization of other wave forms, both components of a derivation are responsible for the attenuation. There is no aspect of this recording suggesting an electrical cancellation of background rhythms in the left posterior region such as might occur with synchronous rhythmic activity. The attenuation extends diffusely throughout the left hemisphere as a moderate spindle attenuation. As usual, V-waves are the wave forms most resistant to unilateral dysfunction. Calibration signal 1 sec, 70μV.

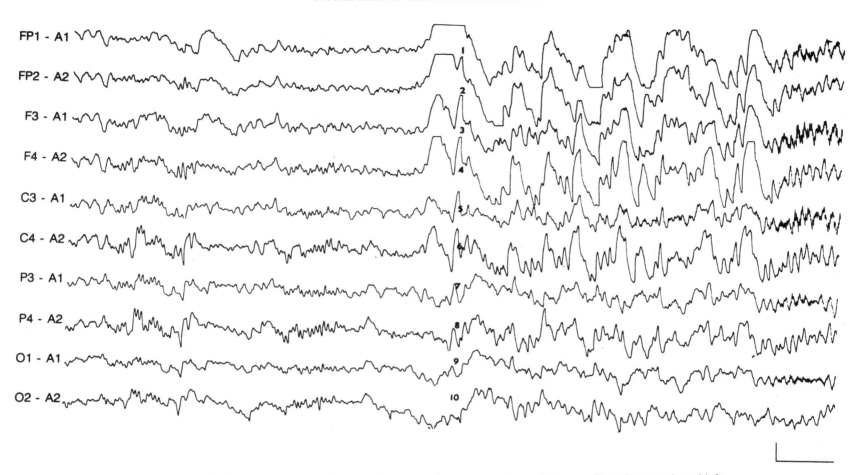

FIG. 7–23. Spindle asymmetry and arousal on ear reference montage. 49 years. The aforementioned left-side spindle reduction is also clearly evident on this ear reference montage. The abnormal arousal pattern, consisting of 2–3 Hz high-voltage diffuse waves, higher in the healthier right hemisphere, likely reflect subcortical (thalamic) dysfunction (49). Once again, an essentially diffuse abnormality, attenuated on the lesioned side, appears primarily in the healthier hemisphere. Calibration signal 1 sec, 50μV.

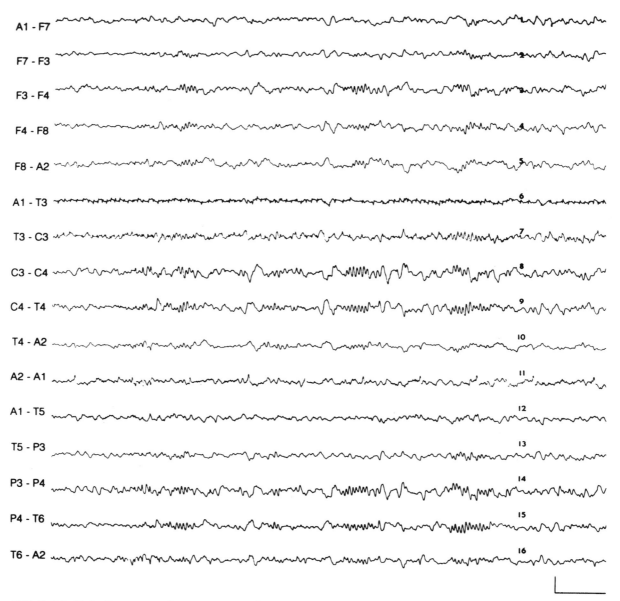

FIG. 7–24. Spindle asymmetry on a coronal montage. 49 years. A prominent reduction of spindles in the left hemisphere is evident when comparing homologous derivations. It is possible that occlusion of the left posterior cerebral artery which created the focal abnormality in Fig. 7–21 also involved the thalamocortical relay cells and therefore obliterated the leftside spindles. Calibration signal 1 sec, 50μV.

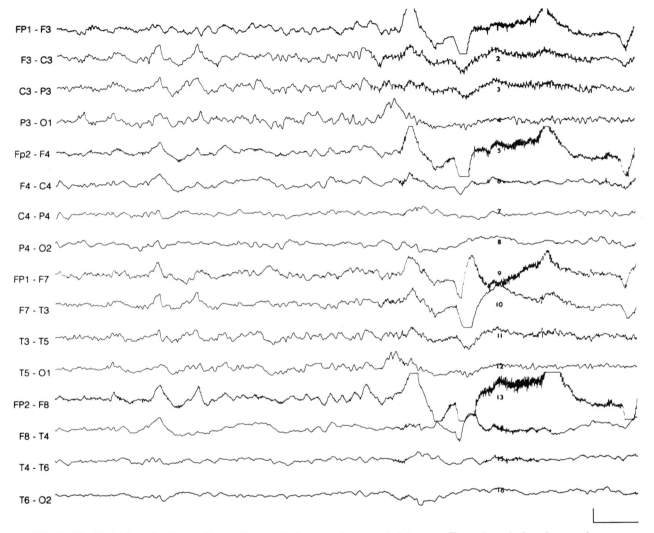

FIG. 7–25. Right hemisphere attenuation and abnormal arousal. 64 years. Even though the abnormal quantity of delta and theta activity accompanying this arousal appears principally on the left, the major abnormality resides in the right hemisphere as a loss of background activity. Normal or abnormal phenomena that are usually symmetrical will appear lower in voltage in the more diseased hemisphere. Note the asymmetry of background potentials posteriorly during the last 3 seconds of this sample, being clearly reduced in the right hemisphere compared to the left. The high-frequency (*darkly colored*) potentials in the bifrontal polar (Fp1, Fp2) and left central (C3) regions are muscle artifact. Their greater expression at C3 may reflect the patient's left hemiparesis consequent to a severe right hemisphere abnormality. Calibration signal 1 sec, 50μV.

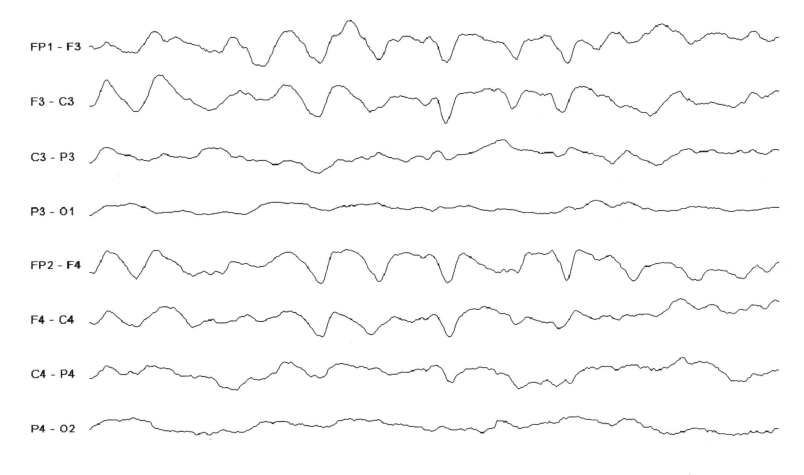

FIG. 7–26. Posterior attenuation—less than apparent? 60 years. A paucity of parietal-occipital activity appears on this bipolar recording, whose principal feature is anterior delta with poorly formed triphasic waves. Calibration signal 1 sec, 30μV.

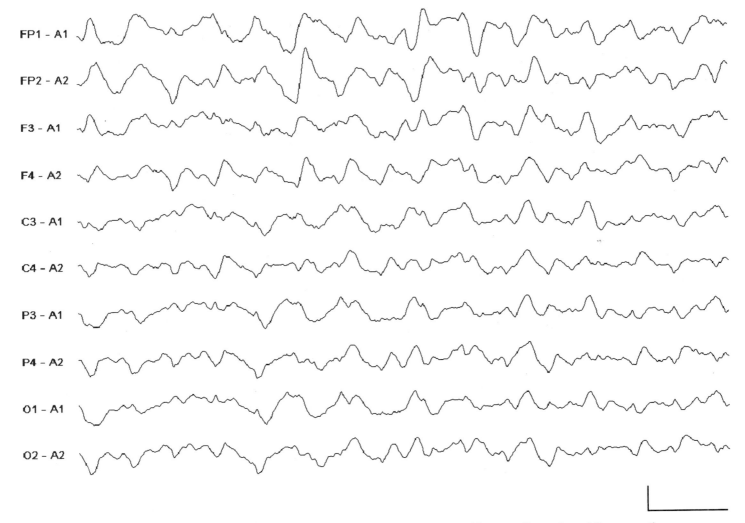

FIG. 7–27. More abundant activity revealed by referential montage. 60 years. Recording at the same time with the same settings as the previous illustration demonstrates considerably more abundant posterior activity, even though the references (A1, A2) may have contributed somewhat to the potentials in posterior derivations. Nonetheless, the montages taken together do reveal a loss of posterior activity, but not as complete as suggested by the bipolar montage. Calibration signal 1 sec, 30μV.

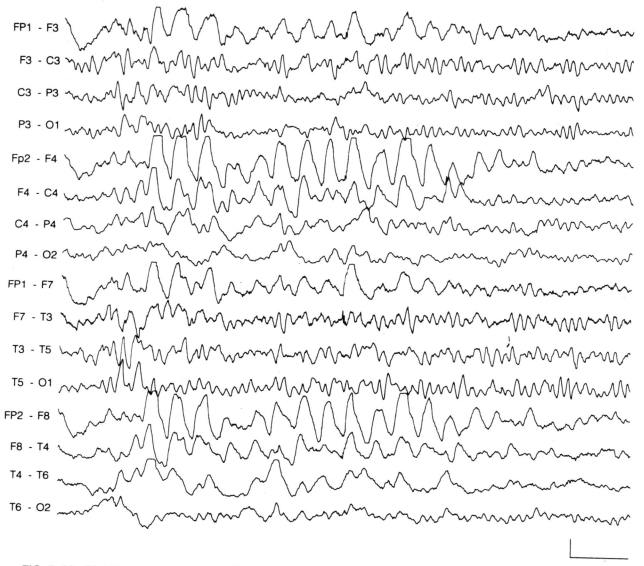

FIG. 7–28. Right hemisphere attenuation; IRDA, principally right. 17 years. Same recording as in Fig. 7–27, but the IRDA is more prominent. Despite this, the principal finding is a diffuse attenuation of background rhythms in the right hemisphere, sparing somewhat the frontal regions. Calibration signal 1 sec, 70μV.

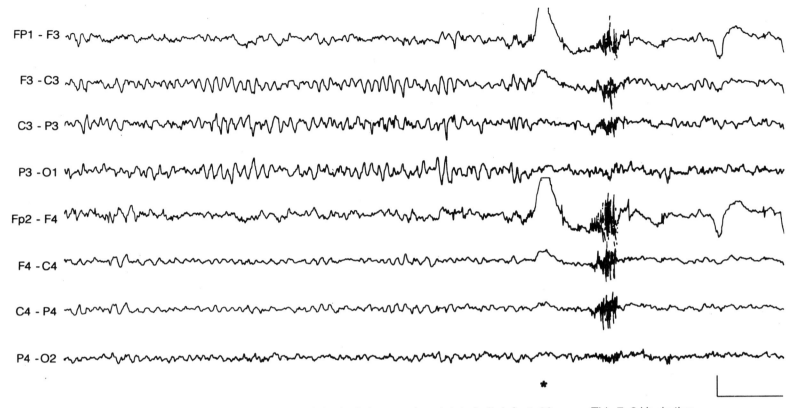

FIG. 7–29. Enhancement of alpha activity by left central-parietal skull defect. 32 years. This 7–8 Hz rhythm occurring principally at P3 is markedly attenuated by eye opening (*asterisk*) and therefore represents an alpha rhythm enhanced by the skull defect (50). Calibration signal 1 sec, 50μV.

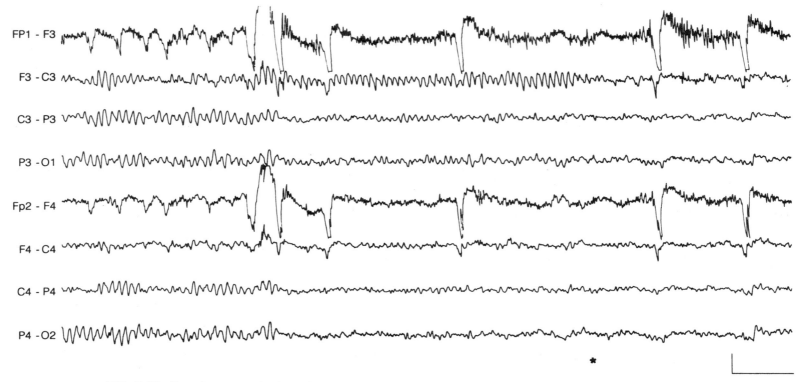

FIG. 7–30. Prominent mu rhythm with skull defect. 30 years. Eye opening in the 4th second blocked the alpha rhythm, revealing a more ample left mu rhythm (breach rhythm) than that of the right, as a consequence of the skull defect (50). Wiggling the right thumb (*asterisk*) abolished this mu rhythm. Calibration signal 1 sec, 50μV.

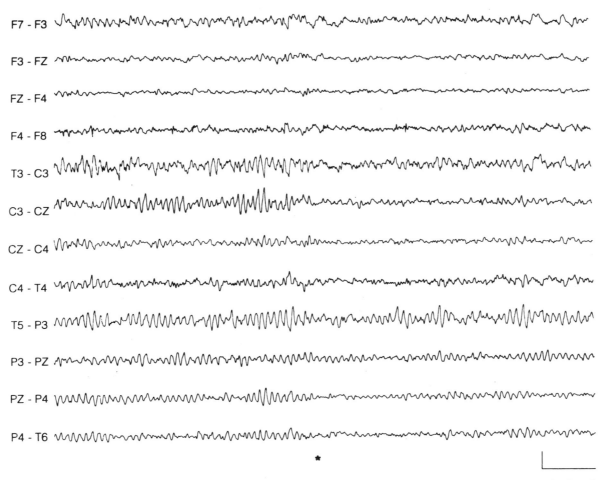

FIG. 7–31. Mu rhythm and alpha with skull defect on coronal montage. 30 years. Wiggling the right thumb with the eyes remaining closed (*asterisk*) attenuated the higher left mu rhythm at C3, revealing that the unattenuated 8 Hz rhythm in the T5-P3 derivation is alpha activity. This higher alpha activity and the undercurrent delta activity at T3 and minimally at T5 are probably not related to the central (C3) skull defect, and suggest dysfunction in the left temporal region (T5, T3). Calibration signal 1 sec, 50μV.

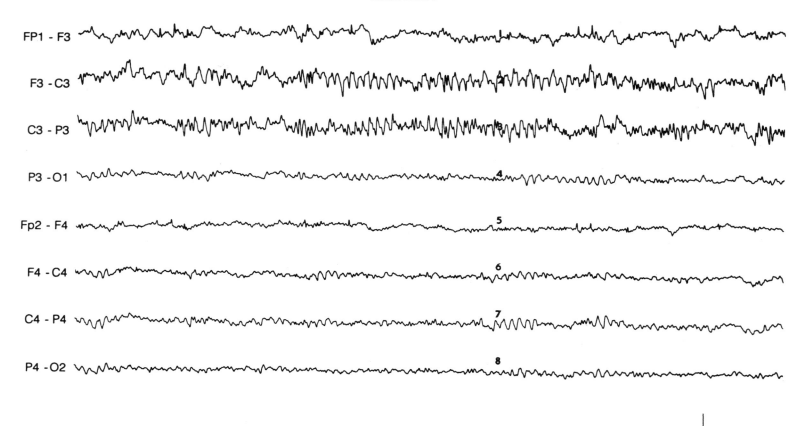

FIG. 7–32. Breach rhythm and delta activity. 40 years. The leftside skull defect is responsible for the greater expression of 20 Hz and 8–9 Hz left central (C3) waves but not the left frontal central (F3, C3) delta activity. Calibration signal 1 sec, 50μV.

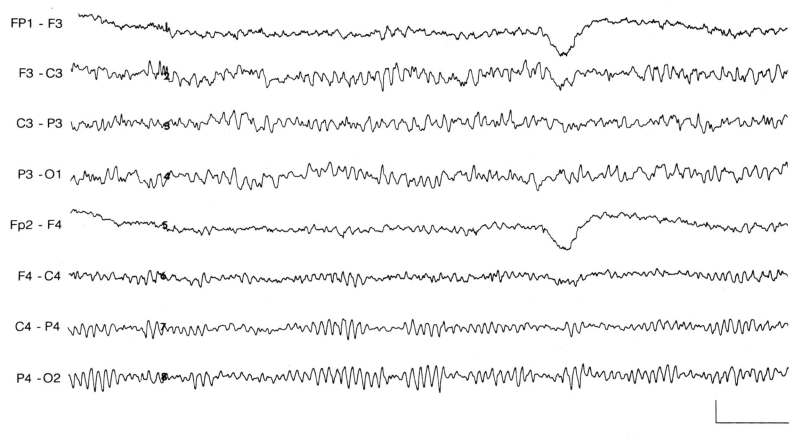

FIG. 7–33. Left central-parietal theta and ipsilateral skull defect. 31 years. Although a test of the responsiveness of this 6–7 Hz left central (C3)—left parietal (P3) rhythm to fist clenching was not performed, it likely represents dysfunction in this area, because its frequency is lower than the 9 Hz rightside rhythms. Calibration signal 1 sec, 70μV.

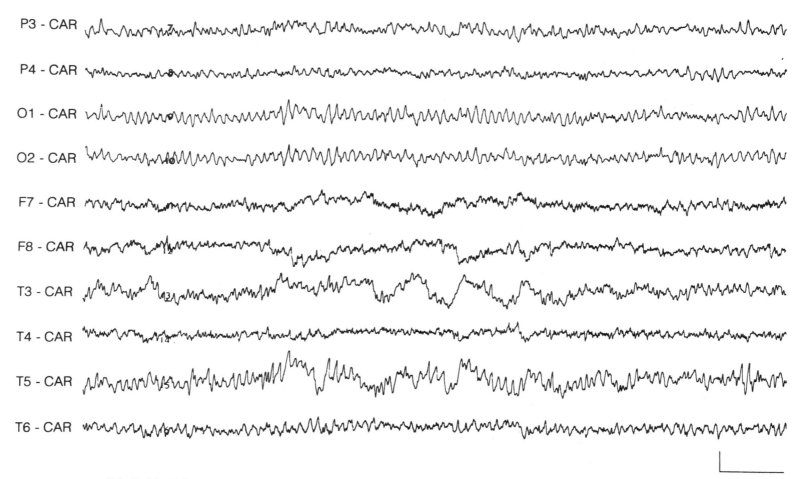

FIG. 7–34. Enhancement of alpha activity with a posterior skull defect. 73 years. Although posteriorly situated delta activity is usually associated with a decrease in higher-frequency background rhythms, the 8 Hz rhythm at T5, within the T5-T3 delta field, is slightly higher in voltage than that at T6. A less prominent increase appears in the left parietal (P3) region compared to the right (P4). The skull defect is largely responsible for this voltage increase. In addition, 15 Hz beta activity is increased at T5 and T3 as the breach rhythm. The arrhythmic delta activity at T3 and T5 represents a focal cerebral abnormality and is not consequent to the skull defect. Calibration signal 1 sec, 50μV.

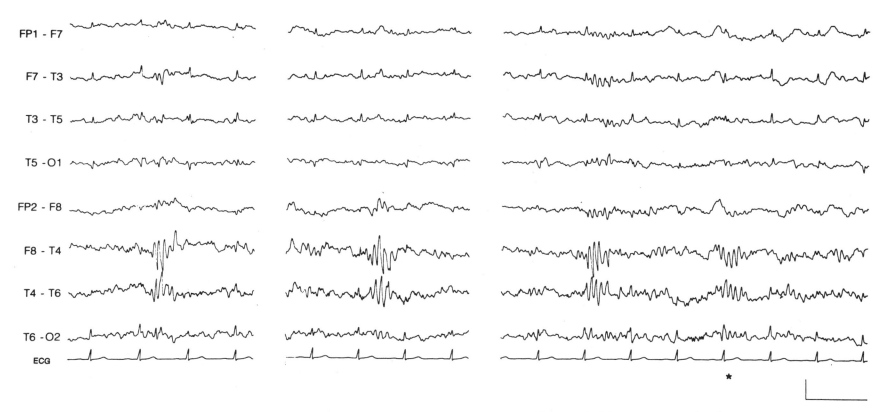

FIG. 7–35. Bursts of spike-like waves with a skull defect. 49 years. These apiculate waves are not spikes, because of their rhythmic nature and the lack of an aftercoming slow wave of the same polarity. Note that the lower-voltage bursts (*asterisk*), similar in morphology to the apiculate higher-voltage ones, do not resemble spikes. Calibration signal 1 sec, 50μV.

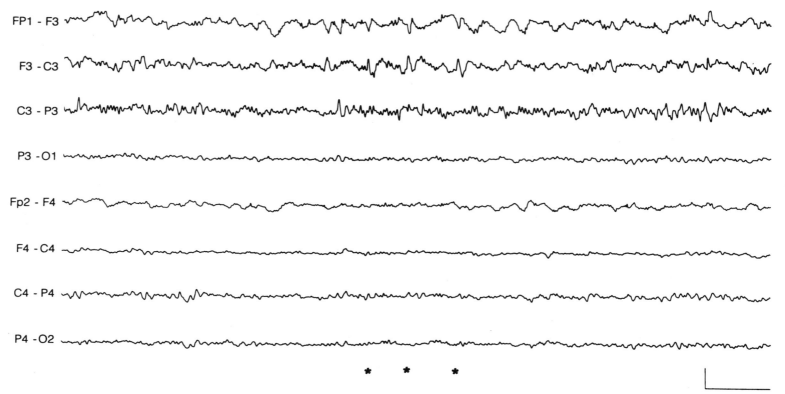

FIG. 7–36. Breach rhythm, focal delta, and spikes. 40 years. A leftside skull defect augments the amplitude of the 20 Hz left central (C3) rhythm; compare with its very-low-voltage right central (C4) counterpart. The combination with 8–9 Hz waves in the same region creates frequent apiculate forms, most of which are not spikes. Identifying any of these potentials as spikes depends on their relationship to background rhythms. Three waveforms (*asterisks*), all left frontal (F3), are sufficiently more apiculate than the background rhythms to be identified as spikes. Calibration signal 1 sec, 50μV.

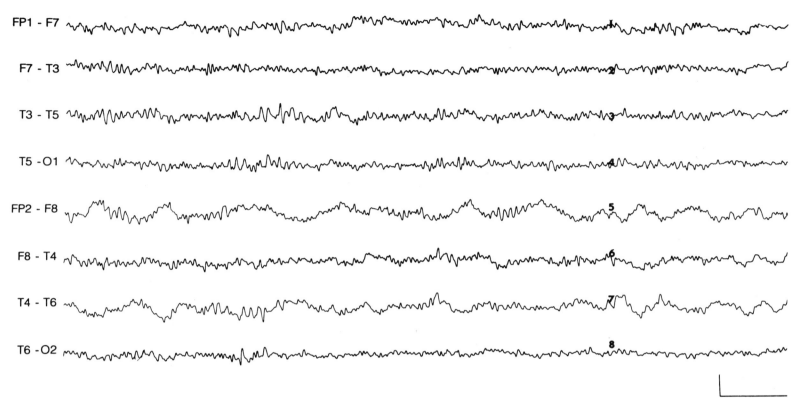

FIG. 7–37. Right temporal delta activity. 39 years. Persistent arrhythmic F8-T4 delta activity. Two remarkable aspects of such activity are the very long duration of some delta waves (up to 1400 msec) and the modest disruption of background activity. Calibration signal 1 sec, 50μV.

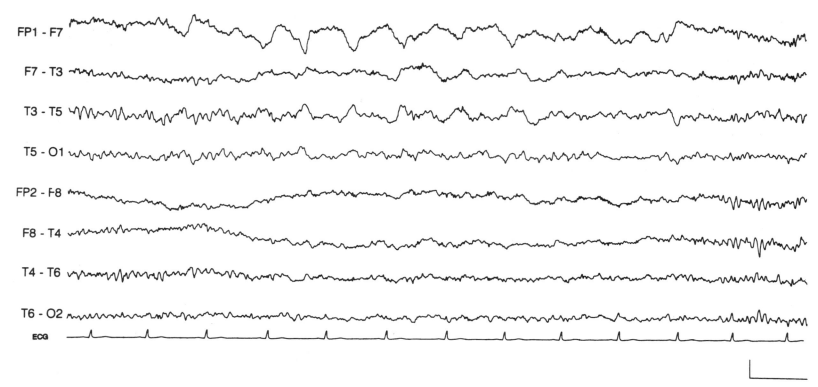

FIG. 7–38. Transient left anterior-midtemporal delta. 39 years. Even though prominent, this temporal delta (F7-T3) appears principally during light drowsiness, as evidenced by loss of alpha. Arousal (*last seconds*) attenuates this delta. Calibration signal 1 sec, 50μV.

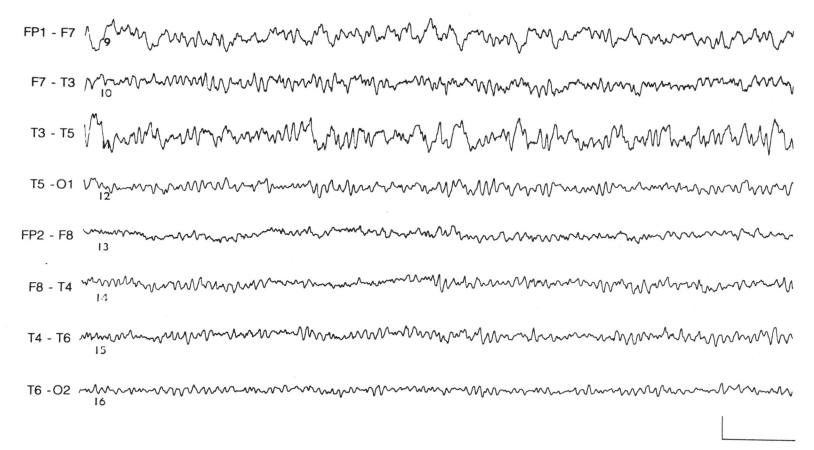

FIG. 7–39. Theta and delta in the left temporal region. 43 years. Background activity is slightly enhanced on the abnormal side. Prominent 3–4 Hz and 1–2 Hz activity appears at F7-T3 in an intermixed fashion. Calibration signal 1 sec, 70μV.

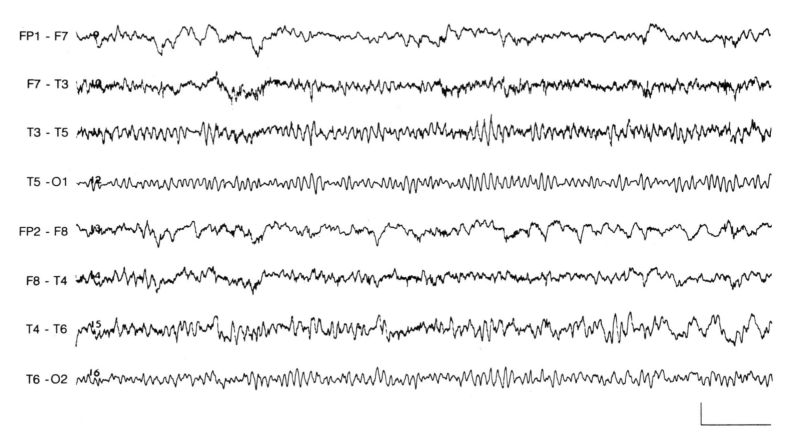

FIG. 7–40. Right temporal delta and theta and muscle and eye movement artifact. 41 years. In practice, many artifacts, particularly eye movements and muscle activity, tend to obscure focal abnormalities, particularly those in the temporal regions. The initial hint of a focal abnormality here might be the less regulated background activity in the T4-T6 derivation compared to that of the homologous T3-T5 derivation. This is due to focal theta activity at T4 and F8 which partially cancels in the F8-T4 derivation. Leaning back, one can appreciate that 500–600 msec delta waves are also present at F8 and T4. The intermittent bilateral delta activity in the third second represents a low-voltage glossokinetic potential from swallowing. Calibration signal 1 sec, 50μV.

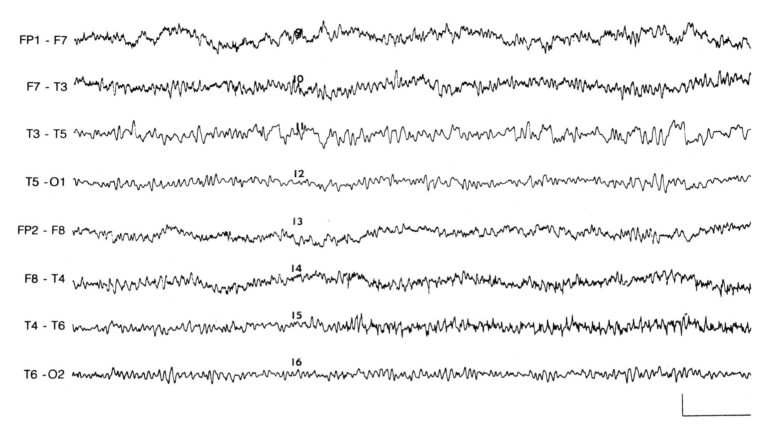

FIG. 7–41. Theta, left temporal. 66 years. This prolonged sequence of left temporal (F7-T3) theta activity, abnormal at any age, is a common finding. Equally common is the modification of its morphology by coexisting potentials such as temporal alphoid (8–9 Hz) rhythm at F7, bilateral beta activity, and slow lateral eye movements as seen in the Fp1-F7, F7-T3, Fp2-F8, and F8-T4 derivations. Calibration signal 1 sec, 70μV.

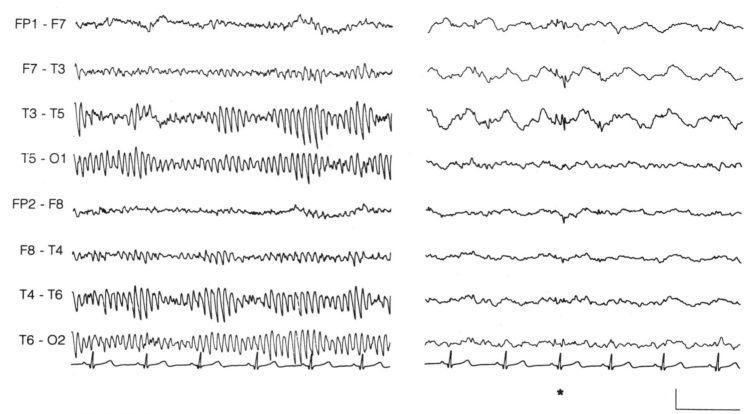

FIG. 7–42. Marked "activation" of delta in light sleep. 29 years. Prominent and persistent delta activity appears in the left temporal (F7-T3) region during light sleep (*right*). The prominent delta in the T3-T5 derivation indicates no spread to T5. Note the left-sided small sharp spike (*asterisk*), a normal phenomenon. Calibration signal 1 sec, 50μV.

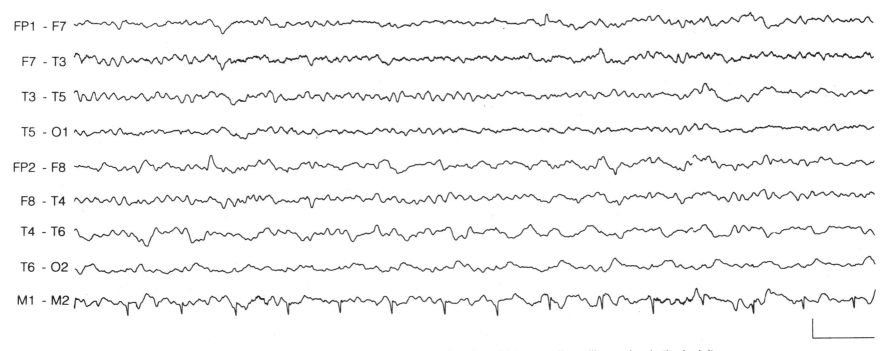

FP1 - F7

F7 - T3

T3 - T5

T5 - O1

FP2 - F8

F8 - T4

T4 - T6

T6 - O2

M1 - M2

FIG. 7–43. Pulse artifact and delta activity. 38 years. Scrutiny of this recording will reveal arrhythmic delta activity involving F8, T4, and M2 (mandibular notch electrode) which is unrelated to the ECG as recorded by the mandibular notch electrodes (M1-M2). In contrast, the rhythmic delta at T6 is timelocked to the ECG and is a pulse artifact. Calibration signal 1 sec, 70μV.

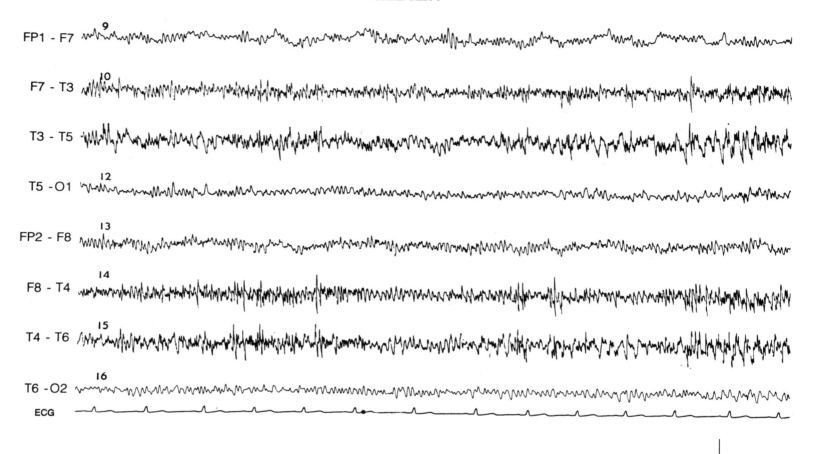

FIG. 7–44. Left temporal delta activity within muscle artifact, beta and eye movements. 23 years. The clue to this focal abnormality at F7-T3 is the delta activity in the T3-T5 derivation underlying muscle and beta activity. Scrutiny of both frontal polar derivations will reveal delta activity in the Fp1-F7 derivation in addition to that produced by eye movements in both Fp1-F7 and Fp2-F8. The diffuse and symmetrical beta activity and other background rhythms further indicate confinement of this dysfunction to the left anterior-midtemporal region. Calibration signal 1 sec, 70μV.

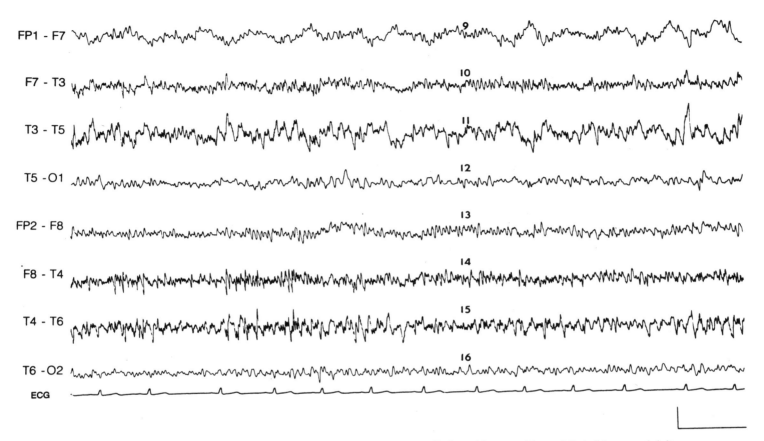

FIG. 7–45. Accentuation of left temporal delta with hyperventilation. 23 years. The subtle left temporal delta in Fig. 7–44 is markedly accentuated by hyperventilation. Calibration signal 1 sec, 70µV.

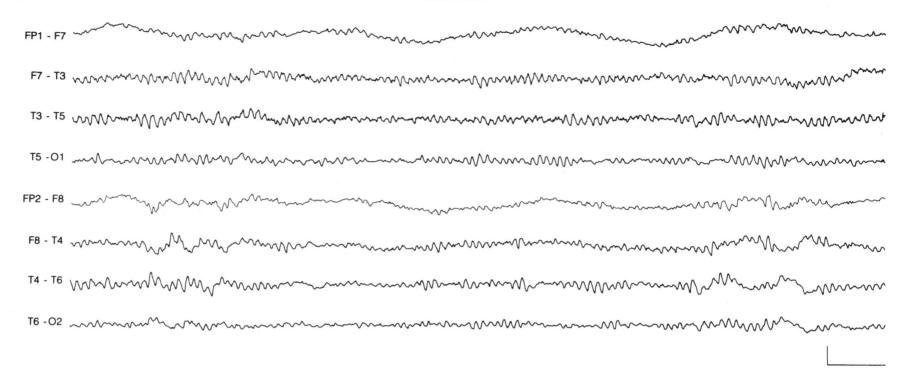

FIG. 7–46. Intermittent temporal delta activity. 55 years. Rarely, focal delta activity can appear intermittently, as in this example. Arenas et al. (51) found temporal delta to occur rarely in the normal elderly and slightly more so in the left temporal region compared to the right. Therefore, this abnormality, occurring in approximately the incidence of the sample depicted here, would indicate a clear focal right temporal abnormality at virtually any age. Calibration signal 1 sec, 100μV.

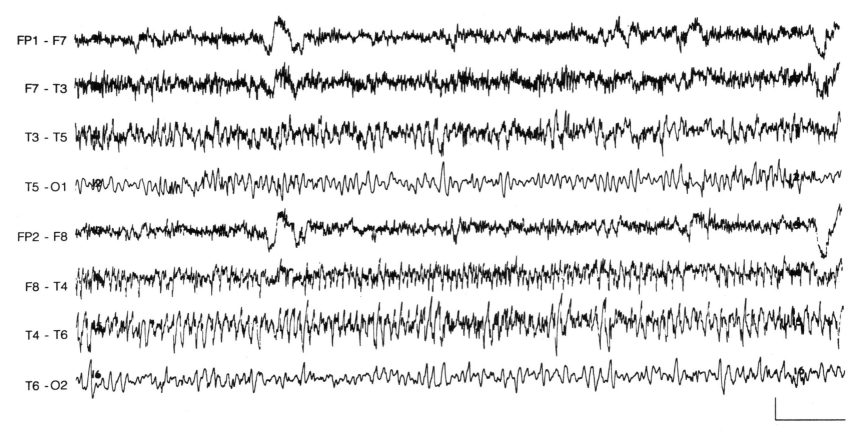

FIG. 7–47. Left temporal delta and theta with bitemporal muscle artifact. 30 years. A mixture of moderately persistent delta and theta activity appears at T3 and F7 as seen through the persistent muscle activity. However, no abnormality is apparent in the right temporal region; the waxing and waning of muscle artifact and intermittent bilaterally synchronous (left maximum) 300–400 msec waves give the false impression of an additional right temporal focal abnormality. Further stretches of the recording would be required to assess whether the right temporal activity was consistently normal, but a clear abnormality appears here only on the left. Calibration signal 1 sec, 50μV.

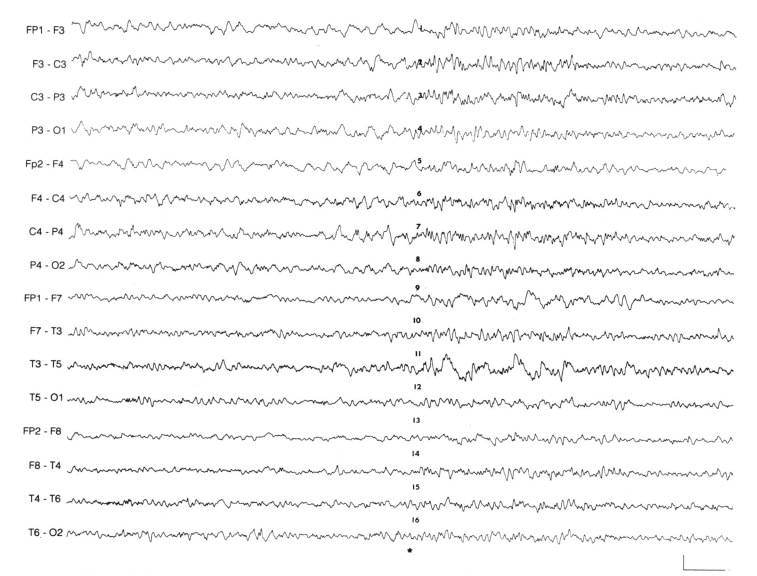

FIG. 7–48. Focal abnormality revealed on arousal. 42 years. No definite regional abnormality can be discerned in the first 7 seconds of this sample. Arousal (*asterisk*) is indicated by an increase in faster rhythms but, more importantly, by 1–2 Hz waves focally at F7-T3. Calibration signal 1 sec, 50µV.

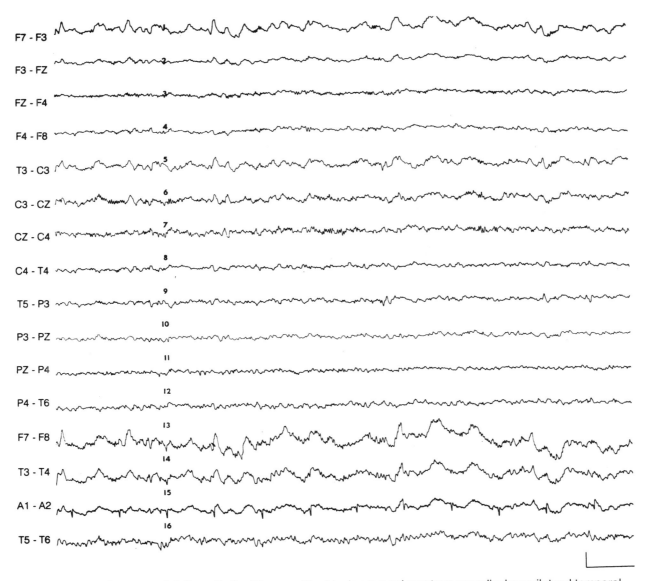

FIG. 7–49. Left temporal delta activity. 32 years. The bipolar coronal montage may display unilateral temporal delta activity, as seen in the F7-F3 and T3-C3 derivations. The lack of in-phase delta activity at F4-F8 and C4-T4 derivations indicates that lateral eye movements are not producing the left temporal delta. Interhemispheric derivations illustrate the anterior-posterior extent of such delta activity, which is seen principally at F7 and T3 with some spread to A1 and minimal spread to T5. Calibration signal 1 sec, 50μV.

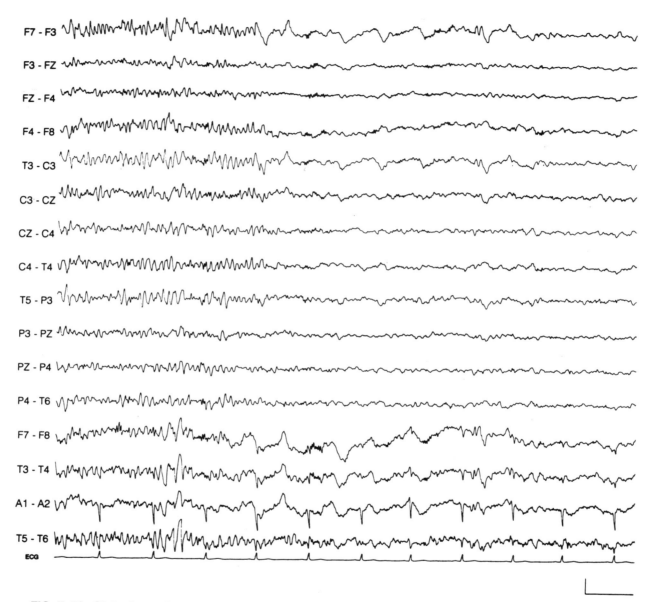

FIG. 7–50. State-dependent left temporal delta. 29 years. This left temporal (F7-T3) delta activity, minimally evident during wakefulness (*first 4 seconds*), is prominently seen during early drowsiness (*subsequent 6 seconds*), only to recede as drowsiness persists. Calibration signal 1 sec, 50μV.

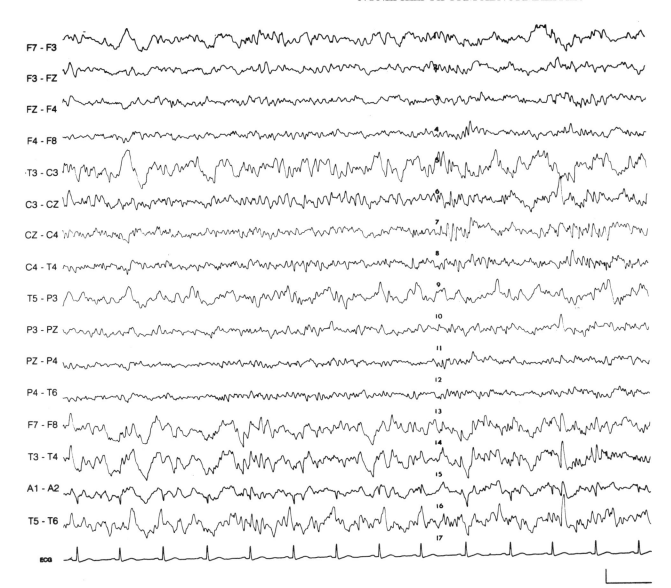

FIG. 7–51. Focal delta activity on coronal montage. 65 years. When the lateralization of focal or regionally accentuated delta activity has already been determined by an anterior-posterior bipolar montage, a bipolar coronal montage may further localize such activity. When the field of such data is discrete—as in this case—a coronal montage alone may describe the distribution. Here the delta appears principally at T5 and T3, with relatively less involvement of F7 and only slight parasagittal spread. The amplitude of delta activity is enhanced by the long interelectrode distances in the interhemispheric derivations. These derivations may confirm a delta or spike localization when complex fields are present. Theta activity is diffuse but is more prominent in the areas of delta. Questionable spikes at T3, T5, and F7 appear in the first and next-to-last seconds. Calibration signal 1 sec, 50μV.

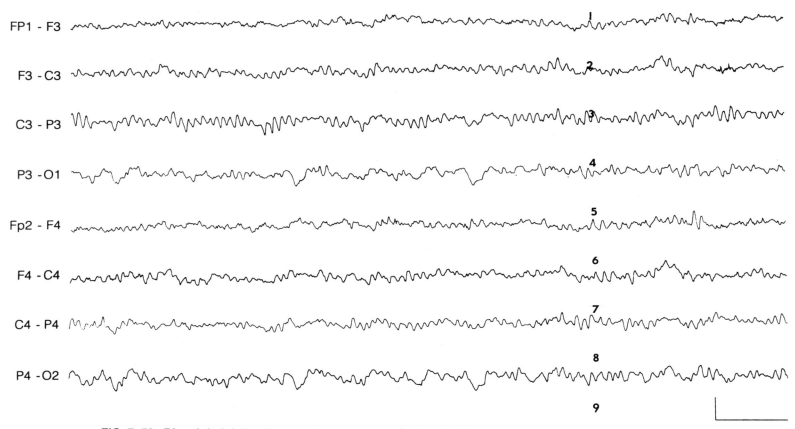

FP1 - F3

F3 - C3

C3 - P3

P3 - O1

Fp2 - F4

F4 - C4

C4 - P4

P4 - O2

FIG. 7–52. Bioccipital delta. 26 years. A recent generalized tonic-clonic seizure may be followed by posteriorly situated and virtually symmetrical delta activity. Most lesion-related delta activity would more clearly and unilaterally disrupt posterior background activity, although a bilateral occipital abnormality cannot be excluded. Calibration signal 1 sec, 70μV.

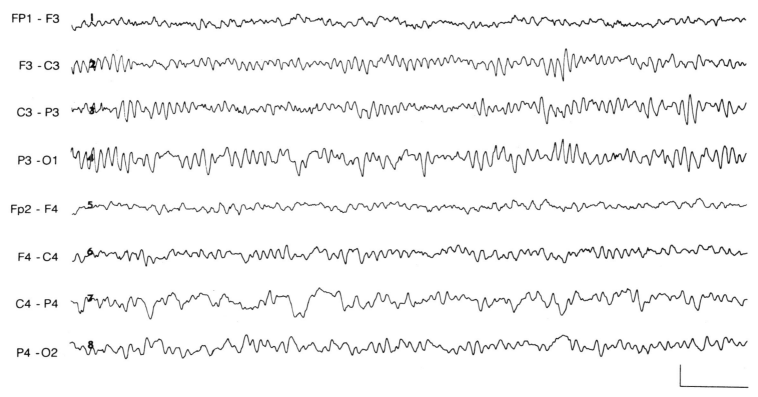

FIG. 7–53. Right parietal-occipital delta markedly disrupts background activity. 18 years. Note the moderate loss of alpha activity on the right in association with this delta activity, which appears principally in the C4-P4 derivation; there is partial cancellation of potentials in the P4-O2 derivation. The occasional slow waves at O1 are normal posterior slow of youth, appearing in the healthier hemisphere. There is only minimal disruption of C4 activity as depicted in the F4-C4 derivation and no abnormality more anteriorly. Calibration signal 1 sec, 70μV.

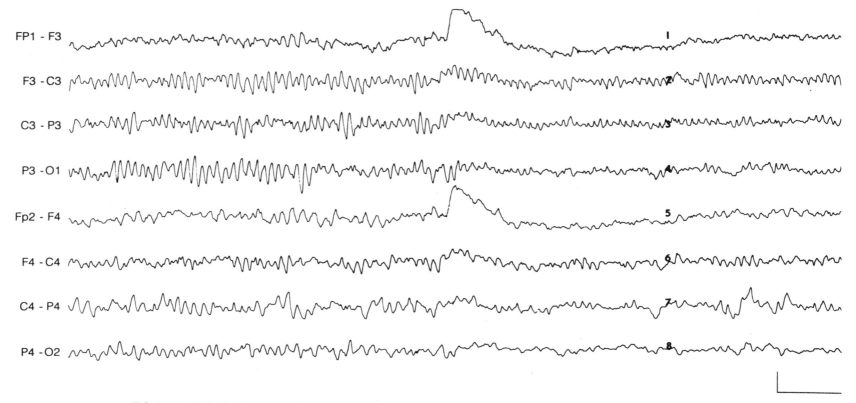

FIG. 7–54. Effect of eye opening on right parietal-occipital delta activity. 18 years. Same patient as in Fig. 7–53. Eye opening somewhat attenuates delta activity, particularly that in the posterior head. Note the greater involvement of C4 by this delta activity compared to that in Fig. 7–53. Right central (C4) background activity is 8 Hz, whereas that of the left central region (C3) is 10 Hz. Similarly, the alpha activity on the left is slightly faster than that on the right. Calibration signal 1 sec, 70μV.

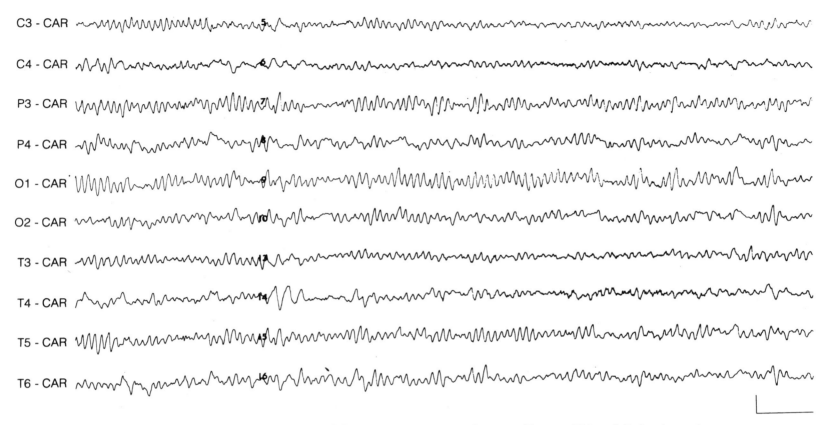

FIG. 7–55. Posterior delta activity and the common average reference. 18 years. This activity involves principally the right parietal (P4) region. The partial sparing of the right occipital (O2) region is attested to by the lower amplitude of delta activity and the moderate preservation of alpha at virtually the same Hz as on the left. Right midposterior temporal regions (T4, T6) are also minimally involved in this delta. The diffuse theta burst in the 4th second has less localizing value, even though it resides principally in the right hemisphere. Calibration signal 1 sec, 70μV.

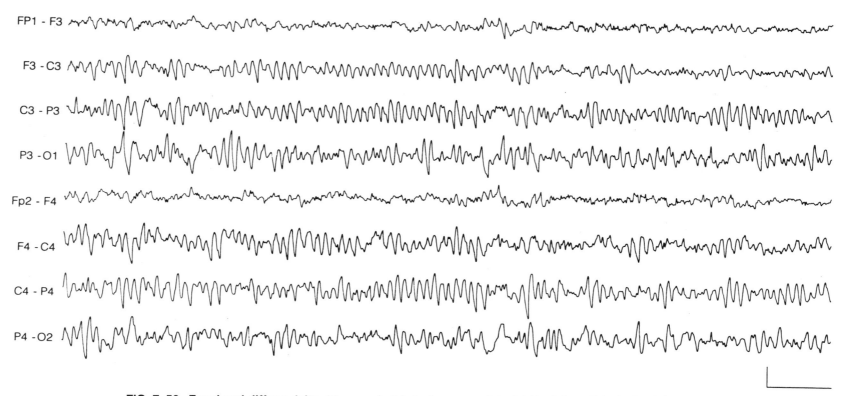

FIG. 7–56. Focal and diffuse delta. 31 years. In this instance, persistent 1 Hz delta activity in the right central-parietal region (F4-C4, C4-P4, and P4-O2 derivations) can be discerned despite the diffuse bursts of intermittent 400–600 msec medium-voltage waves. The C4 and P4 delta is that which is indicative of regional dysfunction because of its lower frequency and persistence. The intermittent delta does not have localizing significance even though it is accentuated posteriorly. Calibration signal 1 sec, 50μV.

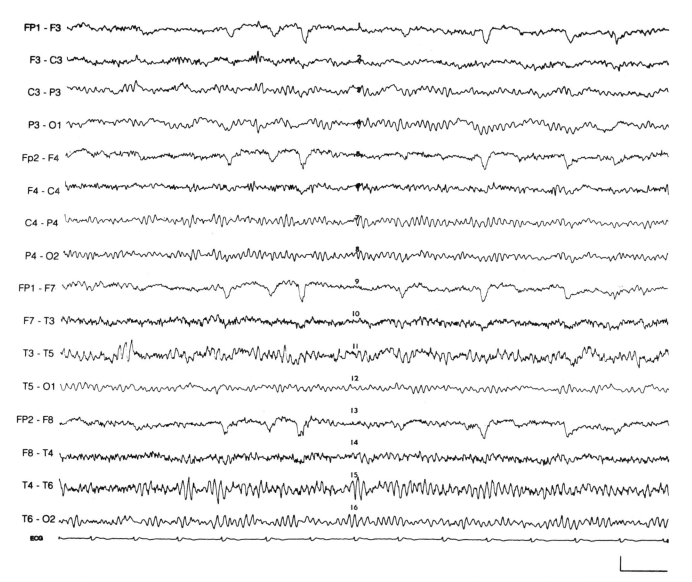

FIG. 7–57. Rhythmic regional delta activity. 67 years. In contrast to most regional delta activity, which interrupts the background rhythms, the regional delta activity seen here does not. Its rhythmicity should immediately raise the possibility of pulse artifact in one or more channels, but the ECG monitor reveals that this is not the case. This delta appears principally in the left parietal (P3), left central (C3), left occipital (O1), and left posterior temporal (T5) areas, producing relative cancellation of such activity in the T5-O1 derivation. Calibration signal 1 sec, 50μV.

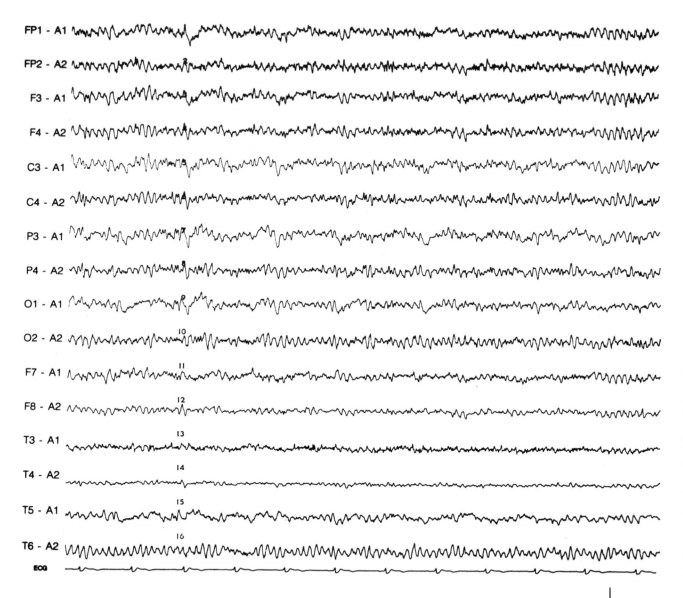

FIG. 7–58. Rhythmic delta activity on an ear reference montage. 67 years. Same patient as in Fig. 7–57. Note rhythmic delta activity in derivations involving P3, C3, T5, and O1 with minimal involvement elsewhere. Without data from the previous anterior-posterior bipolar montage, whether this represents a more anteriorly placed delta activity with referential (A1) involvement could not be fully determined. It is very unlikely that referential involvement with cancellation anteriorly would have produced a delta activity of principal amplitude at the P3-A1 and C3-A1 derivations with slightly less amplitude at the O1-A1 derivation. The partial loss of leftside alpha activity also suggests a more posterior location. A contralateral ear (A2) or common average reference montage would also clearly depict the delta field. Calibration signal 1 sec, 70µV.

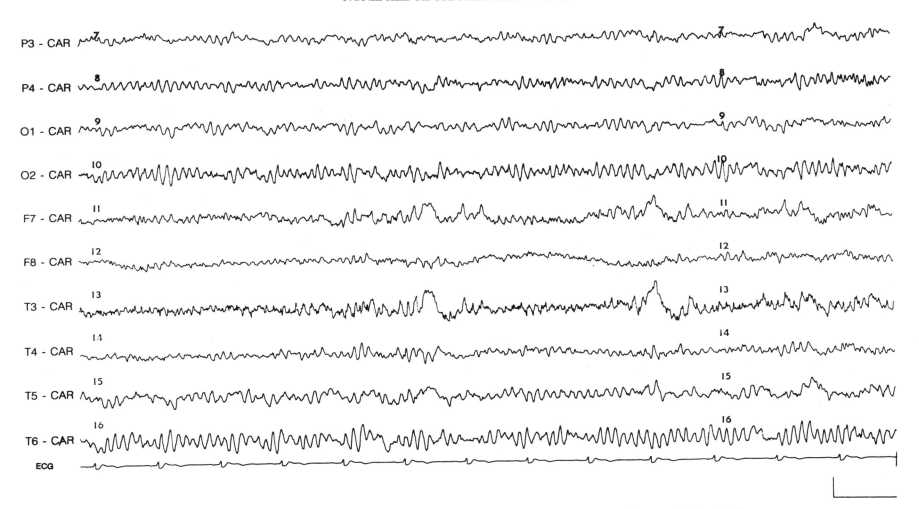

FIG. 7–59. Common average reference and two types of delta activity. 67 years. Same patient as in Figs. 7–57 and 7–58. Once again, the relatively low-voltage, somewhat rhythmic persistent delta activity appears at T5, P3, and O1. Less persistent, higher frequency and higher amplitude delta activity appears more anteriorly at T3 and F7. Persistent regional delta is considered a more reliable indicator of a focal cerebral disturbance than is intermittent delta activity (15). Persistent delta activity also suggests a more recently occurring dysfunction than does intermittent and higher-frequency delta. It is likely that both delta foci here, the persistent and intermittent, each reflect cerebral dysfunction, with the intermittent occurring less acutely than the persistent. Posterior and ipsilateral anterior temporal EEG abnormalities commonly coexist (52). Calibration signal 1 sec, 70μV.

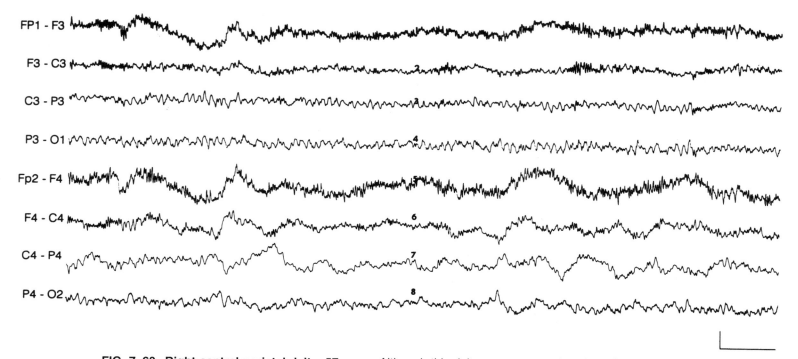

FIG. 7–60. Right central-parietal delta. 57 years. Although this delta appears prominently at C4 and P4, the marked attenuation of alpha activity indicates involvement of the right occipital region. In addition to delta activity, excess theta activity accompanies the slow-wave abnormality. In contrast, the symmetrical frontal beta activity, intermingled with muscle artifact, suggests some sparing of the anterior regions. Calibration signal 1 sec, 50μV.

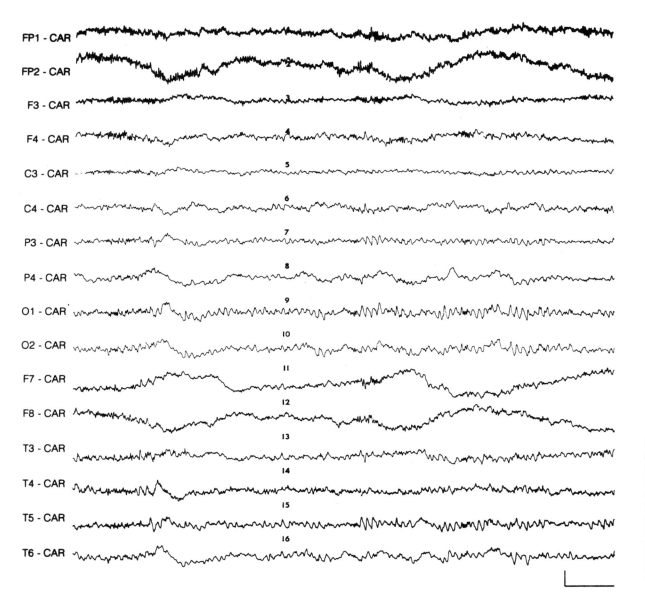

FIG. 7–61. Right parietal-central-temporal delta, and the common average reference. 57 years. Same patient as in Fig. 7–60. The common average reference (CAR) reveals that the delta activity occurs primarily in the right parietal (P4) area with moderate involvement of the right central (C4), right posterior temporal (T6), and right occipital (O2) areas. Note that the CAR depicts slightly better the preserved occipital rhythms than did the bipolar montage. More anteriorly, the slow waves represent oblique eye movements. Calibration signal 1 sec, 70μV.

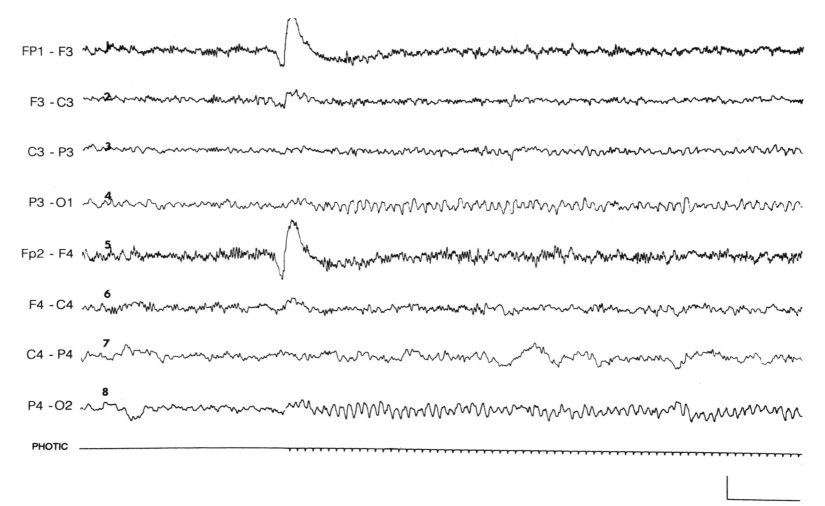

FIG. 7–62. Photic driving is preserved. 57 years. Same patient in Figs. 7–60 and 7–61. Preservation of the photic driving response in symmetrical form suggests intactness of the primary visual pathways and therefore of both the lateral geniculate body and the calcarine cortex (9). Note arrhythmic rightside delta activity. Calibration signal 1 sec, 70μV.

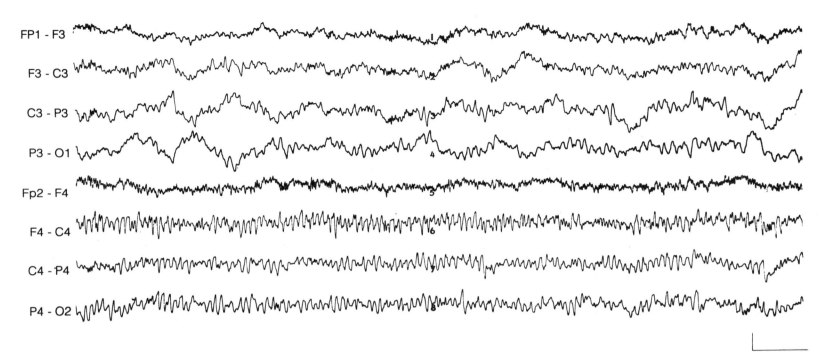

FIG. 7–63. Left central-parietal-temporal delta and attenuation of background rhythms (parasagittal portion). 54 years. Both the leftside alpha and central rhythms are attenuated and slowed in comparison to those of the rightside, which remain unaffected by this left hemisphere process. The process's acuteness is attested to by the arrhythmicity of the delta waves, their low frequency of about 0.5–1 Hz, and their persistence. Although this delta activity appears to involve the entire left hemisphere, further scrutiny reveals phase reversals in several channels, indicating principal involvement of P3, C3, and T5 with some spread to T3. Calibration signal 1 sec, 50μV.

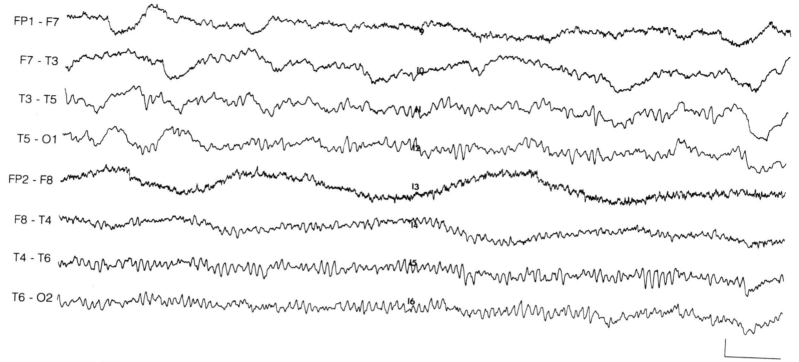

FIG. 7–64. Left central-parietal-temporal delta and attenuation of background rhythms (temporal portion).
Some of the long-duration delta activity in the more anterior leftside derivations represents slow eye movements, which are more clearly seen at the Fp2-F8 and F8-T4 derivations. Further evidence that the frontal lobe is considerably less involved in this delta is the partial preservation of its background activity as 30–35 Hz beta. Despite the high-amplitude delta activity in the left hemisphere, very little appears in homologous regions of the right. Calibration signal 1 sec, 50μV.

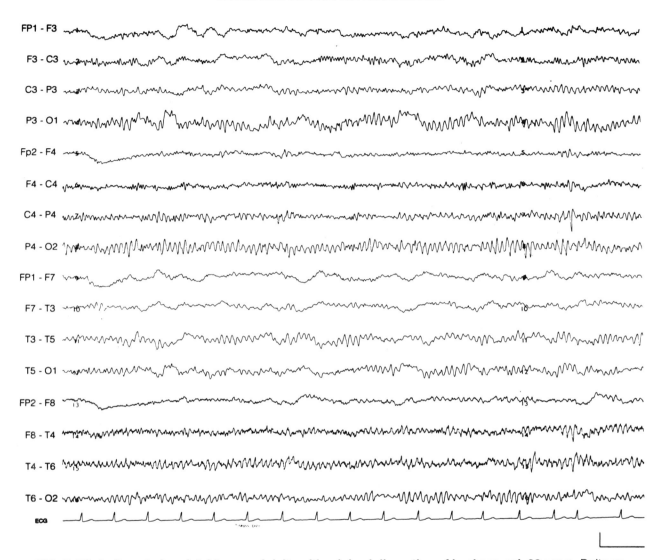

FIG. 7–65. Left central-parietal-temporal delta with minimal disruption of background. 82 years. Delta activity, involving principally T3,T5, C3, and P3 exceptionally causes minimal disruption of background activity. This likely reflects subacuteness of the process. Abundant leftside alpha indicates that the left occipital region is not involved. Calibration signal 1 sec, 100μV.

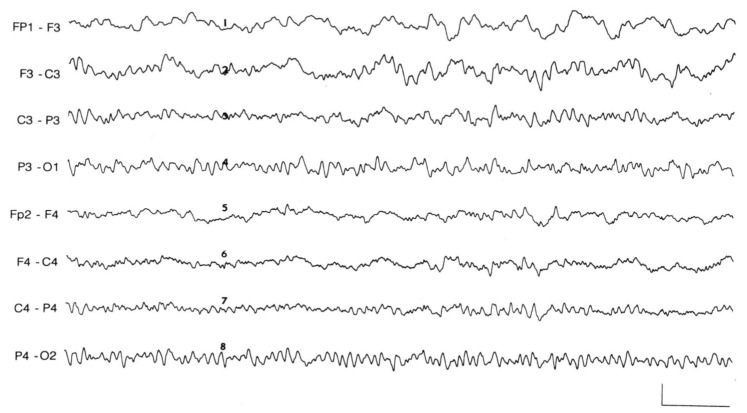

FIG. 7–66. Left frontal and left hemisphere delta activity. 38 years. Arrhythmic 1–1-1/2 Hz delta appears in the left frontal polar and left superior frontal regions (derivations Fp1-F3 and F3-C3) with more modest dysfunction extending posteriorly on the left. Note the diffuse left hemisphere theta activity which accompanies the delta. Delta activity in the right frontal region probably does not reflect an additional process there because of its lower amplitude, the consistent wave-for-wave correspondence with left frontal delta activity, and the lack of associated background abnormalities. Calibration signal 1 sec, 50μV.

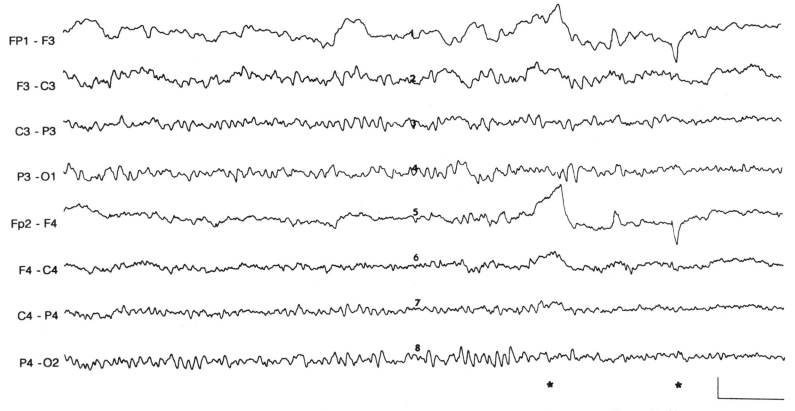

FIG. 7–67. Persistence of left frontal delta with eye opening. 38 years. Same patient as in Fig. 7–66. Note the lack of attenuation of left frontal (Fp1 and F3) delta activity with eye opening (*left asterisk*), which only attenuates some of the background theta. In contradistinction to the delta activity, the eye blink artifact (*right asterisk*) is symmetrical. Calibration signal 1 sec, 50μV.

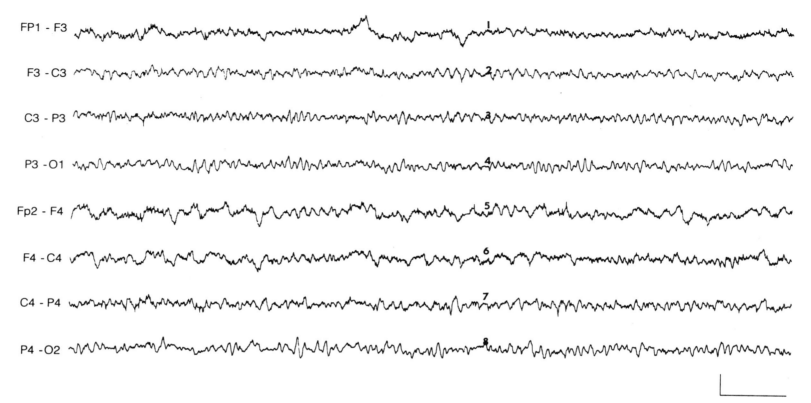

FIG. 7–68. Right hemisphere delta, principally right frontal. 70 years. Delta activity situated anteriorly disrupts the alpha activity less than that situated posteriorly. Lack of phase reversals between Fp2-F4 and F4-C4 indicates that this delta is situated principally in the right frontal polar (Fp2) region with spread to F4 and some spread throughout the right hemisphere. Calibration signal 1 sec, 50μV.

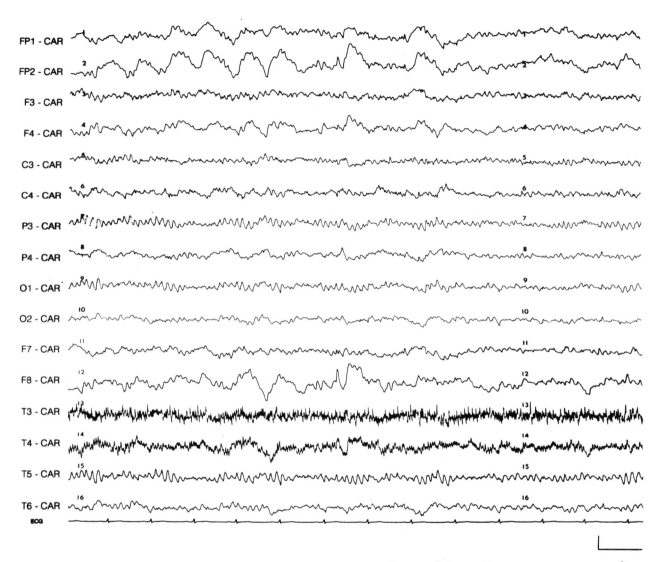

FIG. 7–69. Right frontal temporal delta and right hemisphere abnormalities on the common average reference. 80 years. The common average reference (CAR) is useful in depicting unilateral abnormalities because it (the reference) remains moderately free of "contamination." In this instance, 600–800 msec delta activity appears arrhythmically at F8 and T4 but also prominently at Fp2, with spread to F4 with minimal spread posteriorly. However, the minimal rightside alpha activity indicates involvement of the occipital, parietal, and posterior temporal regions in this process. Note the single right frontal spike at F8, Fp2 with minimal spread to T4. Calibration signal 1 sec, 50μV.

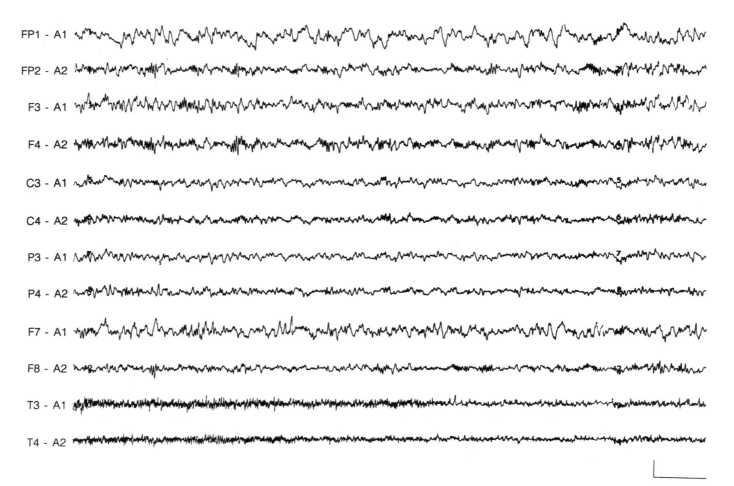

FIG. 7–70. **Left frontal delta activity on an ear reference montage.** 69 years. Because of the usual lack of contamination of the A1 reference by frontal delta activity, this montage clearly depicts the extent of focal delta activity seen here at Fp1 with spread to F7. Note that the degree of 25 Hz beta reduction is greatest in the area of principal delta activity—Fp1 then F7—whereas only minimal beta reduction and delta appear in the left superior frontal region (F3). None of the sharply contoured waves can be identified as a spike. Calibration signal 1 sec, 100μV.

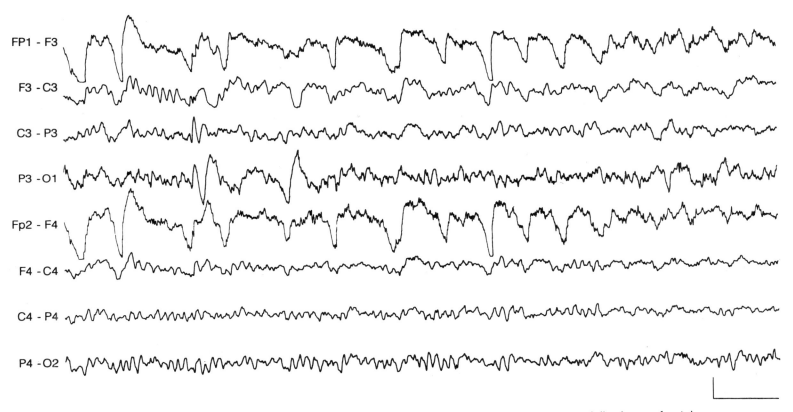

FIG. 7–71. Left hemisphere delta and eye movements. 19 years. Eye movements can partially obscure frontal delta activity, which in this instance is best revealed in the last 3 seconds, which are free of eye movements. Such delta is also revealed by comparing F3-C3 versus F4-C4 and C3-P3 versus the C4-P4 derivations, which illustrate left anterior delta activity. The leftside alpha activity is slightly disrupted by this anterior process. A possible left frontocentral spike appears in the 3rd second, but any downward deflection in the Fp1-F3 derivation is "lost" in an eye blink. Calibration signal 1 sec, 50μV.

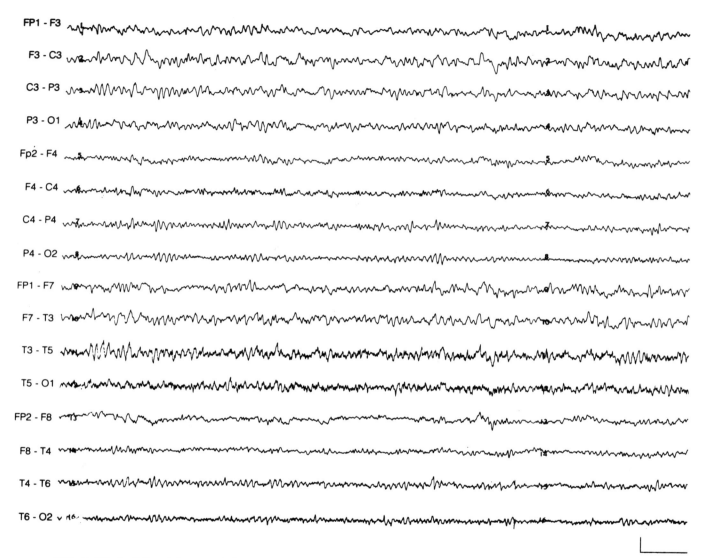

FIG. 7–72. Left frontal-central theta and delta. 76 years. Approximately 5 Hz semirhythmic medium-voltage waves appear continuously in the left frontal (F7, F3, Fp1) derivations, with extension to the left central (C3) region and some extension throughout the left hemisphere. Low-voltage delta underlies the theta. The lack of more prominent midtemporal (T3) involvement suggests principally a frontal as opposed to a temporal abnormality: the F7 and F8 electrodes cover both the inferior frontal and anterior temporal regions. Calibration signal 1 sec, 50μV.

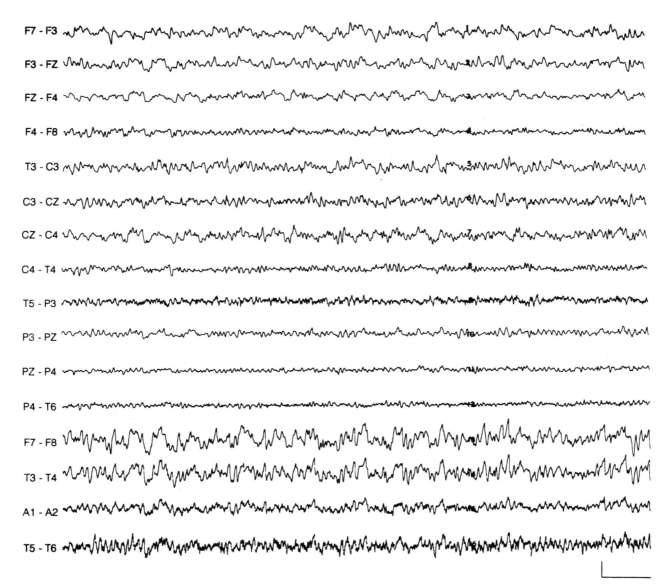

FIG. 7–73. Left frontal-central-temporal delta on a coronal montage. 76 years. Same patient as in Fig. 7–72. In this portion of the tracing, a greater quantity of 2–3 Hz delta activity is evident. The lack of any abnormality on the rightside leads, particularly F8 and T4, indicates that the delta activity in the interhemispheric derivations represents delta activity involving F7 and T3. Therefore, the lack of more prominent delta activity in the T3-C3 and C3-Cz derivations (combined with prominent delta in the Cz-C4 derivation) suggests partial cancellation at these areas and therefore T3, C3, and Cz involvement in the delta activity. The field of the frontally originating delta activity is slightly simpler, with involvement of F7 (F7-F3 and F7-F8 derivations), F3 (F7-F3 and F3-Fz derivations), and Fz (Fz-F4 derivation and not F4-F8). Calibration signal 1 sec, 50μV.

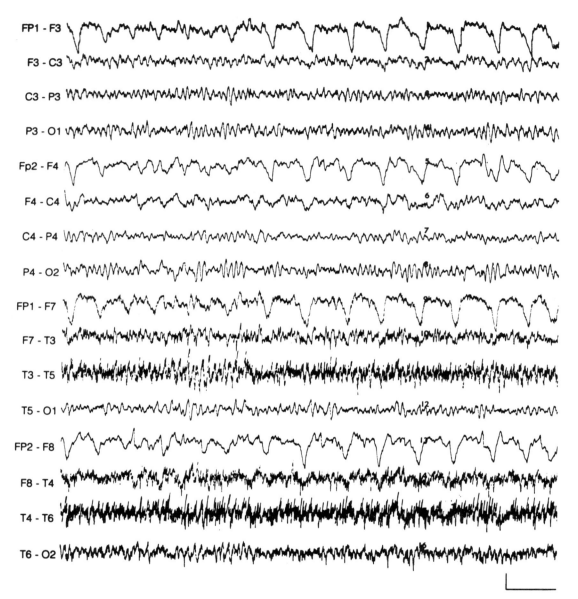

FIG. 7–74. Focal delta activity within eye blink and muscle artifact. 70 years. Frontal delta activity may be partially obscured by vigorous eye blinks, but scrutiny of homologous derivations will reveal its presence. Note the delta activity at Fp2-F4, F4-C4, and F8-T4 derivations and minimally elsewhere: compare with homologous left derivations. Bitemporal theta and muscle artifact complicate the picture. Calibration signal 1 sec, 50μV.

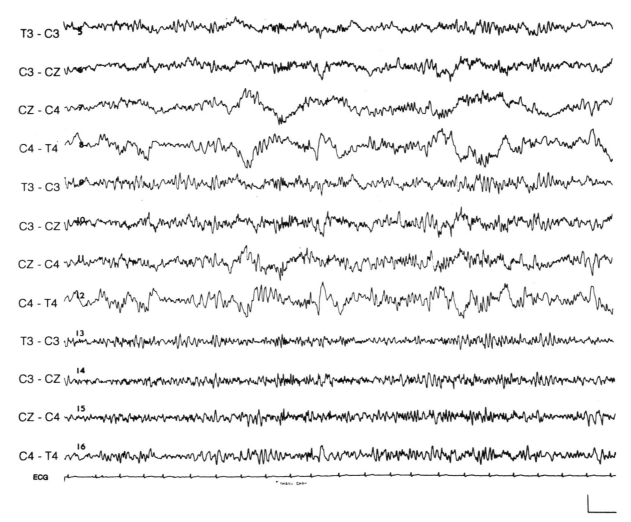

FIG. 7–75. Effect of low-frequency filters (LFF) on delta activity. 75 years. Very-low-frequency delta activity at C4 is moderately attenuated by changing the LFF from 0.3 Hz (*channels 1–4*) to 1 Hz (*channels 5–8*), whereas the higher-frequency delta activity is within both of these LFF ranges. Increasing the LLF to 5 Hz (*channels 9–12*) obliterates the delta. Excess regional theta activity almost always accompanies focal delta and is less attenuated by low-frequency filtering: compare C4 with C3 in each tracing. Note slower paper speed. Calibration signal 1 sec, 70μV.

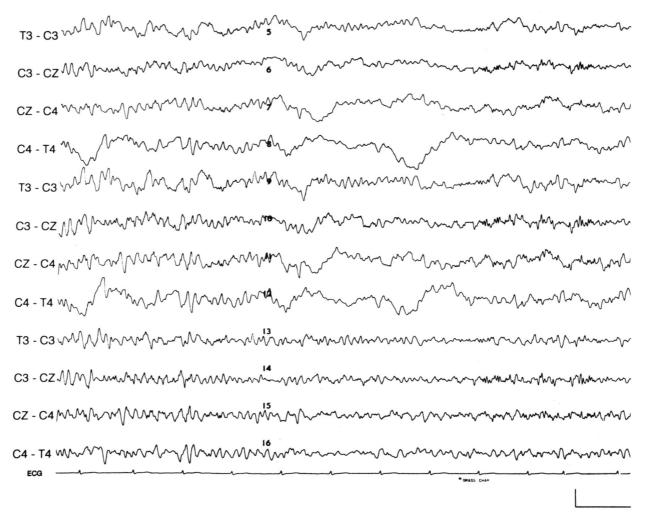

FIG. 7–76. Effect of low-frequency filters on delta activity. 75 years. Usual (3 cm/sec) paper speed. Same filtering sequence as Fig.7–75 has less effect because of higher delta frequency. Only a slight attenuation of the delta activity is evident by increasing the LLF from 0.3 Hz (*top four channels*) to 1 Hz (*middle four channels*), whereas the delta activity is abolished by increasing the LLF to 5 Hz (*lower four channels*). Calibration signal 1 sec, 70μV.

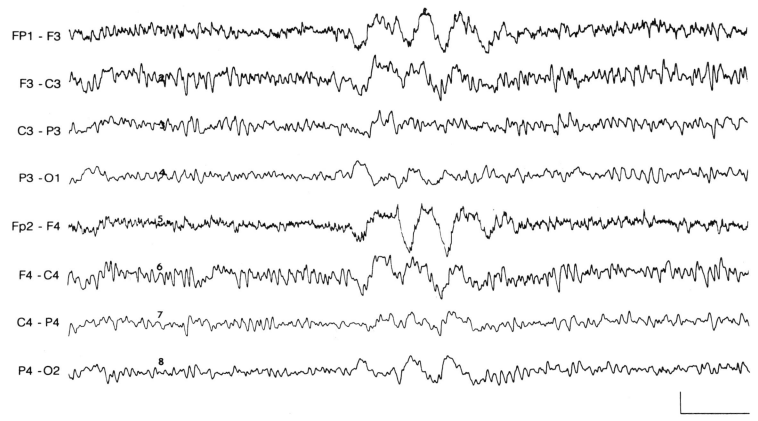

FIG. 7–77. Intermittent rhythmic delta activity (IRDA). 66 years. From a background containing a mild excess of diffuse theta occurs a high-voltage burst of frontally predominant 1.5–2 Hz waves lasting about 2 seconds. This is characteristic of IRDA in adults: a brief burst of diffuse rhythmic delta activity, maximum frontally. Within the frontal region, such activity in this tracing appears principally in the frontal polar region, as in most instances of this phenomenon. However, the superior frontal region also participates moderately, as evidenced by the occasional "phase reversals" at F3 and F4. Calibration signal 1 sec, 50μV.

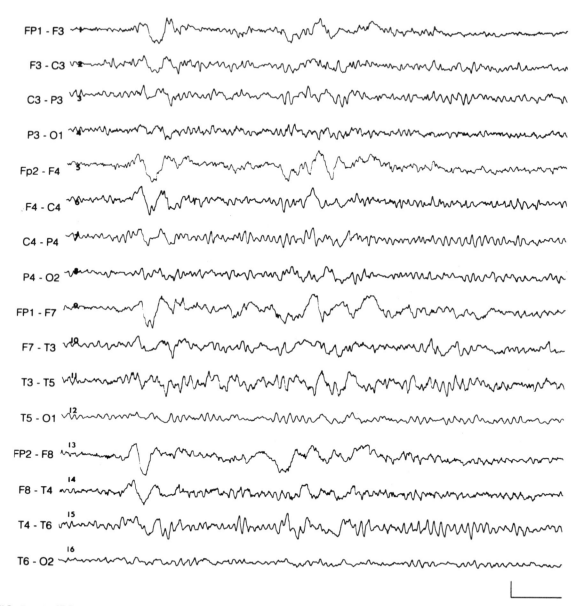

FIG. 7–78. IRDA and focal delta. 74 years. Faced with prominent IRDA, the electroencephalographer should always seek the presence of an accompanying regional abnormality. Note the arrhythmic delta activity in the left anterior-midtemporal (F7-T3) region with left parasagittal spread. Calibration signal 1 sec, 50μV.

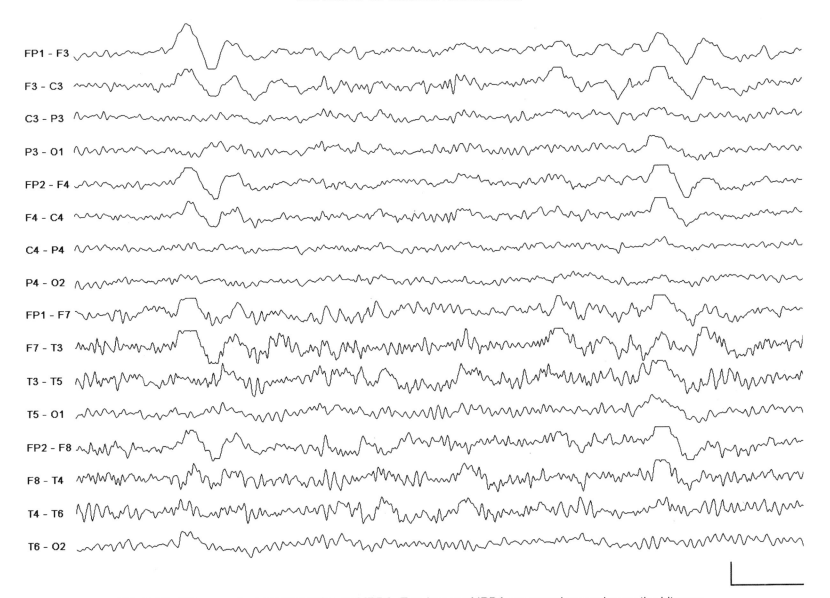

FIG. 7–79. Bitemporal persistent delta and IRDA. Two bursts of IRDA are superimposed upon the bitemporally accentuated, more persistent delta activity. Calibration signal 1 sec, 50μV.

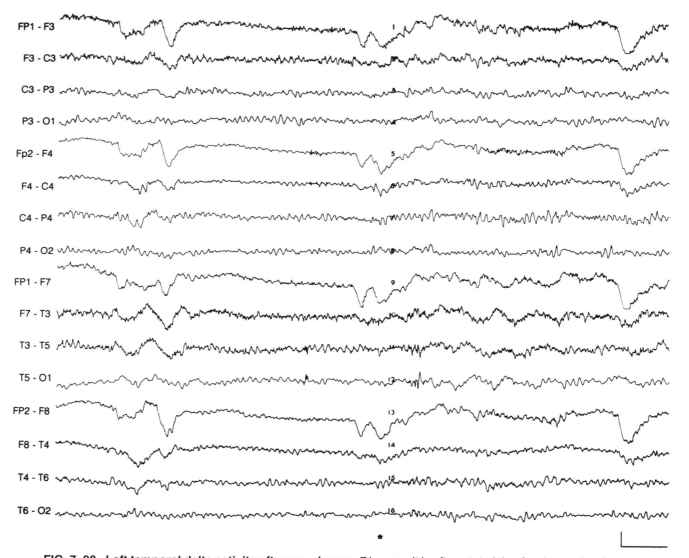

FIG. 7–80. Left temporal delta activity after eye closure. 71 years. It is often stated that focal or regional delta activity is minimally affected by eye opening or closure, but this is often not the case, as illustrated here. With the eyes open, no regional delta activity appears—only the nonlocalizing intermittent rhythmic delta activity (IRDA). Upon eye closure (*asterisk*) regional T3-T5 delta appears, spreads moderately to F7, C3, and P3 and persists. Calibration signal 1 sec, 50μV.

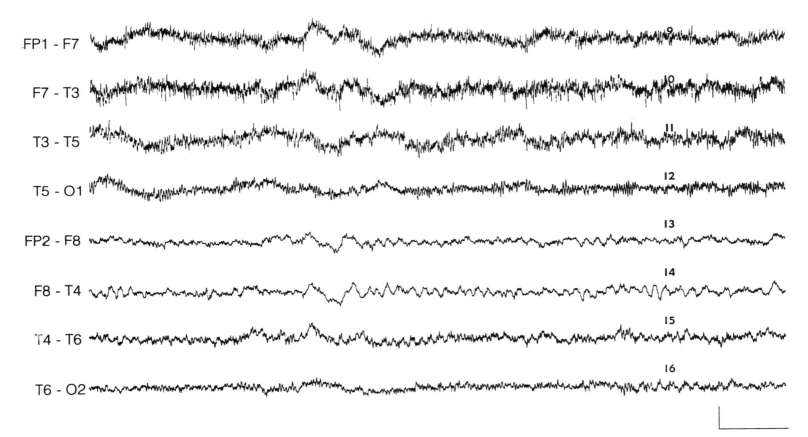

FIG. 7–81. Focal persistent delta and intermittent rhythmic delta activity. 68 years. The existence of nonlocalizing intermittent rhythmic delta activity, seen here in the 4th second, should not impede the recognition of more persistent, usually slower regional delta activity at F7-T3, which is localizing for cerebral dysfunction. Once again, a significant focal abnormality resides in the area of principal muscle artifact; Murphy's Law of EEG. Calibration signal 1 sec, 50μV.

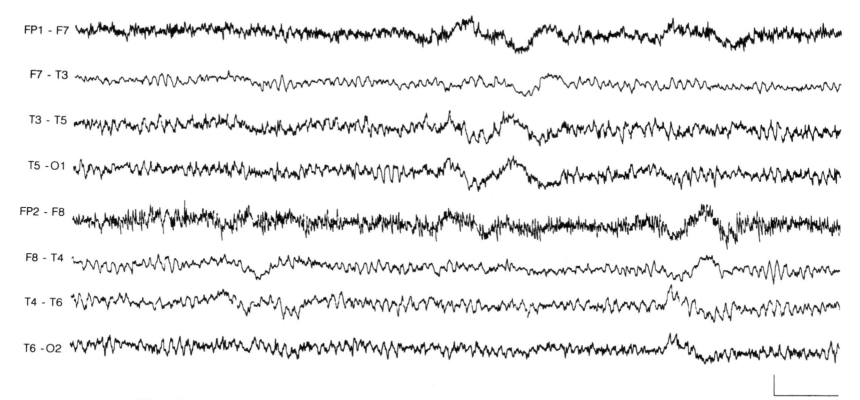

FP1 - F7

F7 - T3

T3 - T5

T5 - O1

FP2 - F8

F8 - T4

T4 - T6

T6 - O2

FIG. 7–82. Intermittent rhythmic delta activity in the temporal regions. 78 years. Intermittent rhythmic delta in the temporal regions is an abnormal finding in the elderly (12). Independently occurring bursts of such activity appear in both the right and left temporal regions in this sample. As does most delta activity, which is rhythmic and intermittent, the background activity is minimally disturbed. Glossokinetic artifact could resemble such waves, but usually a burst of muscle potentials will occur and the slow waves are usually bilaterally synchronous. Calibration signal 1 sec, 50μV.

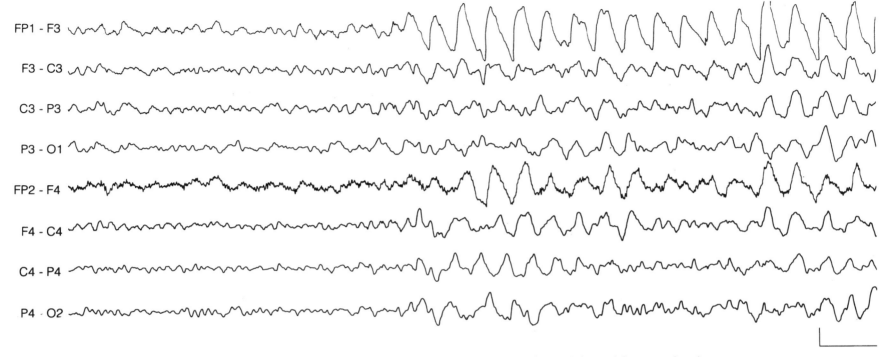

FIG. 7–83. Left hemisphere delta activity, then IRDA. 20 years. Leftside delta activity precedes the more prominent bilaterally synchronous IRDA. Calibration signal 1 sec, 70μV.

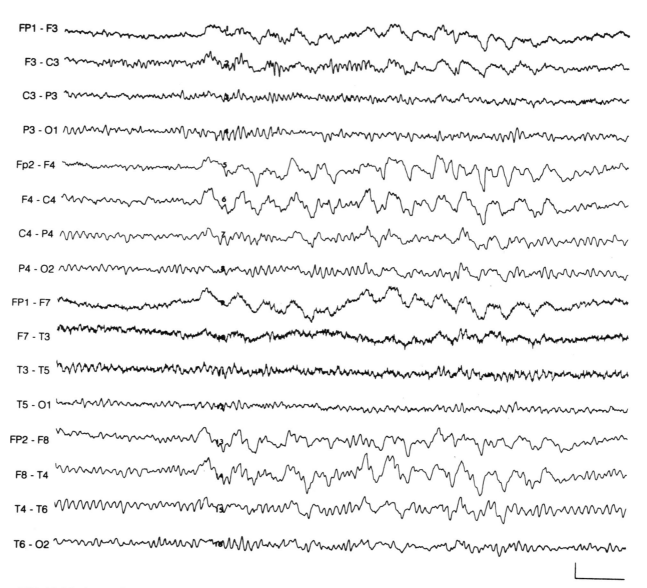

FIG. 7–84. Intermittent rhythmic delta activity (IRDA) and focal delta. 69 years. Bilaterally synchronous rhythmic to semirhythmic medium-high-voltage delta activity of abrupt onset and offset is often associated with diffuse encephalopathies. However, it may also be associated with regional lesions in one hemisphere. Several aspects of this tracing suggest a right frontal focal abnormality underlying the IRDA: (a) its greater amplitude and posterior extension on the right, (b) the attenuation of rightside background rhythms such as mu, and (c) the very low-voltage-theta preceding and following the IRDA burst, as seen principally in the F4-C4 derivation. Calibration signal 1 sec, 50μV.

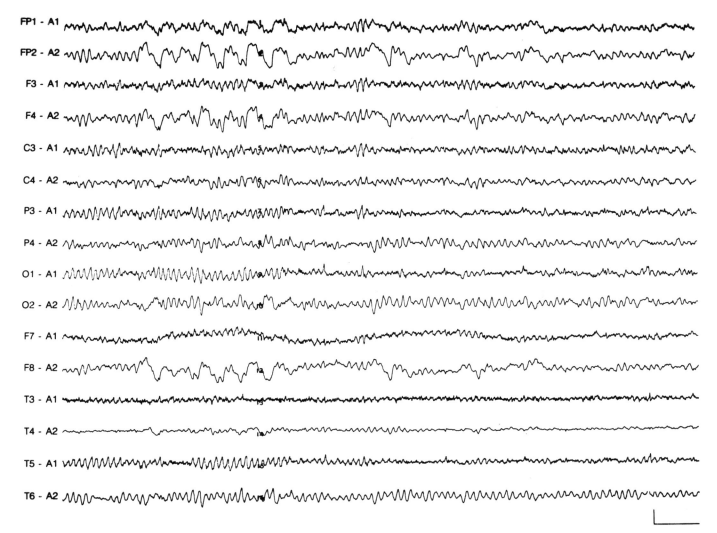

FIG. 7–85. Right frontal IRDA and more persistent delta. 69 years. Same patient as in Fig. 7–84. The IRDA is followed by lower-voltage, longer-duration and more persistent delta waves in the right frontal region (Fp2, F8, F4). The very slow waves in the F7-A1 derivation are slow eye movements. Calibration signal 1 sec, 50μV.

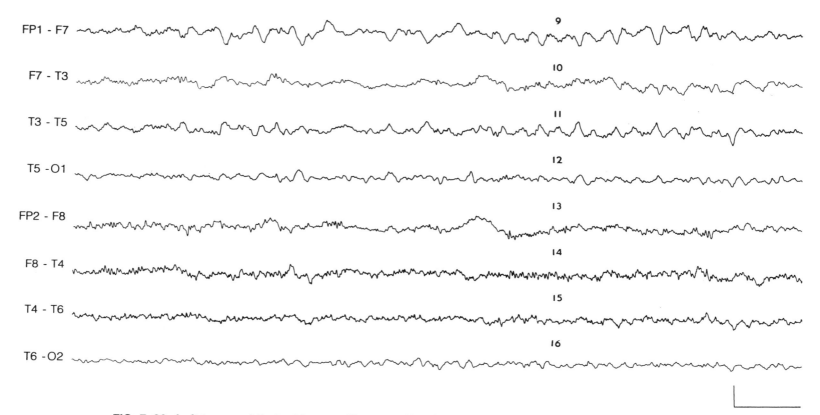

FIG. 7–86. Left temporal theta. 35 years. Here, 4–5 Hz left anterior-midtemporal (F7-T3) theta appears. The contribution of slow eye movements to the delta activity in the F7-T3 derivation is difficult to establish on this montage. Beta activity is appropriately lower in the left temporal region compared to the right (F7-T3 vs. F8-T4 derivations). The patient is drowsy, as evidenced by posterior theta. Calibration signal 1 sec, 50µV.

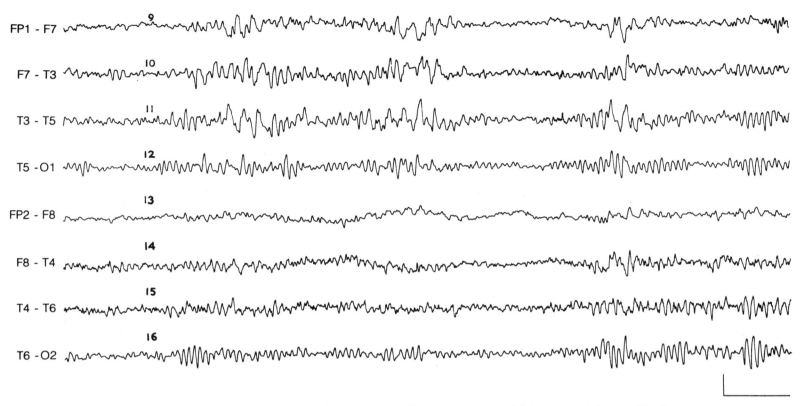

FIG. 7–87. Focal left temporal theta activity. 35 years. The small amount of right temporal theta activity is normal, but that in the left temporal region (F7-T3) is too abundant in incidence and amplitude to be considered normal. Unfortunately, assessing the quantity of theta activity in the left temporal region is more difficult than on the right because of its normally greater quantity on the left. While this quantity of theta activity is clearly abnormal at age 35 years, it would be abnormal even in the seventh decade; Katz and Horowitz (53) found minimal focal slow activity in normal elderly subjects. Calibration signal 1 sec, 70µV.

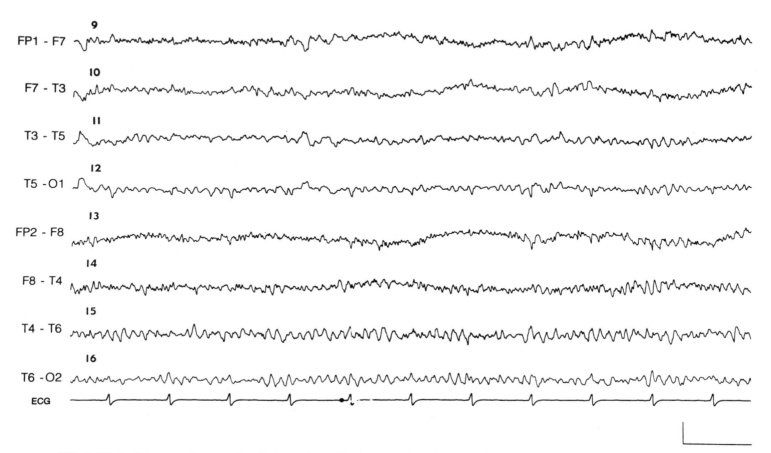

FIG. 7–88. Left temporal excessive theta and amplitude reduction. 68 years. Two focal abnormalities appear in the left temporal region (F7 and T3 with spread to T5): a mild excess of 4–6 Hz theta activity and a reduction of 7–8 Hz activity in the left temporal and (probably) left occipital regions. Calibration signal 1 sec, 50μV.

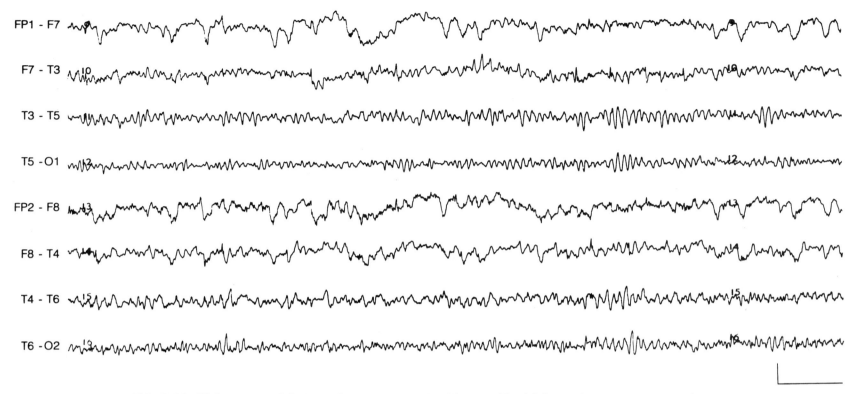

FIG. 7–89. Right temporal theta and eye movements. 44 years. Eye blinks or slower eye movements can sometimes obscure focal abnormalities. However, careful comparison of homologous derivations reveals 4–6 Hz medium-voltage waves at F8 and T4 without spread to T6. The minimal 7–10 Hz waves at F7 are normal. The very brief apiculate waves at Fp1 and Fp2 are eye movement artifacts. Calibration signal 1 sec, 50μV.

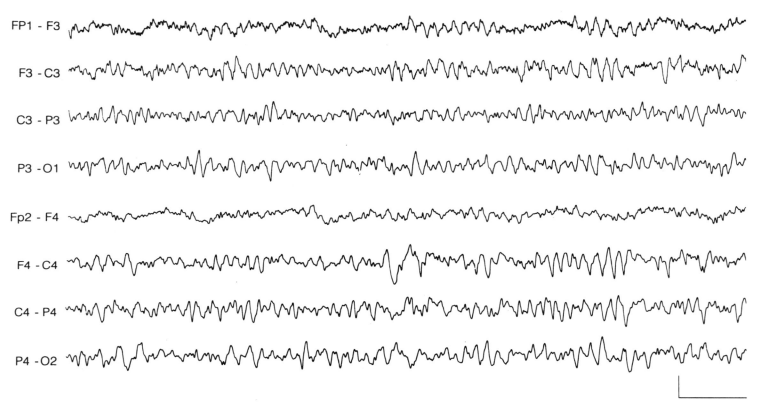

FP1 - F3

F3 - C3

C3 - P3

P3 - O1

Fp2 - F4

F4 - C4

C4 - P4

P4 - O2

FIG. 7–90. Focal and diffuse theta. 29 years. A focal abnormality within a diffuse abnormality is discerned by comparing homologous derivations for the persistence of any excess theta or delta activity in one area throughout most of the tracing. The 6 Hz diffuse theta does not obscure the persistent focal 3–6 Hz theta at C4 and P4. Calibration signal 1 sec, 70μV.

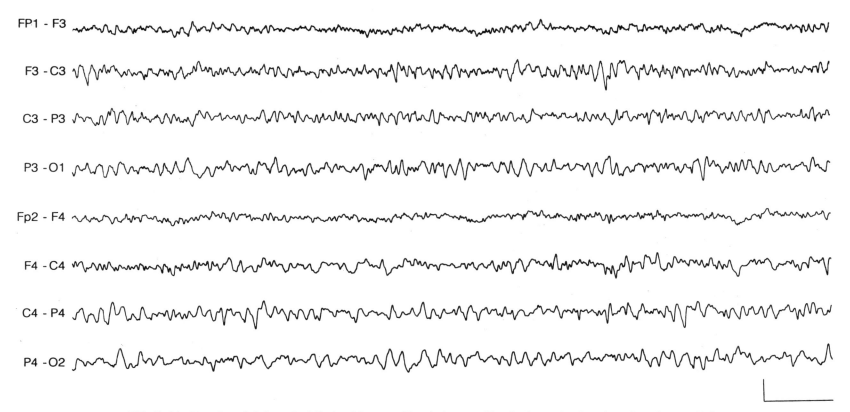

FIG. 7–91. Focal parietal-central theta. 29 years. Focal abnormalities in the parietal region often do not attain high amplitude and therefore can be overlooked. The 5–6 Hz theta is far more persistent at P4 and C4 than at C3 and P3, indicating focal right parietal-central dysfunction. Beta activity extends more posteriorly on the left compared to right. Calibration signal 1 sec, 100μV.

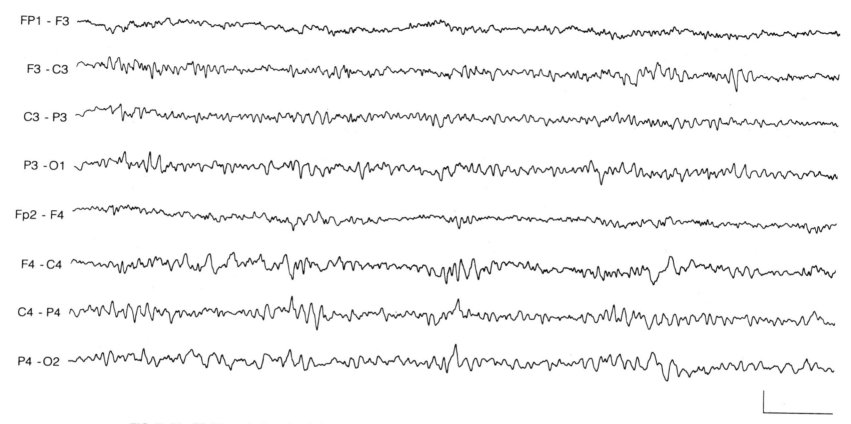

FIG. 7–92. Right central-parietal theta. 29 years. Here, 3–7 Hz theta appears in the right central-parietal (C4-P4) regions. Its minimal expression in homologous areas of the left does not indicate bilateral abnormality. Note the very-low-voltage subtle delta activity underlying such moderately prominent theta, also at C4-P4. Calibration signal 1 sec, 100μV.

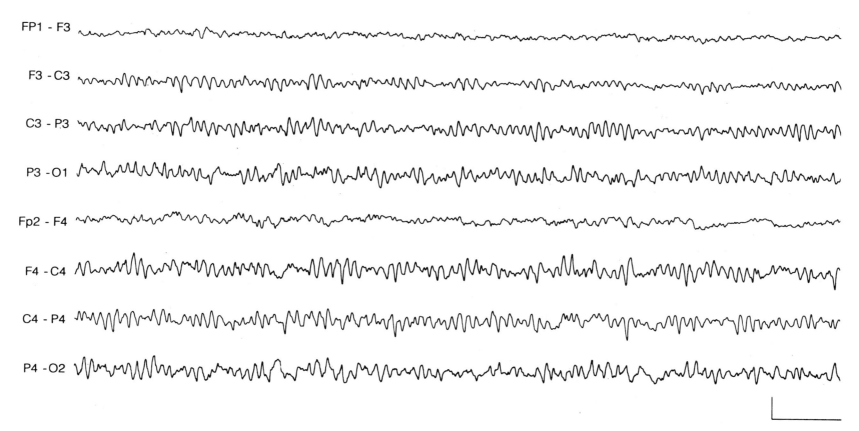

FIG. 7–93. Right central-parietal theta and delta. 31 years. Background activity in the right central-parietal regions (C4 and P4) is slightly interrupted by 5–7 Hz theta and very-low-voltage (approximately 1 Hz) delta activity. The latter can be realized by viewing the tracing from a greater distance. Its minimal presence in the left parietal (P3) region does not indicate an additional abnormality there. The relatively normal alpha activity suggests that the process does not engulf the right occipital lobe. None of the sharply contoured waves is a spike, as they are simply combinations of background rhythms. Calibration signal 1 sec, 70μV.

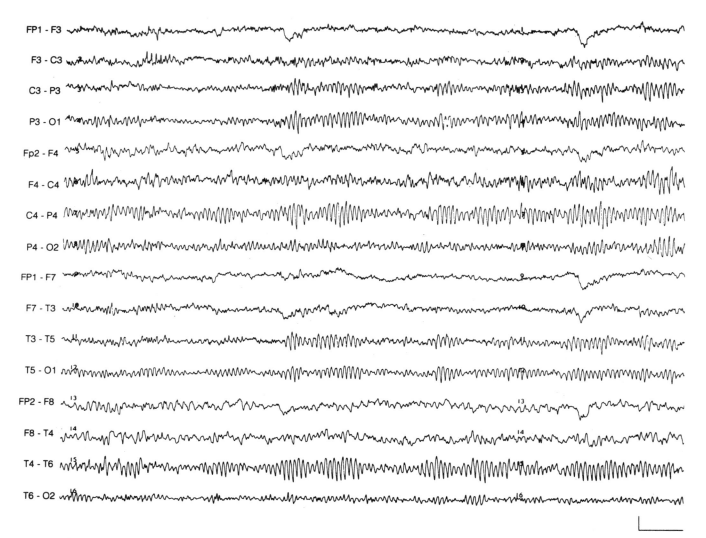

FIG. 7–94. Right frontal theta and delta. 70 years. Although 6 Hz theta is clearly depicted in the right inferior frontal (F8) lead, beta and mu activity involving the Fp2-F4 and F4-C4 derivations hide it well. Lurking underneath the theta is low-amplitude delta activity in the same area. Calibration signal 1 sec, 50μV.

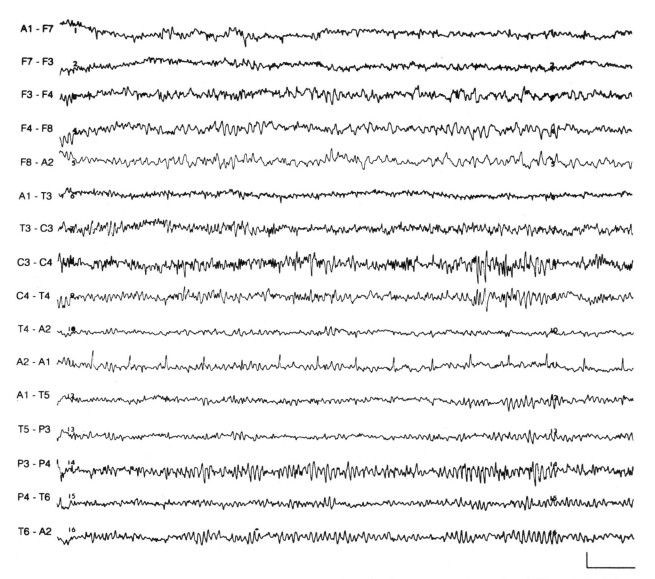

FIG. 7–95. Focal theta on a coronal montage. 70 years. Despite the presence of occasional diffuse theta, this moderately persistent semirhythmic theta at F4 and F8 is well depicted on this coronal montage. Note its virtual absence more posteriorly. The markedly apiculate wave forms at C4 and elsewhere are not spikes but simply combinations of background waveforms. Slow, lateral eye movements produce delta at F7 and F8. Alpha is slightly higher ipsilateral to the abnormality, as may occur with anterior dysfunction. Calibration signal 1 sec, 50μV.

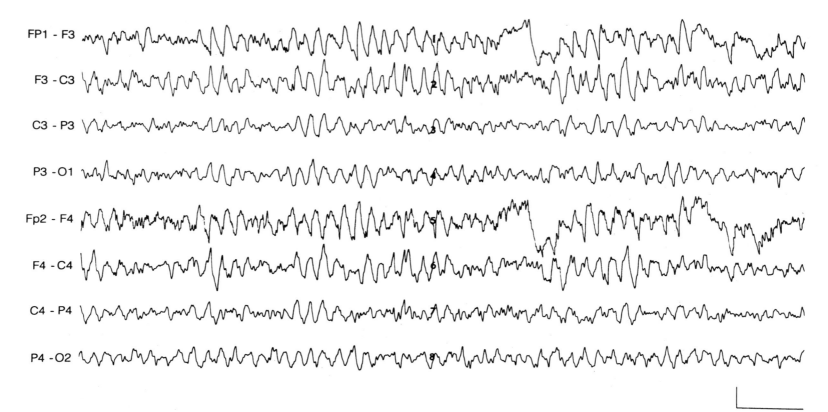

FIG. 7–96. Excess diffuse theta. 22 years. A moderate excess of diffuse 5 Hz theta and a mild excess of frontally dominant 15–20 Hz beta characterize this awake recording. It is unlikely that significant drowsiness creates such diffuse theta, because of the relatively abrupt eye movements seen in the Fp1,2-F3,4 derivations. Nonetheless, drowsiness should always be considered when assessing the quantity of diffuse theta. Calibration signal 1 sec, 50μV.

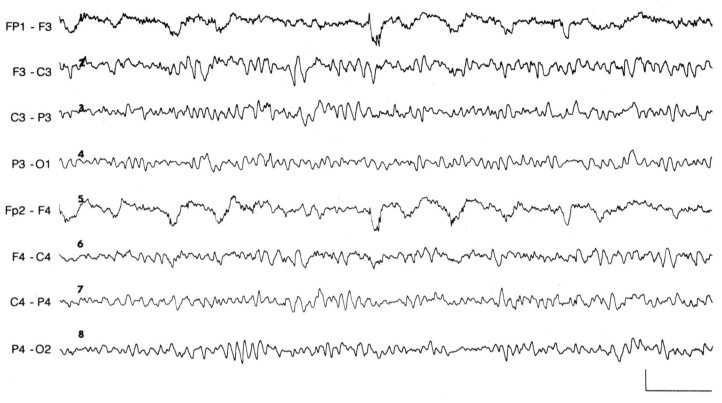

FIG. 7–97. Mild excess theta diffusely. 18 years. Although the alpha activity attains 9 Hz, there is an excess quantity of 3–5 Hz and some 7 Hz theta activity diffusely in this awake tracing. Calibration signal 1 sec, 50μV.

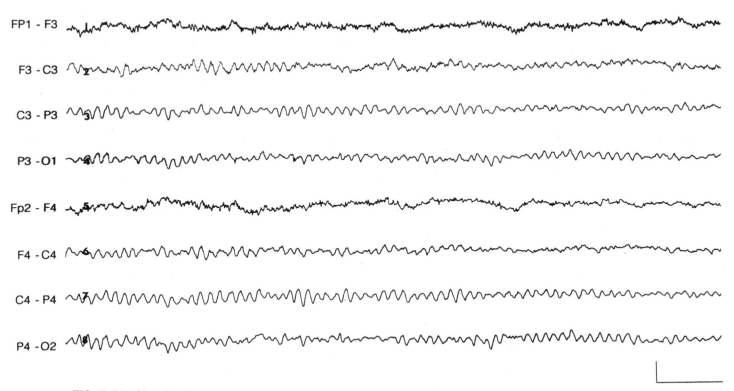

FIG. 7–98. Slow background rhythm. 46 years. At 7–8 Hz, this background rhythm is clearly below the normal alpha frequency (12). As no other abnormality appears in this segment, medication or metabolic factors which could slow the alpha rhythm should be sought such as a high phenytoin serum level and hypothyroidism. Calibration signal 1 sec, 50μV.

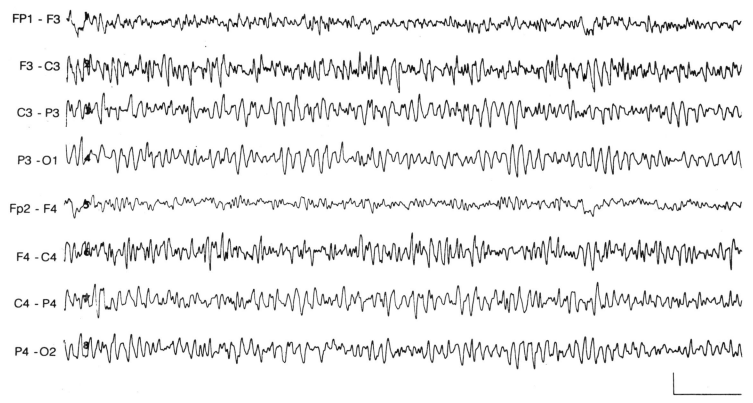

FIG. 7–99. Medication effect. 73 years. Benzodiazepines or barbiturates could be responsible for all the modifications in this sample. The most prominent is frontally dominant, symmetrical, approximately 20 Hz beta activity. The background rhythm posteriorly has slowed to 7–8 Hz. A slight excess of diffuse theta activity also appears. The rich mixture of waveforms produce sharply contoured waves which are not spikes. Calibration signal 1 sec, 50μV.

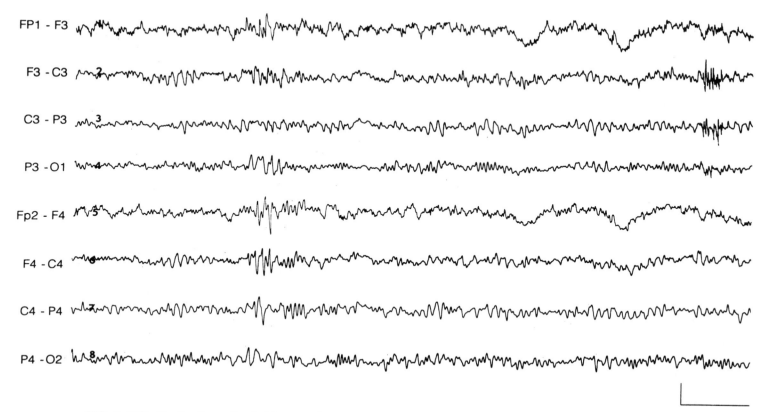

FIG. 7–100. Medication effect. 33 years. Benzodiazepines, barbiturates, and other medications augment the quantity of beta activity and, to a lesser extent, theta. Both these effects are evident here. The complex mixture of frequencies creates sharply contoured waves as seen in the 3rd second. These are unlikely spikes because of this factor and because of the lack of aftercoming slow waves. Therefore, no aspect of this sample suggests cerebral dysfunction beyond the medication effect. Calibration signal 1 sec, 50µV.

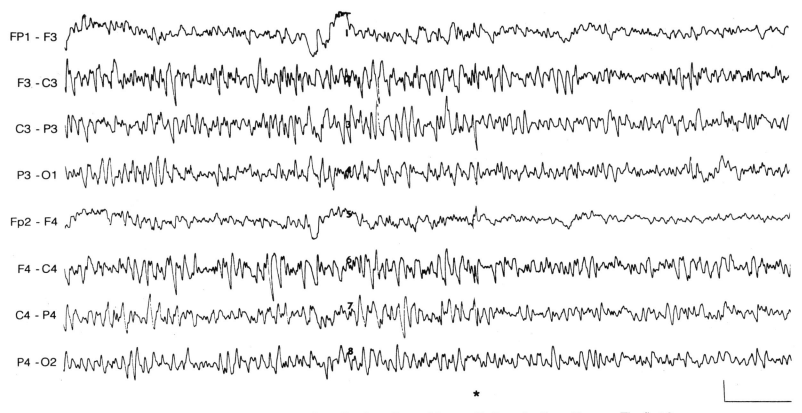

FIG. 7–101. Change in appearance of medication effect with sensitivity reduction. 49 years. The first 6 seconds of this sample show medication effect in abundance: diffuse 20 Hz beta activity, principally anteriorly, intermixed with 4–7 Hz diffuse theta. These features become less striking and certainly less apiculate when the sensitivity is reduced from 50 μV/10mm to 70 μV/10mm (*asterisk*). All of the changes seen here could result from medication effect, and none indicates inherent cerebral dysfunction. Calibration signal 1 sec, 50μV (*left*) and 70μV (*right*).

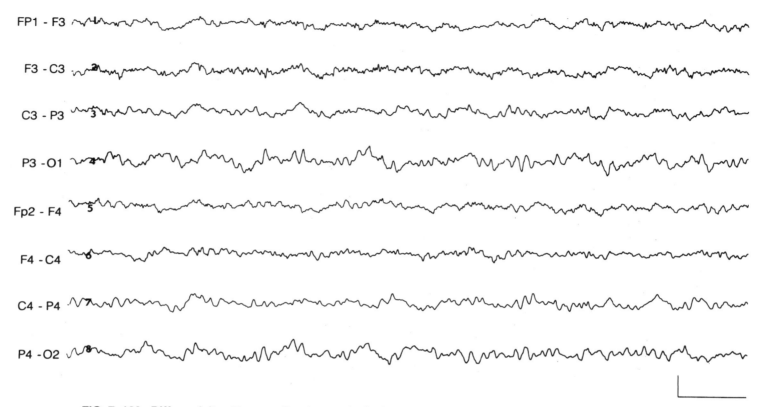

FIG. 7–102. Diffuse delta. 63 years. Continuous rhythmic to semirhythmic medium-voltage diffuse delta activity is abnormal in wakefulness and drowsiness at any age after early infancy. Note the virtually symmetrical background activity in each hemisphere underlying the delta. Calibration signal 1 sec, 50μV.

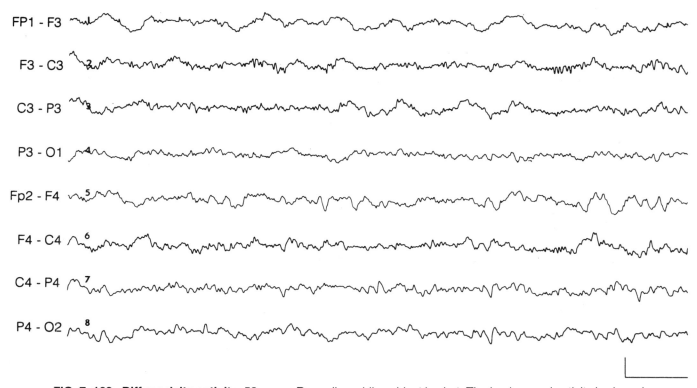

FIG. 7–103. Diffuse delta activity. 53 years. Recording while subject is alert. The background activity is slowed and disorganized. There is an abnormal amount of delta activity diffusely, slightly more in the left hemisphere compared to the right. This would be consistent with a metabolic or toxic encephalopathy with an overriding left hemisphere regional abnormality, or a primary dementing process with initial regional accentuation. Calibration signal 1 sec, 50μV.

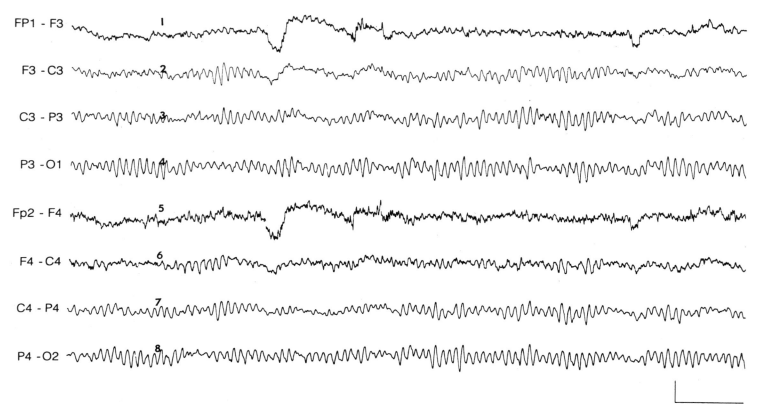

FIG. 7–104. Normal bilateral delta. 18 years. For reasons which are not entirely clear, intermittent or even persistent low-amplitude rhythmic delta activity may appear in the parasagittal regions of normal EEGs as seen principally in the C3-P3 and C4-P4 derivations. The low voltage and bilaterality of the delta and the presence of completely normal rhythms otherwise indicate that such activity is a normal variant. Calibration signal 1 sec, 50μV.

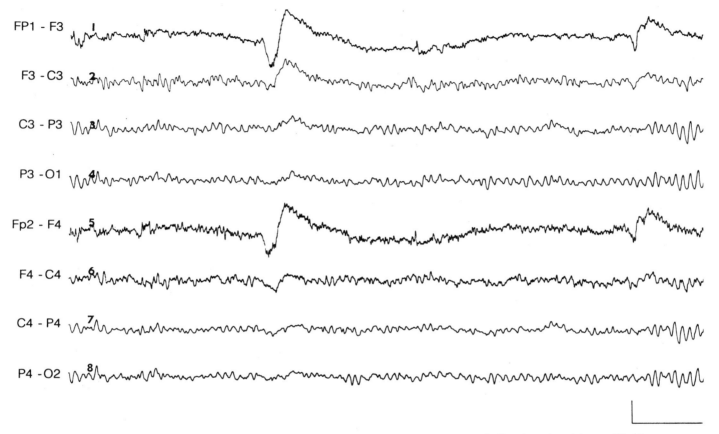

FIG. 7–105. Normal bilateral delta. Continuation of recording in Fig. 7–104. Calibration signal 1 sec, 50μV.

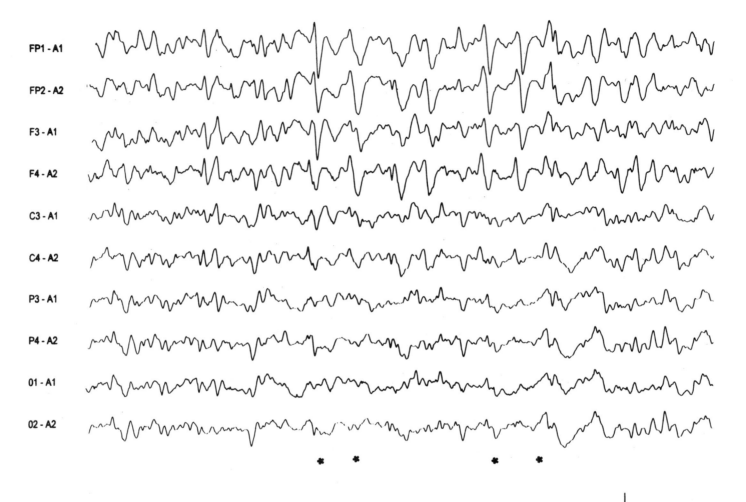

FIG. 7–106. Triphasic waves and diffuse delta. This referential montage depicts the frontally predominant triphasic waves (*asterisks*) together with diffuse delta activity. The low-voltage apiculate waves at A2 may represent ECG. Calibration signal 1 sec, 100μV.

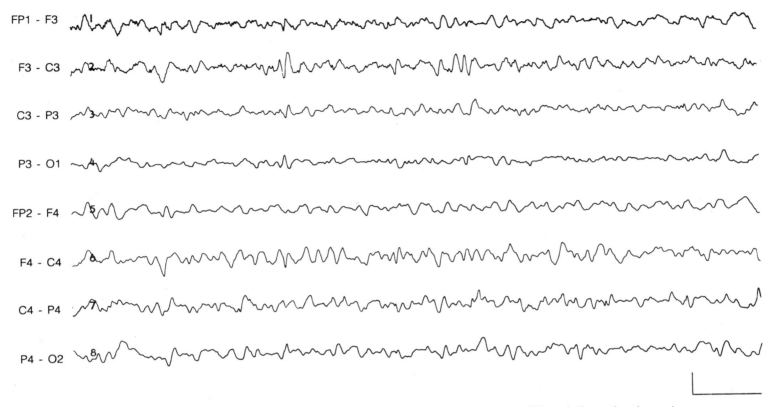

FIG. 7–107. Jakob-Creutzfeldt disease without diffuse discharges. 65 years. Although the patient is awake with eyes closed, the background is slow and disorganized and excess theta and some delta activity appear diffusely. Potentials are generally lower in the left hemisphere compared to the right, but this asymmetry may be seen in some patients with degenerative conditions. This constellation of findings does not distinguish Alzheimer's disease from Jakob-Creutzfeldt disease and can be found in encephalopathies from other causes. However, the low-voltage spike in the left parietal-central (P3, C3) region is a feature seen less commonly in Alzheimer's disease than in Jakob-Creutzfeldt disease (54). Calibration signal 1 sec, 70μV.

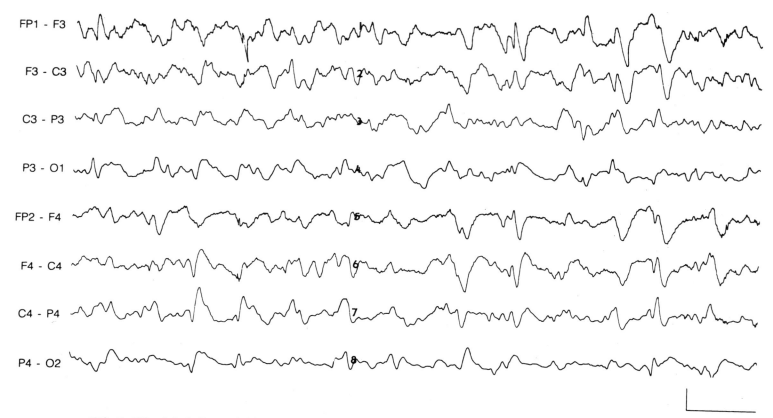

FIG. 7–108. Jakob-Creutzfeldt disease with diffuse discharges. 65 years. Same recording as in Fig. 7–107. Diffuse delta activity has augmented considerably, and bilaterally synchronous spike and slow-wave complexes have appeared. This finding would favor Jakob-Creutzfeldt disease as the etiology of the dementia. Calibration signal 1 sec, 70μV.

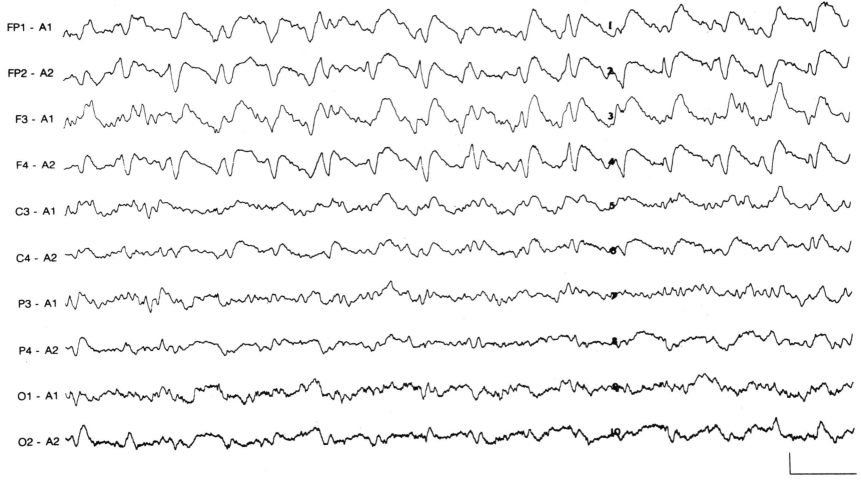

FIG. 7–109. Periodic spikes and diffuse delta; Jakob-Creutzfeldt disease. 67 years. Periodic spikes on ear reference montage. These discharges share some characteristics of triphasic waves and therefore could represent rapidly progressive Alzheimer's disease. Note the diffuse delta and the right frontal (Fp2, F4) accentuation of the periodic discharges. Calibration signal 1 sec, 100μV.

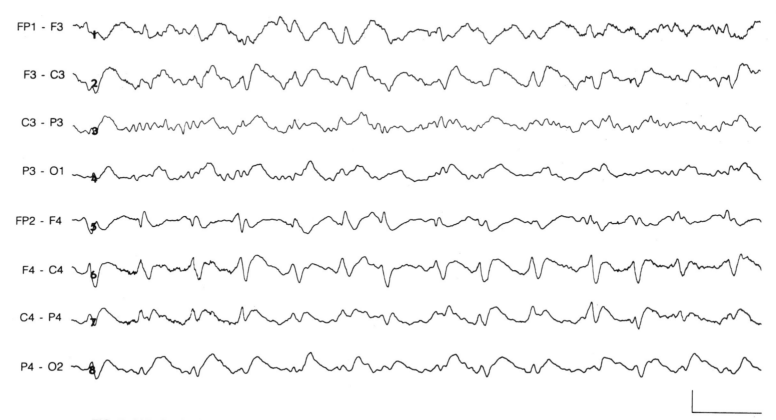

FP1 - F3

F3 - C3

C3 - P3

P3 - O1

FP2 - F4

F4 - C4

C4 - P4

P4 - O2

FIG. 7–110. Periodic spikes in Jakob-Creutzfeldt disease. 67 years. Disorganized background, diffuse delta activity, and periodic broad spikes are all characteristic of this rapidly developing dementia. Such discharges may be asymmetrical or predominate over one region, the right frontal area in this instance (54). This patient was normal until 1 month prior to the recording when forgetfulness, disorientation, apathy, and synchronous twitching of the arms began. Calibration signal 1 sec, 100μV.

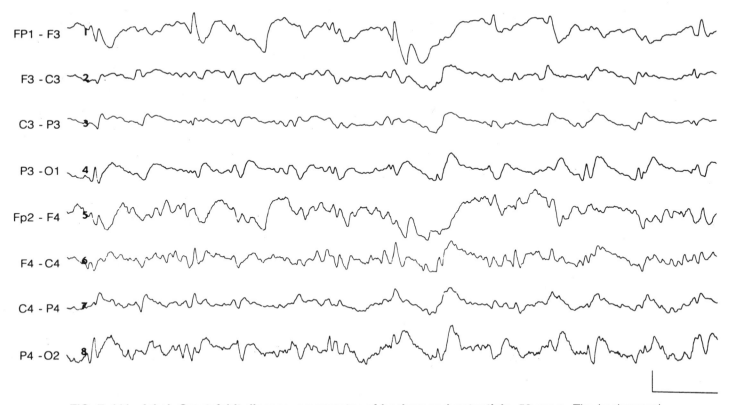

FIG. 7–111. Jakob-Creutzfeldt disease: asymmetry of background potentials. 58 years. The background activity is disorganized and there is an excess amount of diffuse delta activity. As may occur with dementing illness, one hemisphere may be more affected than another; in this instance the background potentials are considerably more attenuated in the left hemisphere compared to the right. A clue to the etiology of the dementia is the frequent multifocal spikes, some of which are synchronous and which repeat at a fairly regular rate. Such discharges suggest Jakob-Creutzfeldt disease, because epileptiform discharges are an unusual feature of Alzheimer's disease (55). This patient had a 1-month history of memory impairment, confusion, rightside visual neglect, and left-right confusion. Calibration signal 1 sec, 70μV.

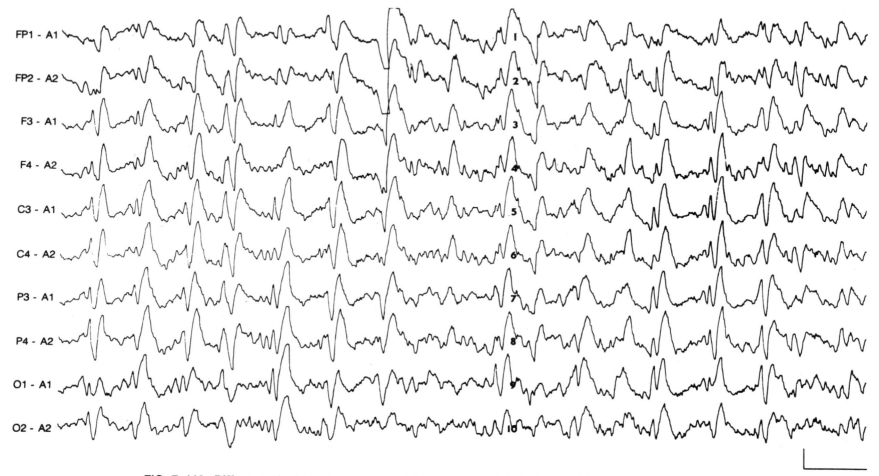

FP1 - A1

FP2 - A2

F3 - A1

F4 - A2

C3 - A1

C4 - A2

P3 - A1

P4 - A2

O1 - A1

O2 - A2

FIG. 7–112. Diffuse periodic spike-waves and delta activity; Jakob-Creutzfeldt disease. 58 years. Same recording as in Fig. 7–111, now in drowsiness on referential montage. The spikes and spike-waves have become more evidently periodic and are more diffuse. Calibration signal 1 sec, 70μV.

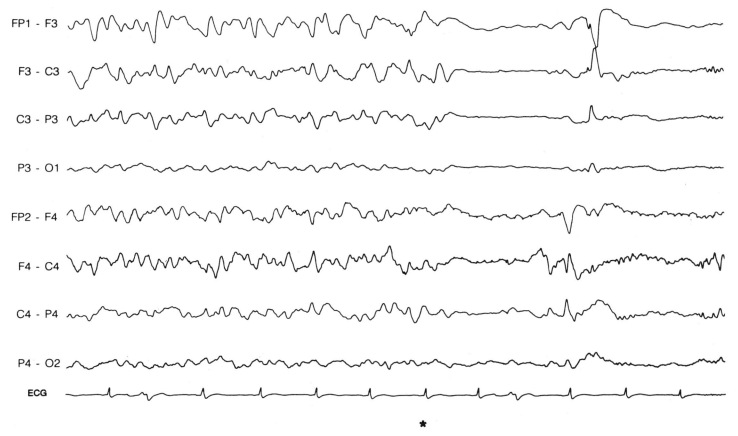

FIG. 7–113. Attenuation with afferent stimuli; Jakob-Creutzfeldt disease. 76 years. This patient became confused and ataxic 1 month prior to this recording. At the time of this awake recording, she was severely demented. Background activity is disorganized and there is diffuse excess delta activity. Afferent stimuli (*asterisk*) attenuated the recording diffusely; right central (C4) and left superior frontal (F3) spikes occurred. The EEG in severe encephalopathies in adulthood may revert in some respects to those of earlier ages. For example, the attenuation with afferent stimuli is similar to that which appears in newborns (56). Calibration signal 1 sec, 100μV.

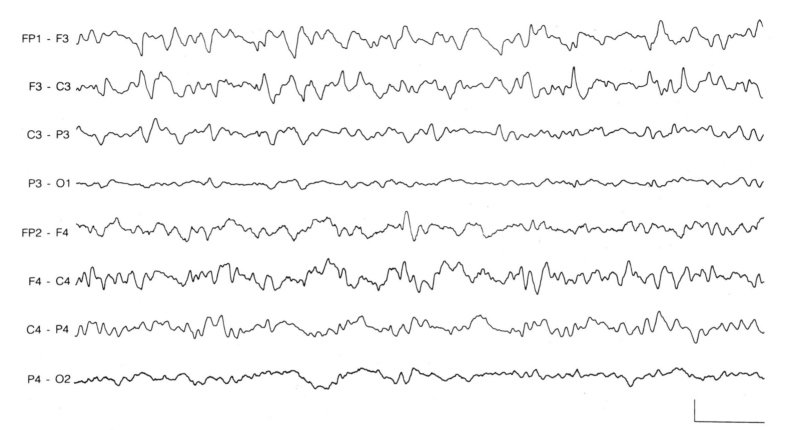

FIG. 7–114. Diffuse delta with dementia. 76 years. In this awake recording, background activity is disorganized and largely replaced by diffuse delta and theta. This pattern is not characteristic of any specific type of encephalopathy: a metabolic encephalopathy or primary dementing process could produce this. Calibration signal 1 sec, 100μV.

Chapter 8

EEG in the Intensive Care Unit (ICU)

Applications of EEG in the ICU (57)
- Assessment of seizures, especially nonconvulsive seizures.
- Monitoring the effects of therapies, for example, treatment of seizures, degree of sedation.
- Appraisal of the severity of illness in various encephalopathies.
- Monitoring the course of brain dysfunction.
- Diagnosis of broad categories of illness, for example, seizures, metabolic encephalopathy, drug intoxications, psychogenic unresponsiveness, and some specific conditions, for example, herpes simplex encephalitis.
- Prognosis of comatose survivors of conditions that can cause neuronal death, especially anoxic-ischemic encephalopathy (58).
- Special studies of sensory pathways and processing: requires computer averaging.

Clinical Uses of Continuous EEG (CEEG) Monitoring

Comatose patient with an unstable but potentially treatable condition:
- Status epilepticus.
- Recurring seizures.
- Conditions in which intracranial pressure is elevated or cerebral perfusion is variable (various neurosurgical conditions including posttraumatic coma, subarachnoid hemorrhage, tumor, postoperative cases, and hydrocephalus).

Monitoring drug effects:
- The depth of anesthesia achieved with barbiturates used in the treatment of status epilepticus.
- Depth of sedation in other patients.

Application of Serial EEGs in the ICU
- Trending, especially when CEEG is not available.

- Prognostication after cardiac arrest.
- Assessment of nonconvulsive seizures.

Application of Quantitative EEG (Power Spectral Analysis) in ICU
- Trending over longer periods of time: objectively examines variability, charts the course of encephalopathies, and detects sudden changes such as those produced by seizures.
- Caveat: Purely quantitative studies may miss major morphologic phenomena in EEG; for example, triphasic waves, some seizures. Hence the "raw EEG" should always be available along with the spectral plot or brain map.

Some Differences in ICU EEGs Compared to Standard Recordings
- Confounders: drugs (narcotics and benzodiazepines) have profound effects on the EEG and can alter rhythms, variability, and reactivity. These have to be taken into consideration, especially in making prognostic judgments.
- Importance of testing for reactivity and trending for variability in assessing the severity of the encephalopathy: electrographic reactivity and spontaneous variability are relatively favorable features.
- Unusual artifacts, especially with CEEG (usually without documentation as technologist is not present).

Classification (59)

Diffuse Encephalopathies:

EEGs should be classified according to the predominant pattern. These are listed below roughly in their order of severity of abnormality:
- Predominant theta/delta, usually rhythmic bilaterally synchronous, symmetrical and frontally predominant, occupying > 50% of the record, with variability and, usually, reactivity. There is a gradation of severity, as shown in the sequential figures (**Figs. 1–7**). Sometimes there is an association with

469

suppression in the posterior head, an unfavorable feature, if it is not due to scalp edema (**Figs. 8, 9**).

- Triphasic waves: Three phases of increasing duration, with total duration 150–500 msec. The larger-amplitude positive wave is preceded and followed by smaller negative waves. Bilaterally synchronous, usually frontally predominant against an attenuated background; often occur in runs of several (**Fig. 10**). Although triphasic waves are not pathognomonic of any specific encephalopathy, they are most common in hepatic and renal failure and sepsis. They can also be seen in aluminum intoxication, but intervening spike-waves are more characteristic of this condition (**Fig. 11**).
- Spindle coma: Abundant sleep spindles, yet the patient is in coma rather than Stage II sleep, and the EEG does not show normal reactivity. This usually implies that there is some preservation of integrated thalamocortical function. The prognosis tends to be more favorable than that of the alpha/theta coma pattern. However, some patients may not recover if there is severe, concomitant brainstem damage (**Figs. 12, 13**).
- Alpha/theta pattern coma (60): Diffuse, persistent rhythms while patient is in a comatose state, with lack of reactivity. The predominant frequency is in the alpha (8–13 Hz), theta (> 4 but < 8 Hz) or, more commonly, a mixture of both frequency bands. Most often the rhythms are more prominent frontally, except in some cases of brainstem stroke, where they may be more in the posterior head. These patterns are most commonly found in anoxic-ischemic encephalopathy after cardiac arrest. Other causes include trauma, brainstem stroke and intoxications. With the latter, the encephalopathy may be completely reversible. With other causes, the prognosis is usually but not invariably unfavorable (**Figs. 14, 15**).
- Burst-suppression: Generalized flattening at standard sensitivity for 1 second at least every 20 seconds, either without (**Fig. 16**) or with (**Figs. 17–19**) epileptiform discharges within the bursts.
- Suppression: This is usually generalized (lateralized suppression is a special category). Suppression can be moderate (< 20 μV, but > 10 μV) or severe (10 μV) (**Figs. 20, 21**).

Epileptiform Activity:

- This can be focal, multifocal, or generalized. Periodic complexes against a suppressed background constitute a special category, most commonly found in severe anoxic-ischemic encephalopathy (**Figs. 22, 23**).
- Epileptiform discharges can be interictal (**Fig. 24**) or can be components of seizures.
- Seizures follow an evolutionary pattern for > 10 seconds, usually as generalized or focal spikes, sharp waves, periodic lateralized epileptiform discharges (PLEDs), or spike-and-wave at > 3/second (**Figs. 25–27**). If such discharges are at < 3/second, they should show an incrementing or decrementing pattern or abolition following an antiepileptic drug. Some seizures consist not of spikes or sharp waves but of rhythmic waves that show an incrementing onset, decrementing offset, or postdischarge slowing or attenuation.

EEG Artifacts in the ICU (61)

- Faulty electrode: single or multiple scalp, ground, or reference electrodes (see Chapter 2).
- Faulty connections: generalized abnormality that may resemble ground or reference artifacts.
- Exogenous artifacts:
—electronic devices: periodic, short-duration potentials or 60 Hz.
—nonelectronic artifacts (**Figs. 28, 29**).

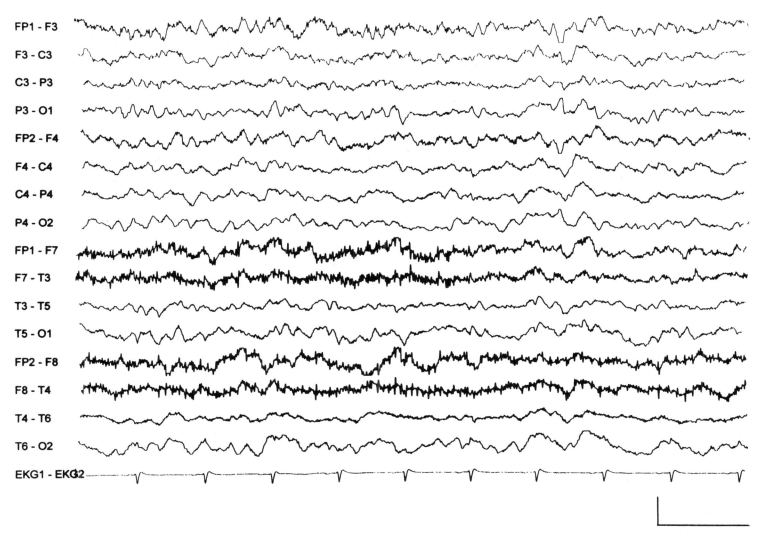

FIG. 8–1. Excessive, diffuse theta. 80 years. Mild septic encephalopathy. The predominant rhythm is theta with some intermittent delta activity, in a diffuse, symmetrical and variable pattern. There is muscle artifact, especially in the 9th, 10th, 13th and 14th channels. Calibration signal 1 sec, 50μV.

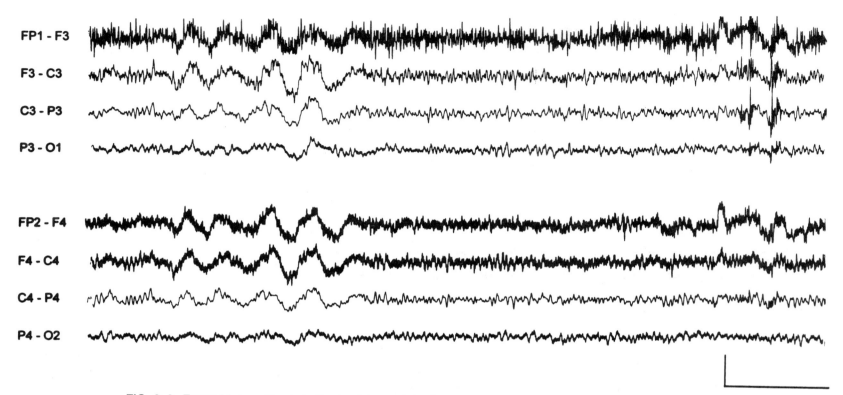

FIG. 8–2. Frontal intermittent rhythmic delta activity (FIRDA). 50 years. Lithium toxicity and mild toxic encephalopathy. There are bursts of FIRDA superimposed on fairly normal background (beta from comedication with benzodiazepines). The patient also showed an abnormal arousal response with FIRDA on arousal. Calibration signal 1 sec, 50μV.

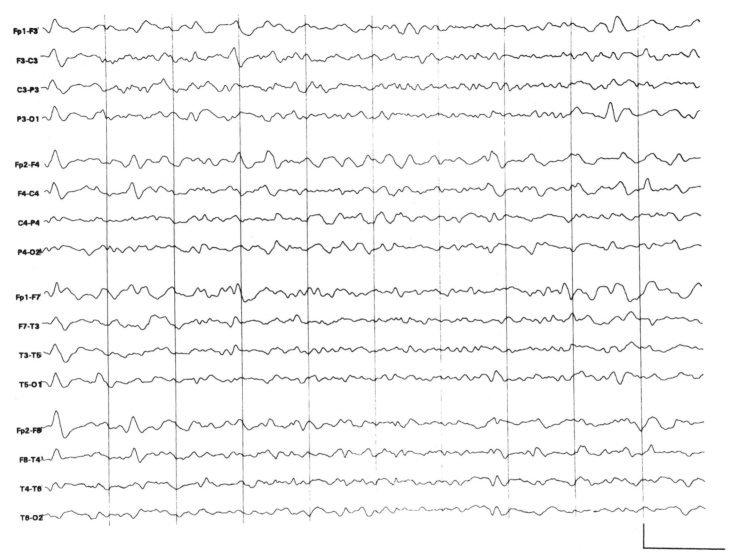

FIG. 8–3. Focal and generalized abnormalities. 62 years. The patient had a ruptured right middle cerebral artery aneurysm and superimposed septic illness. The right cerebral hemisphere has slower frequencies, and a relative absence of the faster frequencies found in the left cerebral hemisphere. It is common in the intensive care unit to find such mixtures of focal and diffuse brain dysfunction. With increasing severity of the metabolic or septic illness, focal abnormalities may not be apparent. Calibration signal 1 sec, 50μV.

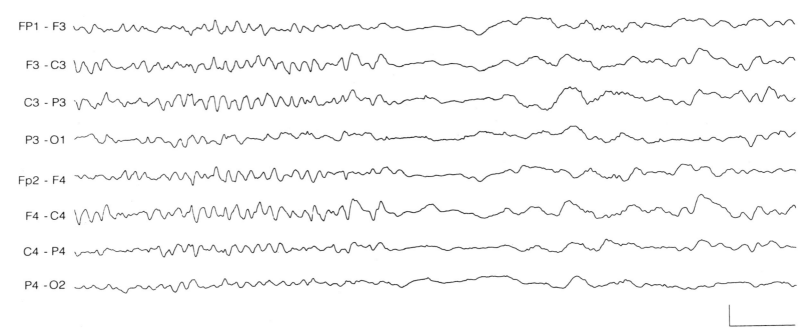

FIG. 8–4. Encephalopathy with abnormal reactivity. 36 years. Halfway through the recorded segment an auditory stimulus was given, followed immediately by attenuation of the previous diffuse theta rhythm and then a very-low-voltage spindlelike pattern with superimposed delta followed by a return to theta rhythm. While such reactivity indicates an encephalopathy, the prognosis is more favorable than if no electrographic response occurred. Calibration signal 1 sec, 70μV.

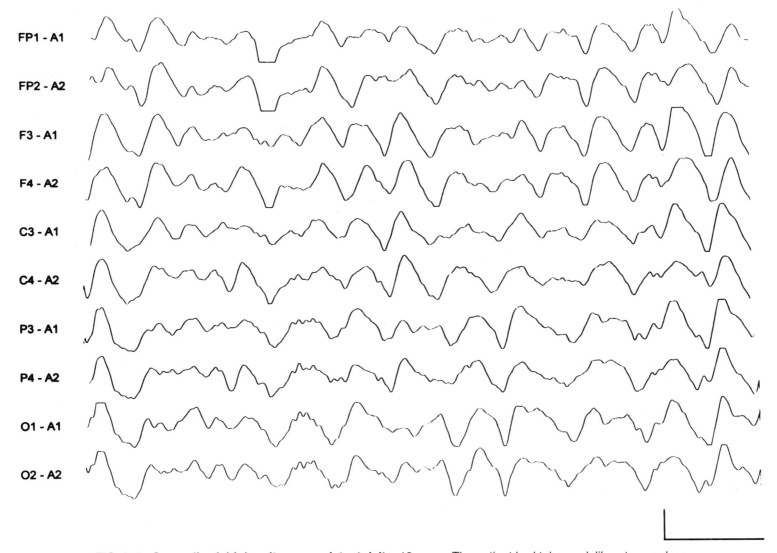

FIG. 8–5. Generalized, high voltage, persistent delta. 19 years. The patient had taken a deliberate overdose of valproic acid. The recording is dominated by diffuse, high-voltage rhythmic delta activity with a minimum of faster frequencies superimposed. The relative lack of mixtures of frequencies with little variability and no reactivity to stimulation indicates a severe encephalopathy. She recovered completely. Calibration signal 1 sec, 70μV.

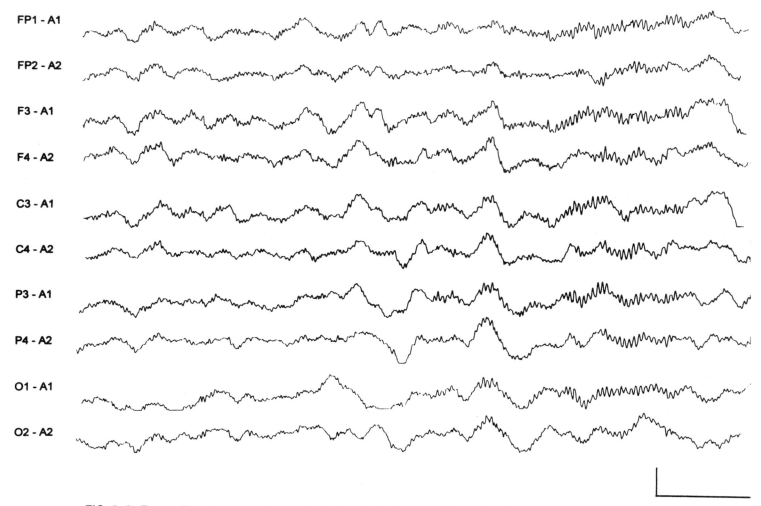

FP1 - A1

FP2 - A2

F3 - A1

F4 - A2

C3 - A1

C4 - A2

P3 - A1

P4 - A2

O1 - A1

O2 - A2

FIG. 8–6. Benzodiazepine overdose and skull defect. 17 years. This patient had a previous craniotomy in the left frontal central region for a vascular malformation and presented with status epilepticus. He was given large doses of various benzodiazepines and barbiturates to stop the seizures. This recording, done the next day, shows diffuse delta with superimposed beta activity, suggestive of benzodiazepines and/or barbiturate intoxication. The asymmetry is likely due to the skull defect on the left. In patients who fail to awaken after treatment of convulsive seizures, it is important to perform an EEG to determine the cause, for example, differentiation of drug toxicity, nonconvulsive status epilepticus and metabolic encephalopathy. Calibration signal 1 sec, 70μV.

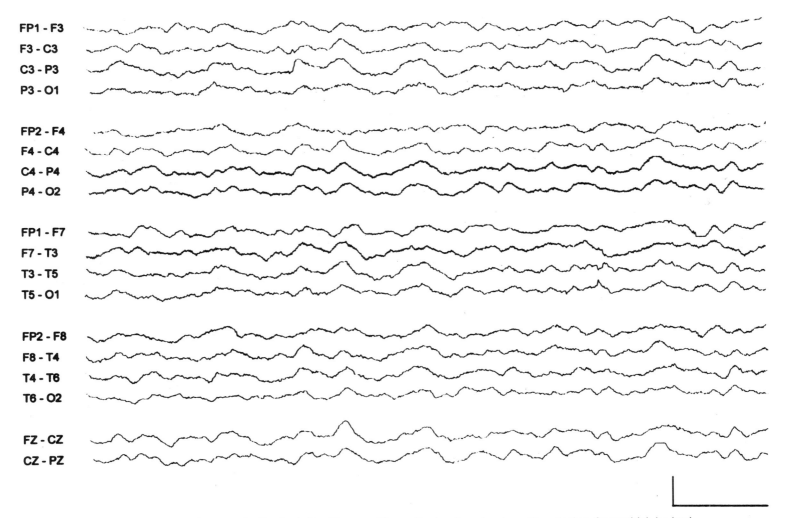

FIG. 8–7. Low-voltage arrhythmic delta. 29 years. The patient suffered a closed head injury from which he had recovered enough to follow commands, but then developed sepsis a week later and became comatose, at which time this recording was performed. Both medium-voltage arrhythmic delta and low-voltage higher-frequency rhythms were present. The pattern was invariant and without reactivity. Nonetheless, the patient recovered awareness after his septic condition resolved. Most often, even severe sepsis produces an encephalopathy that is largely reversible, providing that the patient recovers from the systemic illness. Calibration signal 1 sec, 50μV.

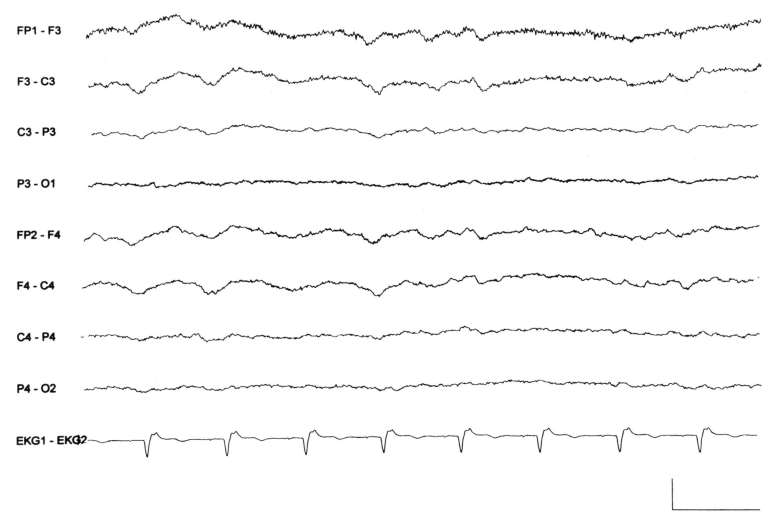

FIG. 8–8. Suppression in posterior head. 70 years old. The patient was comatose, with intact brain stem reflexes, following a cardiac arrest 4 days earlier. The posterior head (C3-P3, P3-O1, C4-P4, and P4-O2) is markedly suppressed in voltage, whereas there is poorly maintained delta and intermittent theta in the anterior head (FP1-F3, F3-C3, FP2-F4, and F4-C4). This was invariant and unreactive. The technologist and electroencephalographer should ensure that suppression in the posterior head is not due to physical factors, especially scalp edema (common in ICU patients in a supine position). Calibration signal 1 sec, 50μV.

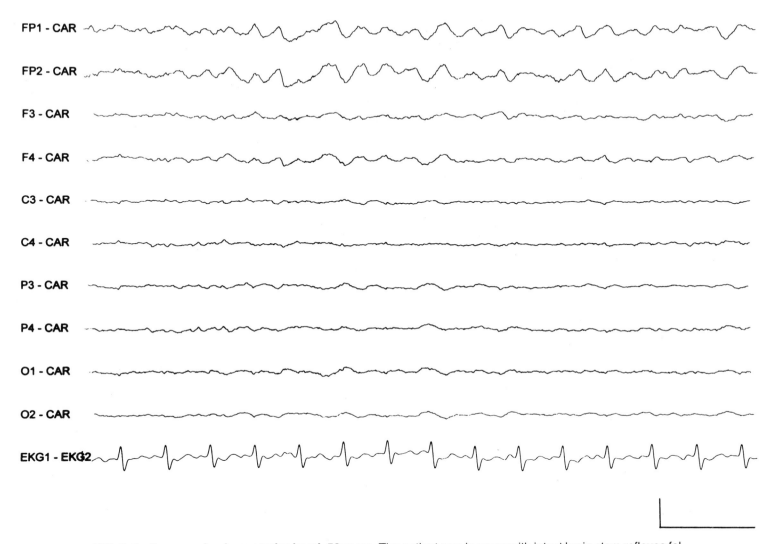

FIG. 8–9. Suppression in posterior head. 52 years. The patient was in coma with intact brain stem reflexes following a cardiac arrest the day before. As in Fig. 8–8, there is suppression in the midposterior head and only some arrhythmic delta in the anterior head. It is wise to consider eye movement artifact in this situation, but that is not the case here, as the wave forms (morphology and relative amplitudes) in the first and second channels would be better preserved in the 3rd and 4th channels if the waves were due to eye movements. In difficult cases, eye movement electrodes could be applied or the patient could be given a muscle relaxant. Calibration signal 1 sec, 70μV.

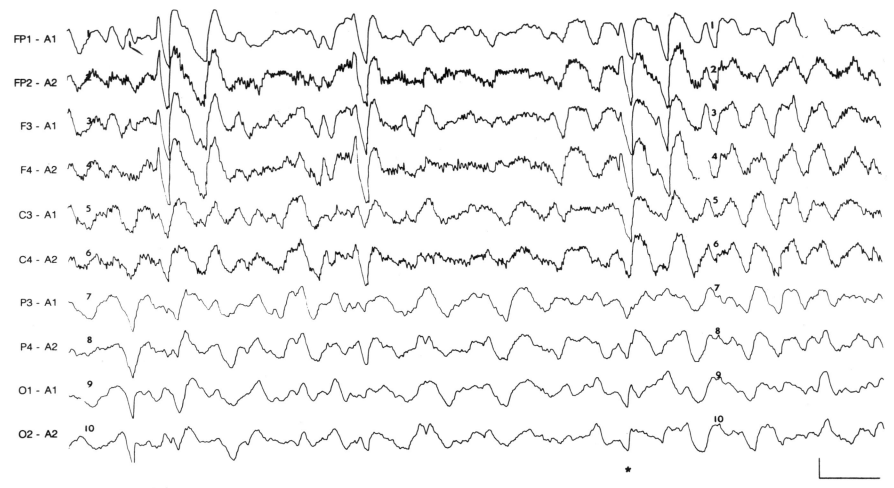

FIG. 8–10. Triphasic waves in metabolic encephalopathy. 68 years. The fully developed triphasic waves in this tracing begin with an initial, brief, negative wave (upward deflection), followed by a prominent, electropositive, sharply contoured wave, and then a broader negative wave. The duration of each succeeding wave of the complex is greater than the one before. Most of the waves have no anterior-posterior lag, but is evidenced in one (*asterisk*). In addition to their three phases, triphasic waves are bilaterally synchronous and usually frontally predominant. In metabolic encephalopathies, the case here, they usually appear in groups. Note the diffuse and persistent delta activity. Muscle artifact appears at FP2, F4, and C4. Calibration signal 1 sec, 70μV.

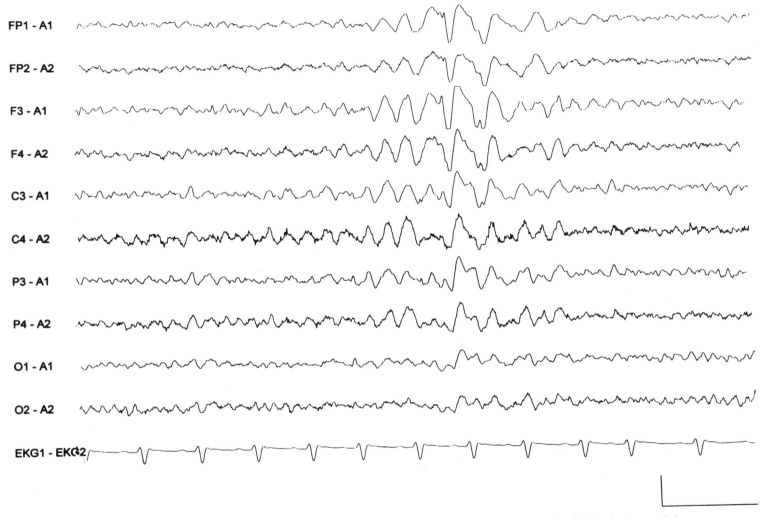

FIG. 8–11. Subtle spike waves mimicking triphasic waves in dialytic encephalopathy (dialysis dementia).
56 years old. Patient had very high serum aluminum levels and was showing features of dialysis dementia: impaired cognitive function, aphasia, slowing of speech, myoclonus, and ataxia. Note the very sharp initial spike in what appears to be a triphasic wave. In a later complex within the burst, a smaller spike is present at F3, F4, C3, and C4 is near the trough of a wave. Calibration signal 1 sec, 100μV.

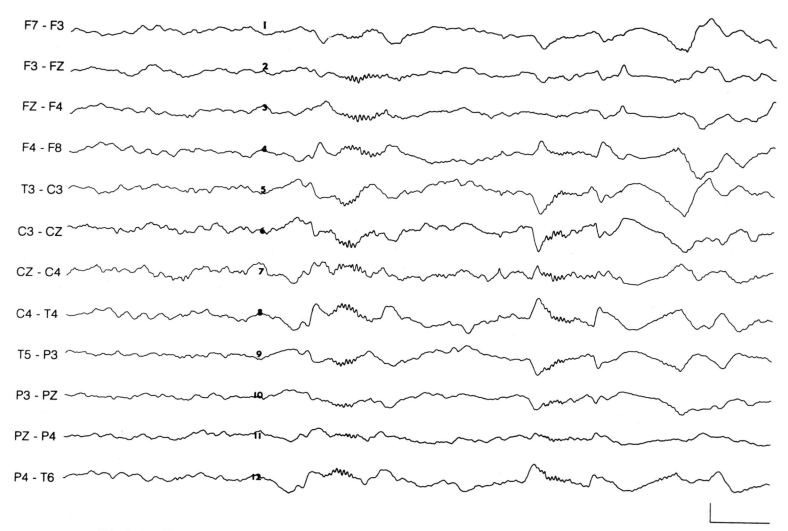

F7 - F3

F3 - FZ

FZ - F4

F4 - F8

T3 - C3

C3 - CZ

CZ - C4

C4 - T4

T5 - P3

P3 - PZ

PZ - P4

P4 - T6

FIG. 8–12. "Spindle coma pattern." 89 years. The coronal montage illustrates prominent normal-appearing spindles and V-waves together with diffuse delta of fluctuating amplitude, and theta. All of these aspects suggest a favorable outlook. However, the spindle coma pattern has an equivocal prognosis and depends on etiology, reactivity, and the integrity of brain stem function. Calibration signal 1 sec, 50μV.

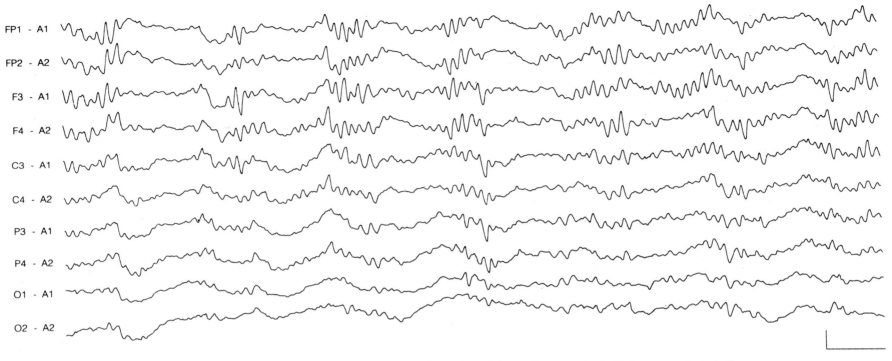

FIG. 8–13. "Spindle-like bursts." 54 years. Intermittent theta (slower than usual spindle frequency but similar in distribution and morphology) in bursts upon a diffuse delta background. Calibration signal 1 sec, 50μV.

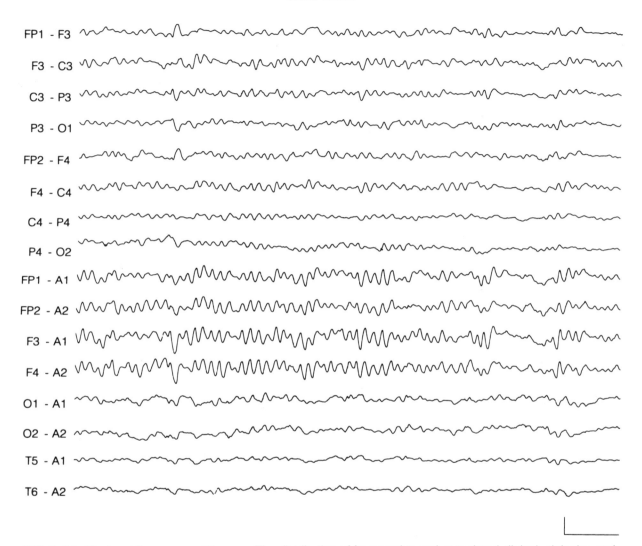

FIG. 8–14. Theta pattern coma. 54 years. The distribution of frequencies and associated clinical etiologies and outcomes of theta pattern coma are identical to those for alpha pattern coma. Note the distinctly greater amplitude of diffuse frontal theta activity on the referential portion of this recording compared to the bipolar component. Electrical cancellation occurs on bipolar montages when rhythms are synchronous and diffuse. Calibration signal 1 sec, 50μV.

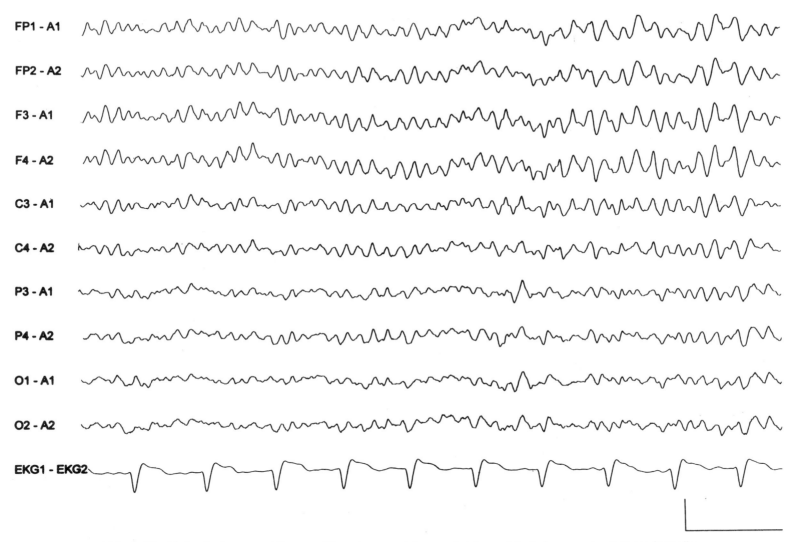

FIG. 8–15. Alpha-theta coma. 55 years. There is a coexistence of alpha and theta frequencies that are frontally predominant and invariant. Calibration signal 1 sec, 100μV.

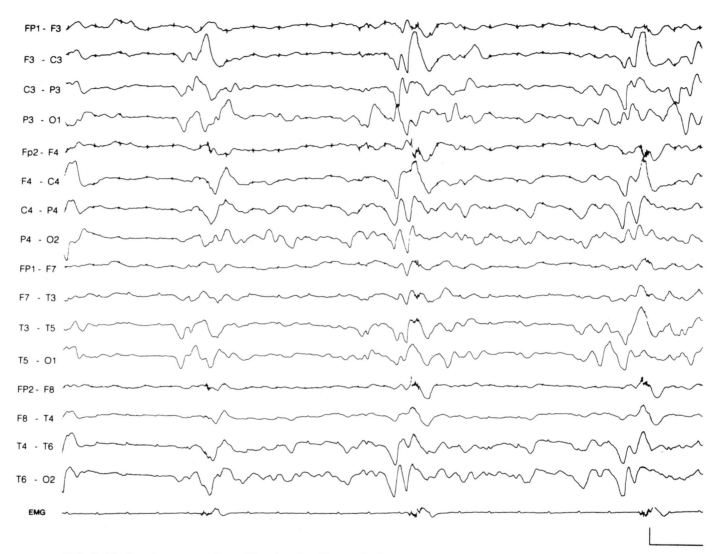

FIG. 8–16. Burst-suppression without epileptiform discharges. 66 years. Periodic bursts of delta and theta are separated by periods of relative inactivity, more marked in the left hemisphere. The EMG trace records brief tonic contractions of the right forearm which are invariably preceded by at least one element of each EEG burst. Transformer artifact creates the periodic low-voltage brief potentials seen principally at FP1 and FP2. Calibration signal 1 sec, 50μV.

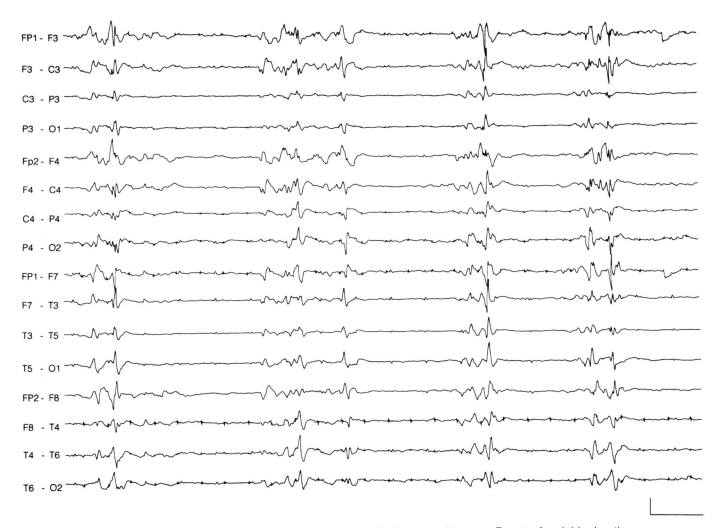

FIG. 8–17. Burst-suppression containing epileptiform discharges. 29 years. Bursts of variable duration contain spikes that are usually bilaterally synchronous and are separated by almost complete, generalized suppression. When associated with anoxic-ischemic encephalopathy, the prognosis tends to be worse than when bursts do not contain epileptiform discharges. Other, potentially more reversible conditions associated with this pattern include drug intoxication (e.g., carbamazepine or penicillin intoxication), certain general anesthetics, and advanced status epilepticus. Calibration signal 1 sec, 50μV.

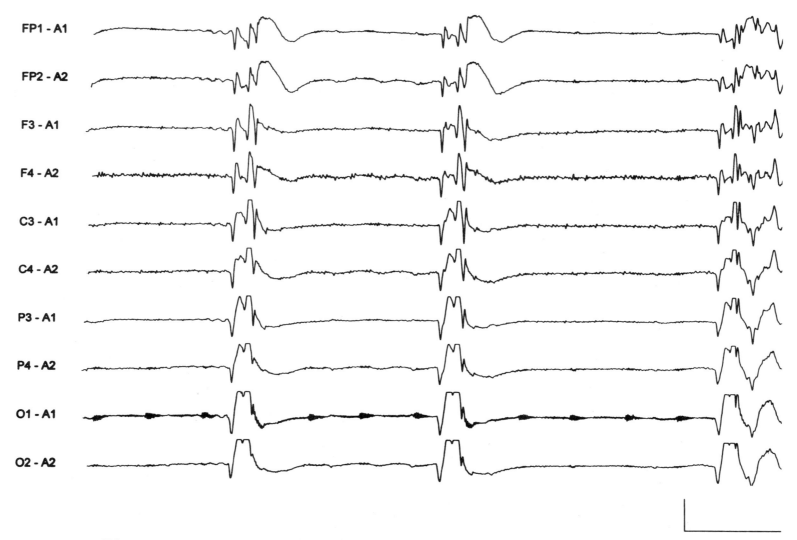

FIG. 8–18. Burst-suppression containing epileptiform discharges. 66 years. The patient suffered a cardiac arrest 1 day earlier and showed myoclonus of eyelids and jaw muscles coincident with the bursts. Somatosensory evoked potentials showed no cortical response. The bursts contain polyspikes and waves, sometimes mixed with theta activity. Note the low amplitude. Calibration signal 1 sec, 20μV.

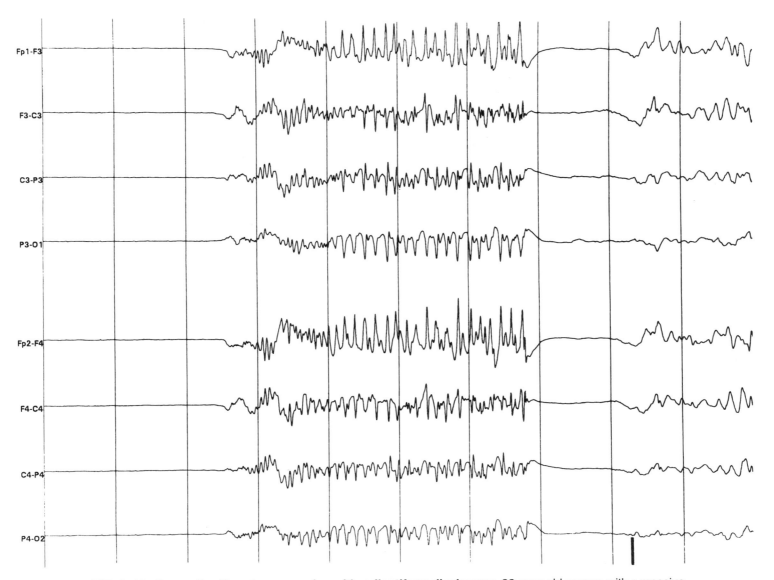

FIG. 8–19. Generalized burst-suppression with epileptiform discharges. 32-year-old woman with a massive carbamazepine overdose. Bursts contain runs of rhythmic waves followed by sequential, bilaterally synchronous spikes without intervening slow waves. Between the bursts, the recording is completely suppressed. With falling carbamazepine serum concentrations, the patient regained continuous EEG rhythms and epileptiform activity disappeared. Calibration signal: dark vertical line 100μV, distance between other vertical lines: 1 second.

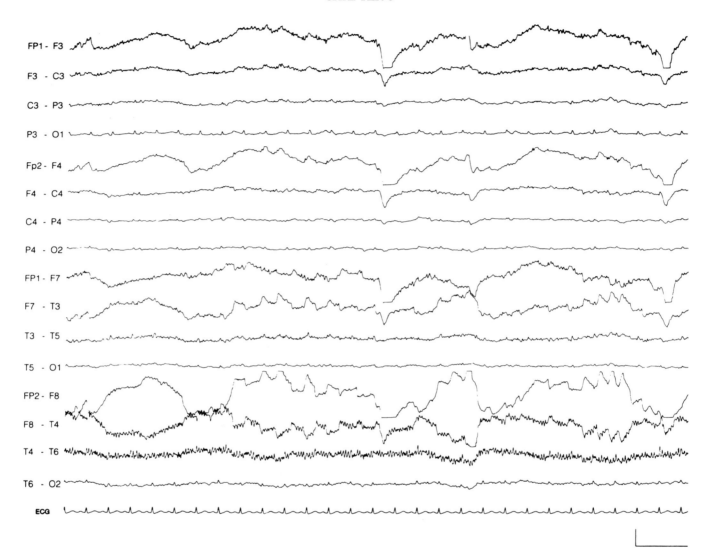

FIG. 8–20. Generalized suppression and eye movements. 42 years. Almost all the deflections in this recording can be attributed to horizontal and vertical eye movements, ECG contamination, and muscle artifact. Muscle relaxant drugs would remove the eye movement and EMG artifact. Calibration signal 1 sec, 20μV.

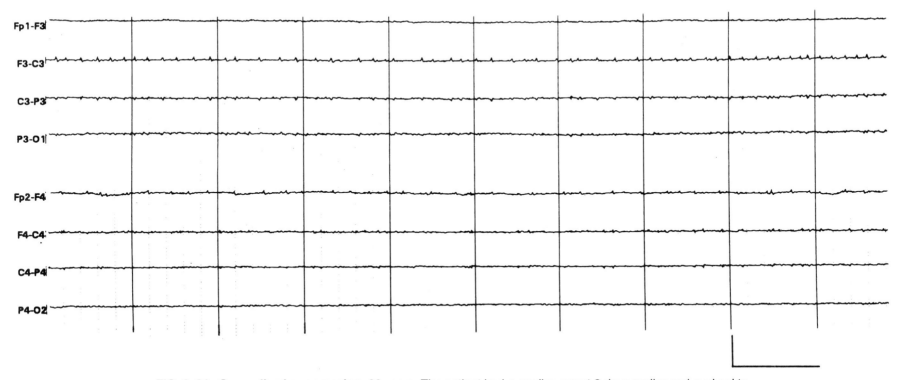

FIG. 8–21. Generalized suppression. 66 years. The patient had a cardiac arrest 2 days earlier and evolved to the clinical picture of brain death. The recording shows complete suppression at this sensitivity, with only low-voltage muscle spicule artifact. Calibration signal 1 sec, 20μV.

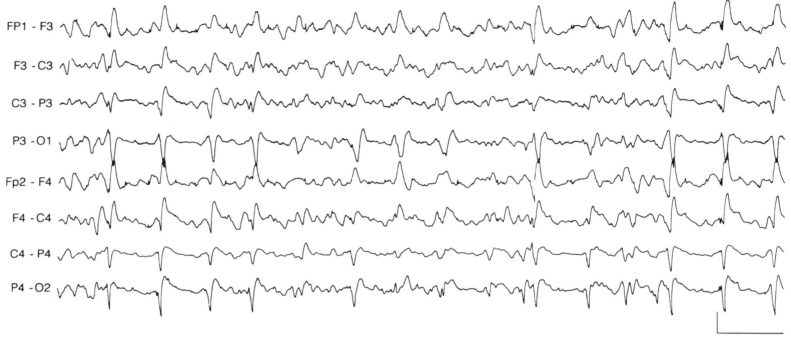

FIG. 8–22. Bilaterally synchronous periodic spikes. 66 years. The patient had suffered a cardiac arrest and was in a coma. Such discharges are bilaterally synchronous, persistent, pseudoperiodic, and typically show intervening attenuation of voltage (only intermittent in this case). The pattern is unreactive to stimulation. The prognosis is usually poor, confirmed by serial EEGs. Calibration signal 1 sec, 50μV.

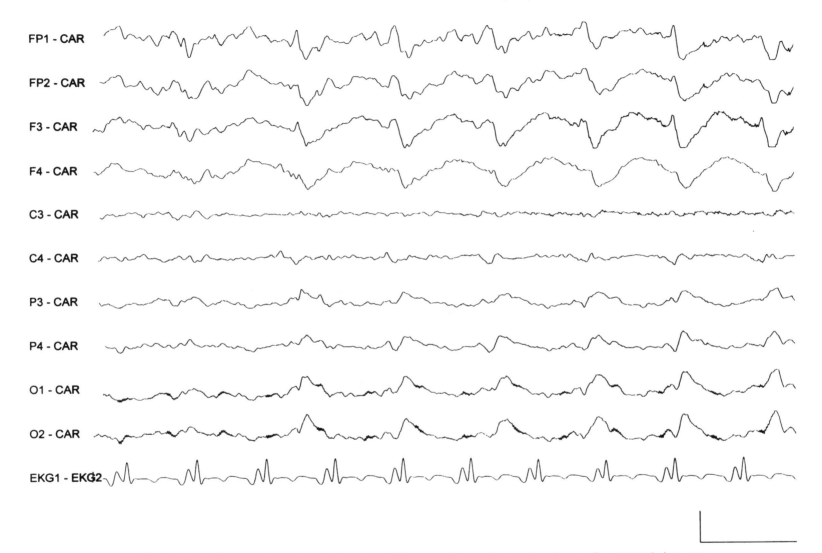

FIG. 8–23. Periodic complexes in anterior head. 36 years. This patient suffered a cardiac arrest 2 days earlier. Note the periodic biphasic complexes followed by delta waves in the first 4 channels. The bottom 4 channels show complexes related to contamination of the common average reference (CAR). Note the abnormal EKG. Calibration signal 1 sec, 100μV.

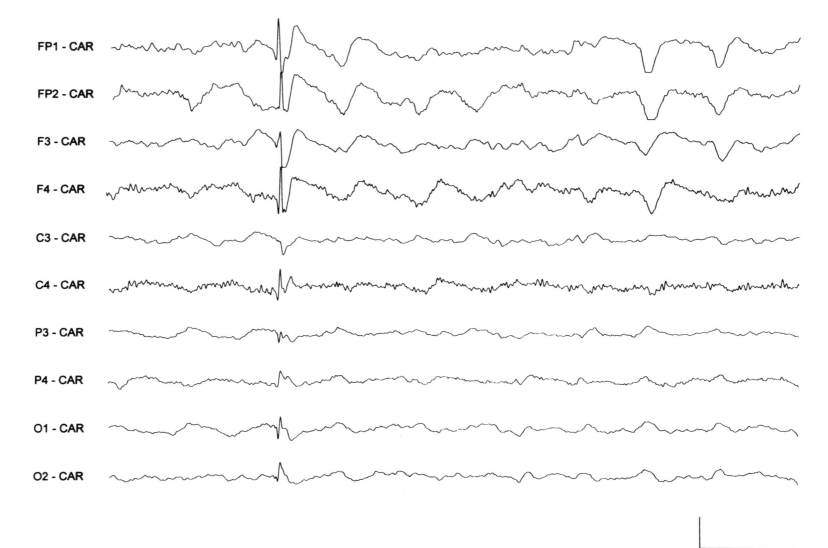

FIG. 8–24. Combination of epileptiform activity and encephalopathic features. 60 years. The patient had a history of primary generalized epilepsy and developed a metabolic encephalopathy with multiorgan failure. Note the discrete, bilaterally synchronous spike in the first half of the page and the bilaterally synchronous delta and blunted triphasic waves in the remaining part of the tracing. The downward deflections in the bottom 5 channels reflect contamination of the common average reference. The clinical features are in keeping with the EEG; there are two processes: residual spikes from an underlying seizure disorder and a severe metabolic encephalopathy. Calibration signal 1 sec, 70μV.

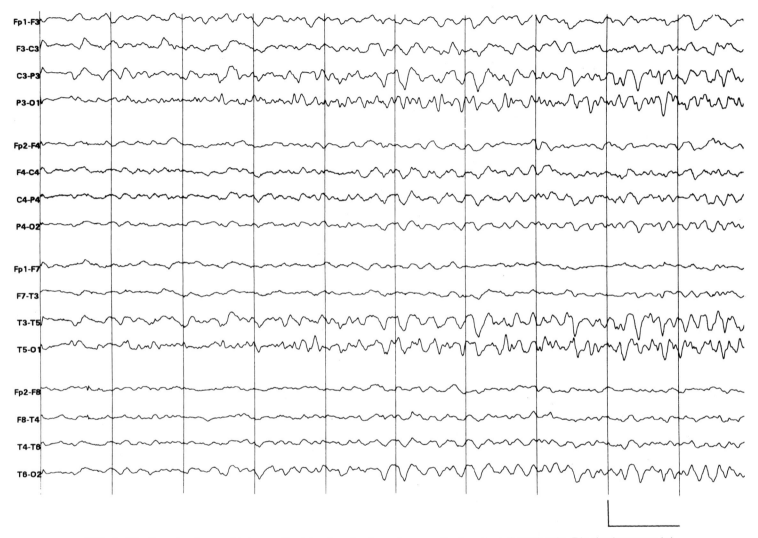

FIG. 8–25. Focal seizure. 51 years. Evolving focal seizure from cortical venous thrombosis. Rhythmic waves initially in the alpha frequency range at P3-O1 and T5-O1 slow in frequency and spread to adjacent electrodes (T5 and P3, as shown by the involvement at C3-P3 and T3-T5 derivations). Note that the slower frequencies of non-ictal rhythms are more prominent in the left hemisphere than the right. Calibration signal 1 sec, 70μV.

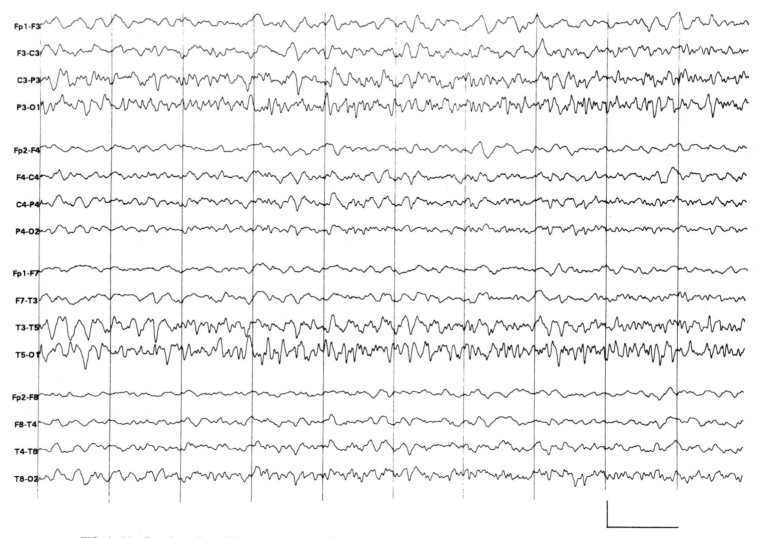

FIG. 8–26. Continuation of the seizure from Fig. 8–25. The seizure shows a continuous change of frequency, morphology and amplitude of waves in the left posterior head (C3-P3, P3-O1, T3-T5, and T5-O1), associated with sequential spikes at O1. Calibration signal 1 sec, 70μV.

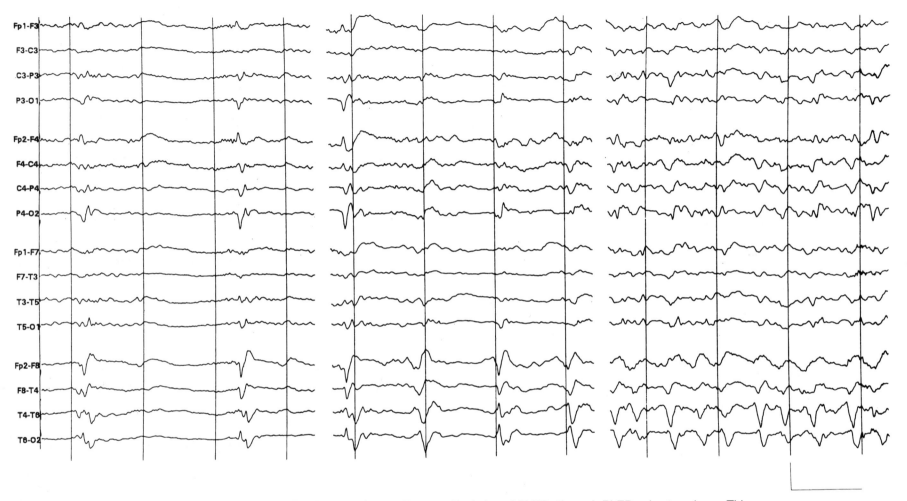

FIG. 8–27. PLEDs evolving into a seizure. 58 years. Evolution of PLEDs through PLEDs plus to seizure. This composite shows PLEDs in the first section, an acceleration in the second section, and an electrographic seizure in the third section. The seizure consists of 2–3 per second sharp waves in the left posterior head, with intervening continuous ictal rhythms. Calibration signal 1 sec, 100μV.

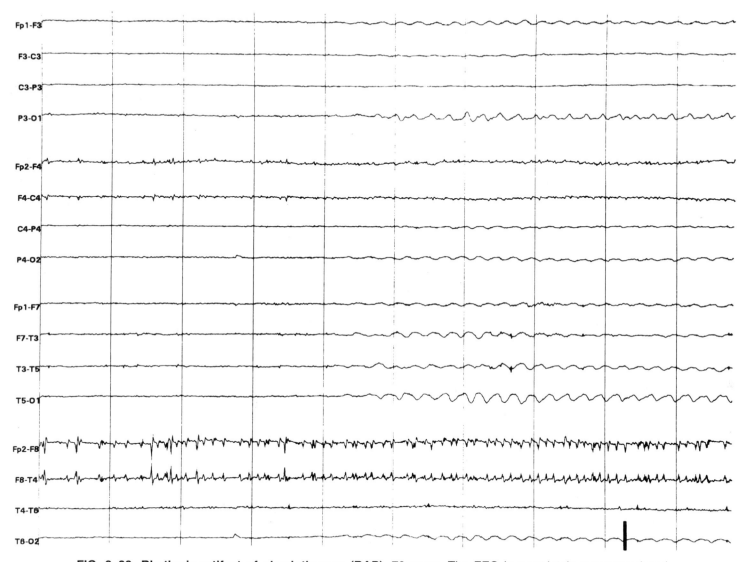

FIG. 8–28. Rhythmic artifact of physiotherapy (RAP). 70 years. The EEG is completely suppressed and shows intermittent 4 Hz, rhythmic delta activity, seen mainly in the 1st, 4th and 7th through 9th channels. This was produced by chest physiotherapy. Calibration: bold vertical line: 20μV, distance between other vertical lines = 1 second.

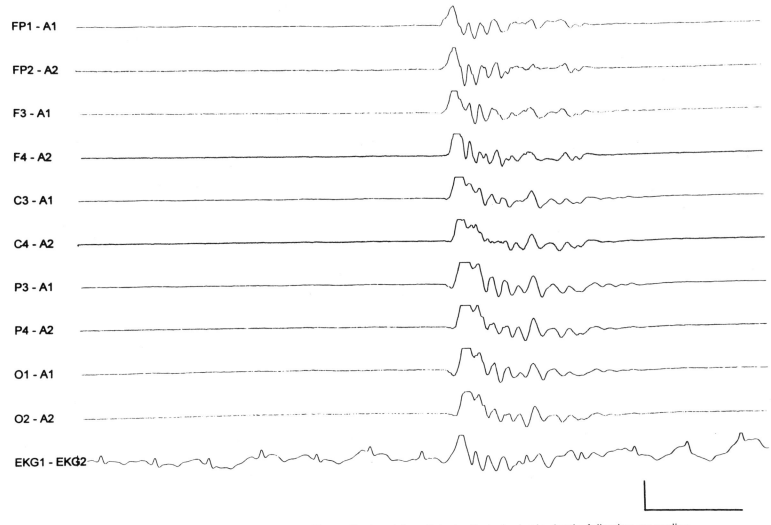

FIG. 8–29. "Jiggle" artifact. 25 years. The patient met the clinical criteria for brain death, following an earlier cardiac arrest. The EEG was completely suppressed except for occasional rhythmic complexes that occurred due to mechanical bed movements (note the simultaneous involvement of the EKG channel). Note that the amplitude of the waves progressively lessens, as would be expected with a mechanical perturbation. This initially gave the erroneous impression of a generalized burst-suppression pattern. Calibration signal 1 sec, 30μV.

Chapter 9

Digital Electroencephalography

Modification of viewing parameters by digital EEG creates several advantages and a few pitfalls compared to analog recordings. This chapter treats some of these aspects under four categories: (a) montage reformatting for focal and regional spikes, (b) reformatting for diffuse, bilateral phenomena, (c) alteration of sweep speeds, and (d) frequency filtering. Each group of figures illustrates its particular EEG epoch by two or more display parameters.

Montage Reformatting for Focal and Regional Spikes

- Localization of potentials, particularly spikes, accomplished by reformatting montages.
- See advantages/disadvantages of principal montages in Chapter 1.
- The several montages variably succeed in displaying focal spikes, temporal in this instance.
- Less relevant portions of some montages are omitted for clarity of display.

Figs. 1–11: The same temporal spikes and delta activity displayed by different reformatted montages.

Figs. 12–17: Varying ability of several montages to localize widespread occipital parietal spikes.

Figs. 18–20: Multifocal spikes illustrated by a bipolar and a referential montage with a regular and a shorter time constant.

Reformatting for Diffuse, Bilateral Phenomena

Figs. 21–22: Triphasic waves and delta activity on longitudinal bipolar and ear reference montages.

Alteration of Sweep Speeds

- Identification and more precise evaluation of complex or partially hidden diffuse wave forms by referential montage and fast sweep speeds.
- Appreciation of repetitive or reactive events by slow sweep speeds.

Figs. 23–25: 6 Hz spike-waves better illustrated by ear reference montage, enhanced sensitivity, and faster sweep speed.

Figs. 26–27: Repetitive potentials better assessed at slower sweep speed.

Fig. 28: Modification by afferent stimuli in a comatose patient better depicted by slower sweep speeds.

Frequency Filtering

- Elimination of muscle potentials by high-frequency filtering.
- Better appreciation of focal spikes by low-frequency filtering, that is, a shorter time constant.

Figs. 29, 30: Lowering high linear filter setting eliminates muscle artifact to better depict focal spikes.

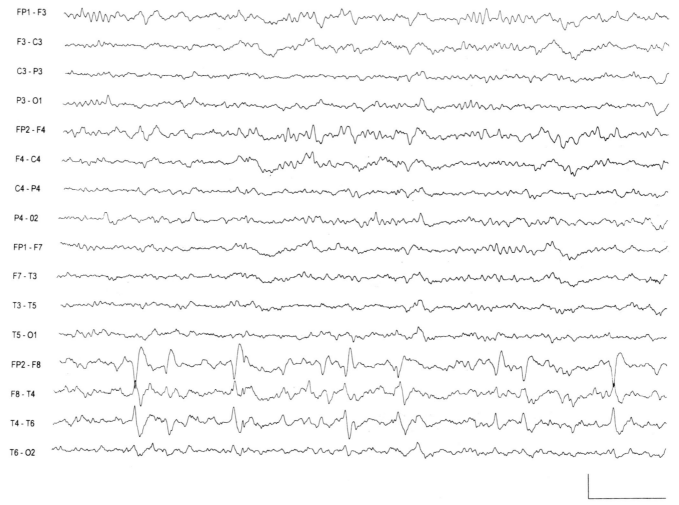

FIG. 9–1. Anterior-posterior bipolar. Right temporal delta in light sleep with frequent principally electronegative right temporal (F8-T4) spikes. In some patients, such spikes could spread to the right frontopolar region (Fp2). Light sleep recording. Calibration signal 1 sec, 50μV.

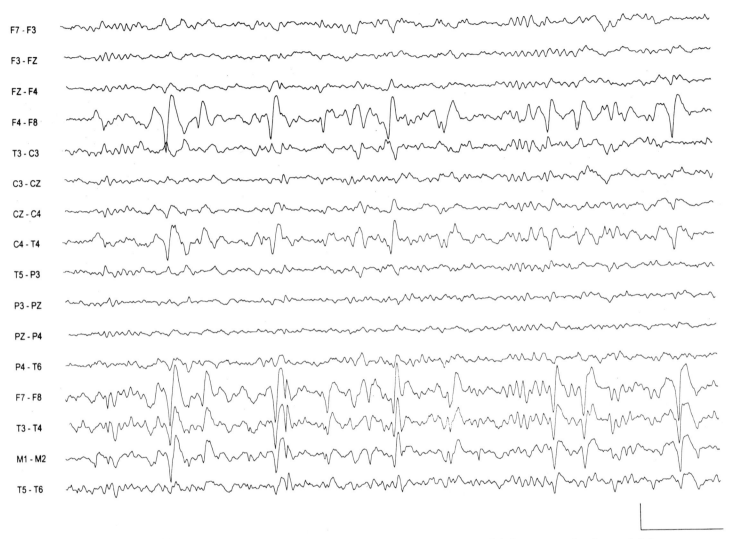

FIG. 9–2. Coronal bipolar montage with sagittal leads. This confirms that: (a) the temporal spike and delta fields do not significantly involve parasagittal regions, and (b) their anterior-midtemporal location as T6 is minimally involved. Note the M2 involvement of these anterior-mesial temporal spikes and delta. Calibration signal 1 sec, 50μV.

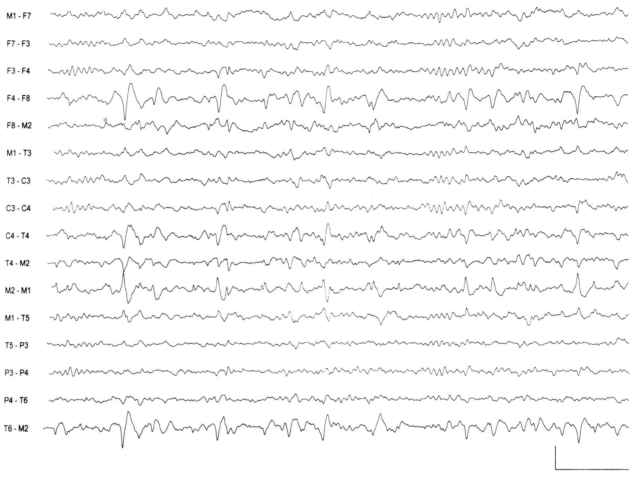

FIG. 9–3. Coronal bipolar without sagittal leads. These electronegative spikes appear principally at the right anterior mesial temporal (F8, M2) region. The occasional downward deflection in the T4-M2 derivation indicates that the midtemporal area is sometimes less involved; note the variability of spike field in this respect. The prominent and consistently downward deflection in the T6-M2 derivation and lack of deflection in the P4-T6 derivation indicates lack of right posterior temporal (T6) involvement. Confinement of the delta and spike fields to the right temporal lobe is indicated by the aforementioned derivations, and also by the minimal to no deflections in F3-4, C3-4, and P3-P4 derivations as well as the consistently downward deflections in the C4-T4 derivation. Finally, the consistently upward deflections in the M2-M1 linkage indicates, with other data, the lack of prominent crossfiring to the left inferior temporal region. Whether the slight upward deflection at the M1-T5 derivation suggests minimal M1 involvement in this respect or whether this represents a dipole with some positivity in the left hemisphere and parasagittal areas is not clear from this montage. Calibration signal 1 sec, 70μV.

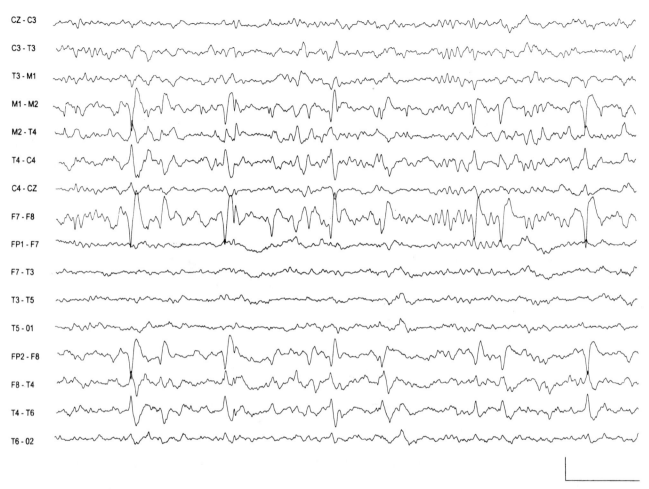

FIG. 9–4. Coronal-bitemporal bipolar. Right anterior temporal spikes have a slightly variable field involving M2, T4, and F8. Calibration signal 1 sec, 50μV.

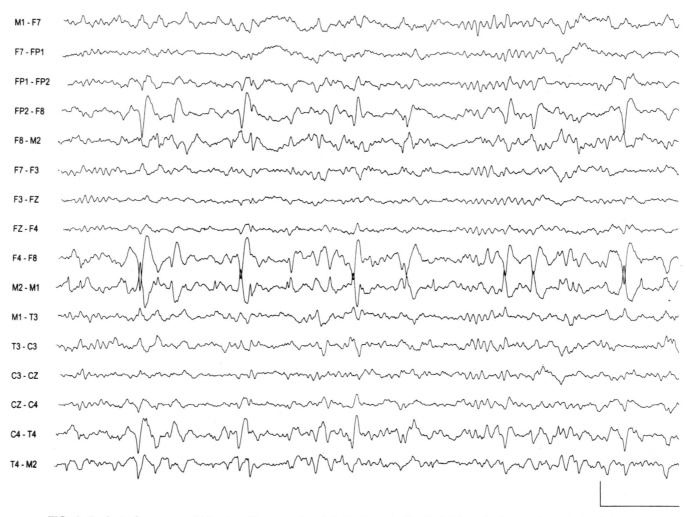

FIG. 9–5. Anterior coronal bipolar. The prominent deflections in the Fp2-F8 derivation and the lack of phase reversals around Fp2 indicate that the right frontopolar region is not involved in this temporal spike field. Calibration signal 1 sec, 50μV.

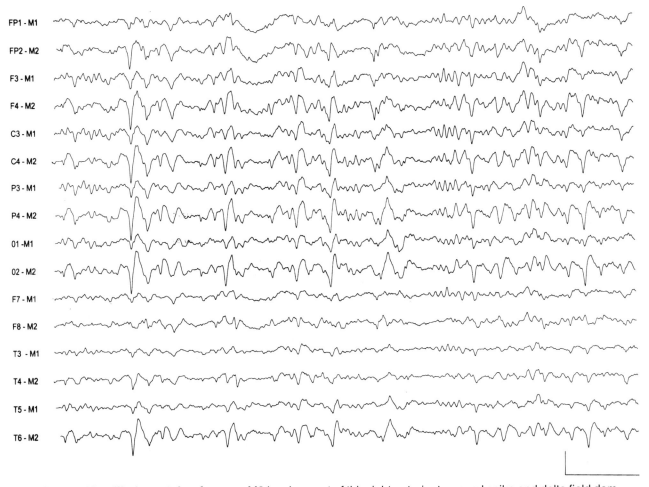

FIG. 9–6. Mandibular notch reference. M2 involvement of this right anterior temporal spike and delta field dominates many channels here. The lack of an upward deflection in the principal spike component in any channel suggests that no region exceeds M2 in negativity. The complete cancellation in the F8-M2 derivation indicates equal involvement of these electrodes in that field; the minimal downward deflections in the T4-M2 derivation indicates slight T4 involvement. The less downward spike deflection in the Fp2-M2 derivation compared to other parasagittal derivations reflects slight propagation of temporal spikes to the frontopolar region. In contrast, the prominent deflections in derivations involving posterior leads reflect the restriction of the potentials anteriorly. The slight downward deflections in the derivations involving left parasagittal leads suggest either slight negativity at M1 or positivity parasagittally, as suggested by an earlier montage. Calibration signal 1 sec, 70μV.

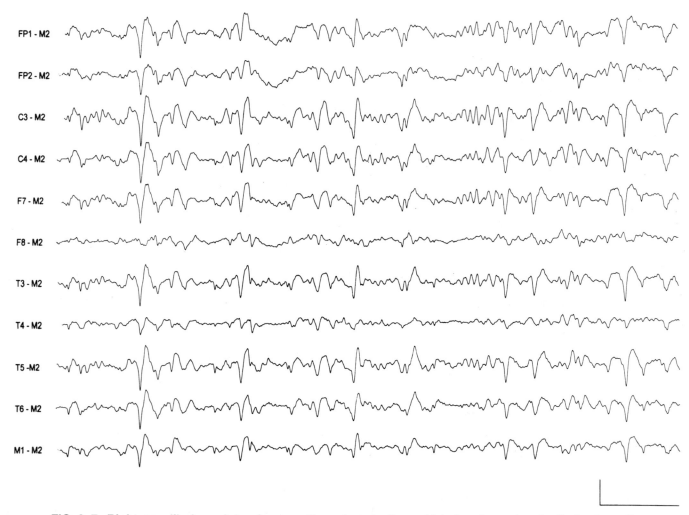

FIG. 9–7. Right mandibular notch reference. The only derivations which do not prominently display the spike and delta fields are those (F8-M2, T4-M2) that are considerably involved in the fields. Again, the lack of any upward deflection of the principal spike component suggests that no position exceeds M2 in negativity. Not the best montage to display these spikes. Calibration signal 1 sec, 70µV.

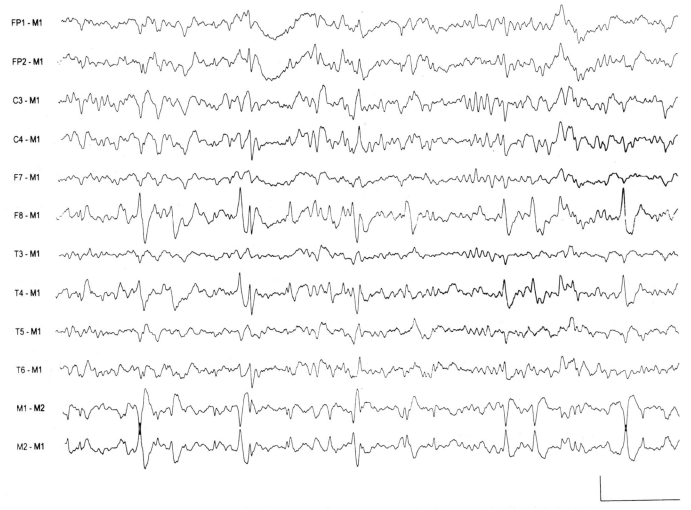

FIG. 9–8. Left mandibular notch reference. Although this montage clearly depicts the right anterior inferior temporal spikes, the long interelectrode distances of many of the derivations allow depiction of large fields as well as the more restricted right temporal ones, impeding spike assessment. Calibration signal 1 sec, 50μV.

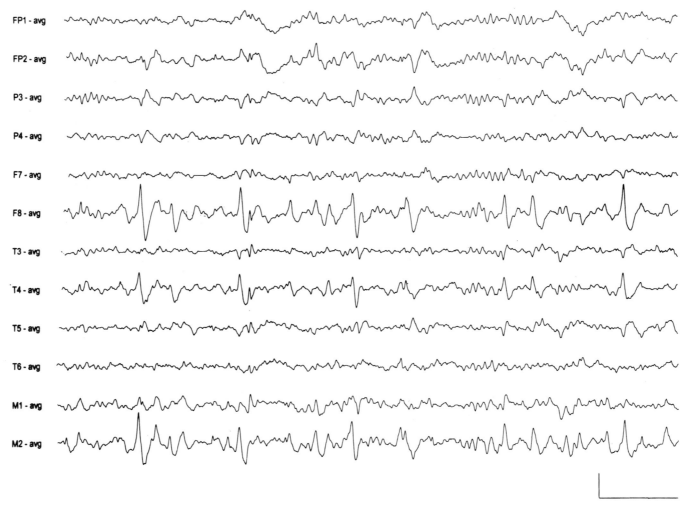

FIG. 9–9. The average reference (common average reference). The restricted fields of these anterior temporal spikes and delta fail to involve the average reference, allowing the spike field and its variations to be displayed clearly and accurately. Average reference involvement is assessed by including electrodes distant from presumed field, based on bipolar montages; thus, P3 and P4 are included. Calibration signal 1 sec, 50μV.

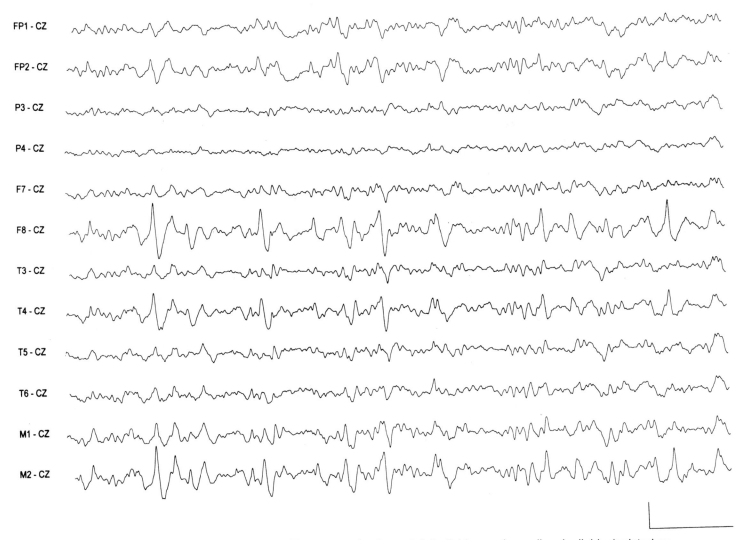

FIG. 9–10. Central sagittal reference. The temporal spike and delta fields are also well and reliably depicted on this montage. Calibration signal 1 sec, 70µV.

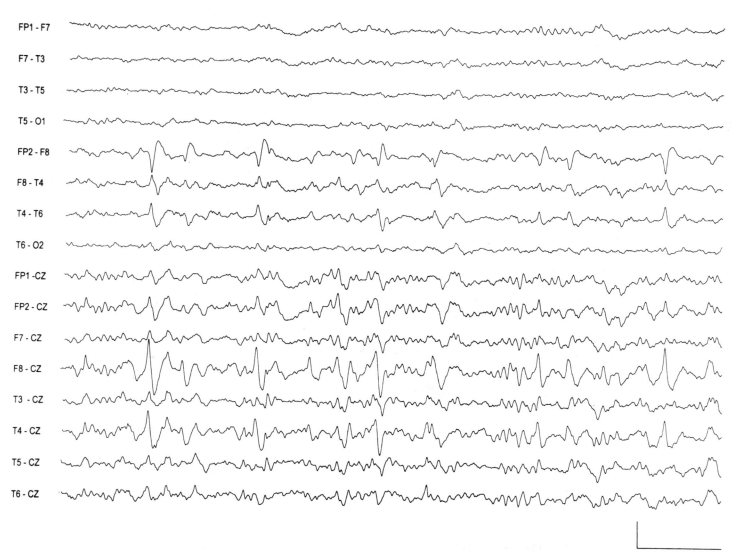

FIG. 9–11. Combined longitudinal temporal bipolar and central sagittal reference. The principal involvement of F8 (lacking M2) is depicted in both sections of this combined montage. Calibration signal 1 sec, 70μV.

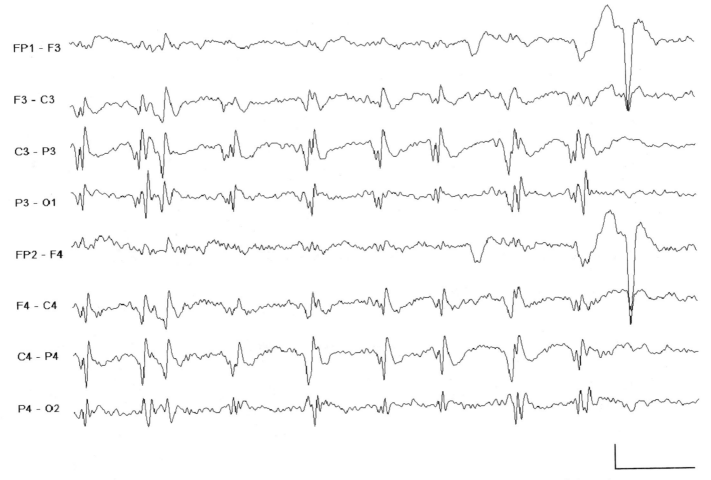

FIG. 9–12. Bisynchronous posterior spikes. Lack of frontal involvement and the absence of clear phase reversals, except possibly involving the right parietal (P4) region suggest that these spikes involve the occipital regions bilaterally but do not clearly lateralize their onset. Calibration signal 1 sec, 50μV.

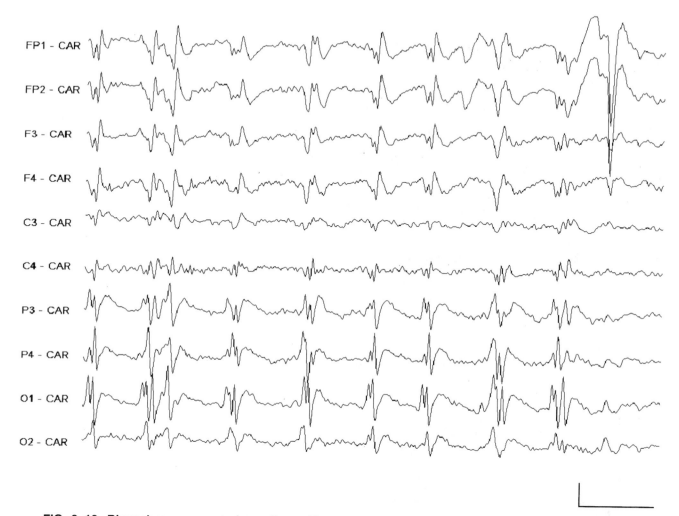

FIG. 9–13. Bisynchronous posterior spikes with common average reference. The widespread and synchronous nature of these discharges creates common average reference "contamination" so that they appear prominently in derivations involving the frontal leads. This represents an example of prominent apparent field distortion by an involved reference. Calibration signal 1 sec, 70μV.

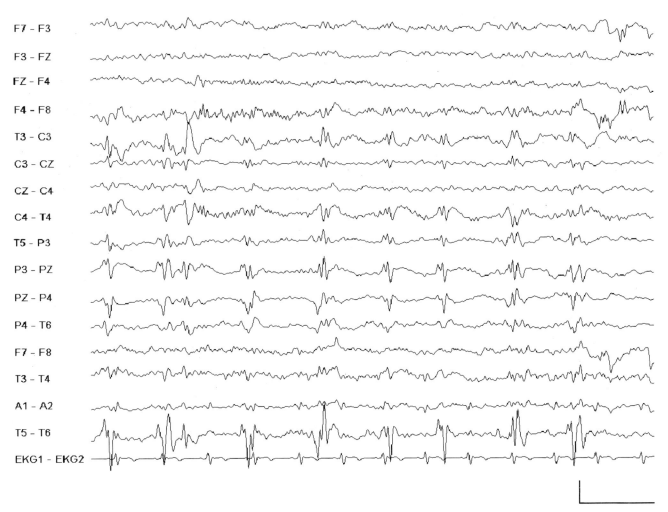

FIG. 9–14. Posterior bisynchronous spikes on coronal montage. The lack of distinct involvement of these spikes in any linkage involving the frontal or anterior midtemporal leads confirms the posterior situation of these discharges. Note particularly the lack of A1-A2 involvement. Cancellation of spike potentials among all of these derivations, with varying interelectrode distances, would be highly unlikely. Calibration signal 1 sec, 70μV.

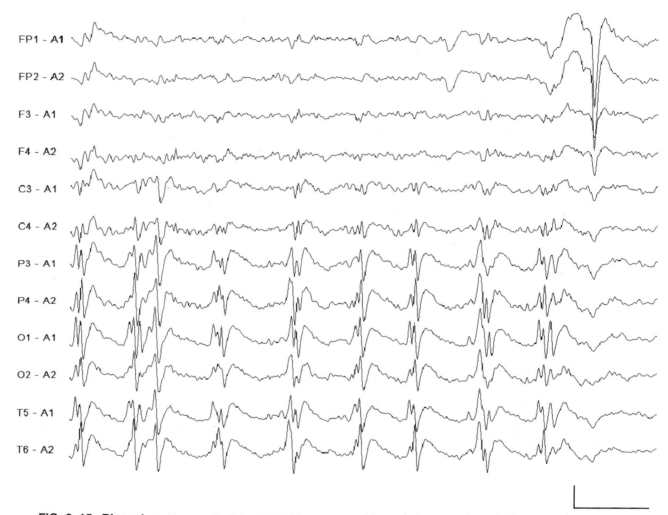

FIG. 9–15. Bisynchronous posterior spikes on ear reference montage. The lack of involvement of A1 and A2 allows this reference to accurately depict the spike field and confirms its posterior situation. Calibration signal 1 sec, 100μV.

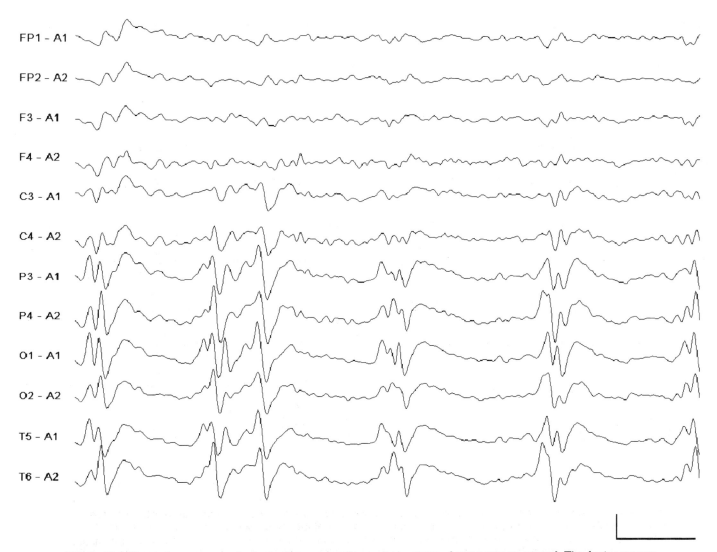

FIG. 9–16. Bisynchronous posterior spikes, ear reference montage, faster sweep speed. The faster sweep speed suggests that these discharges, in some instances, may originate slightly earlier in the left occipital posterior temporal parietal (O1, T5, P3) region, but this origin is less apparent in other discharges. Calibration signal 0.5 sec, 100μV.

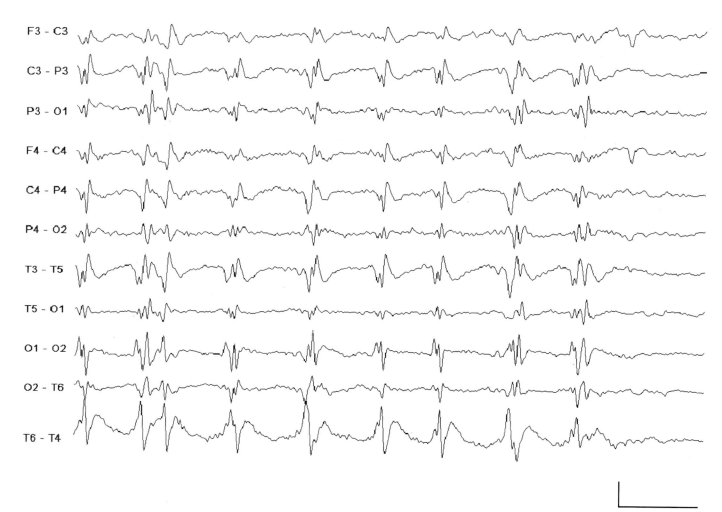

FIG. 9–17. Posterior synchronous discharges with a posterior coronal and longitudinal bipolar montage. Phase reversals in the coronal portion of this montage suggest that the left posterior temporal-occipital (T5, O1) region is principally involved in most discharges. Moreover, usually the zone with the greater number of phases is the originating one: note the greater number of phases in discharges involving left posterior leads compared to those of the right in this complex field. Calibration signal 1 sec, 100μV.

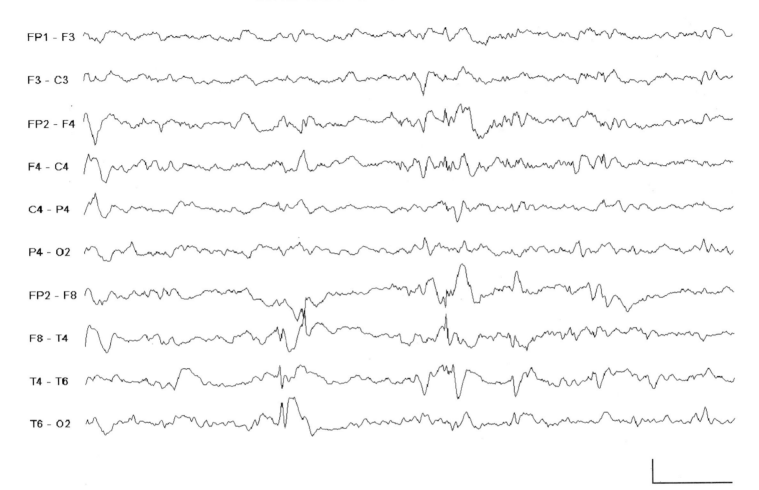

FIG. 9–18. Multifocal spikes, display with montage and time constant modifications. Relevant portions of this montage illustrate the multifocal nature of these right hemisphere epileptiform discharges and the right hemisphere accentuation of diffuse delta in this sleep recording. Calibration signal 1 sec, 100μV; low linear filter (LLF) = 0.3 Hz.

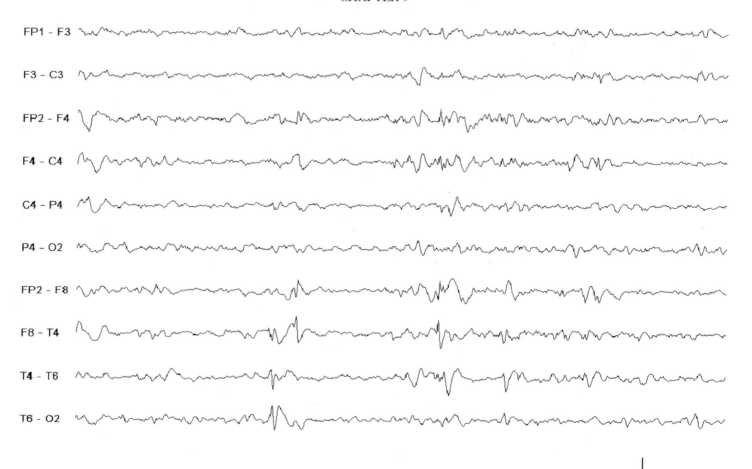

FP1 – F3

F3 – C3

FP2 – F4

F4 – C4

C4 – P4

P4 – O2

FP2 – F8

F8 – T4

T4 – T6

T6 – O2

FIG. 9–19. Clearer depiction of multifocal spikes with shorter time constant. Same instance as in previous figure with clearer depiction of spikes by diminishing the delta activity by changing the LLF from 0.3 Hz to 3 Hz. Calibration signal 1 sec, 100μV.

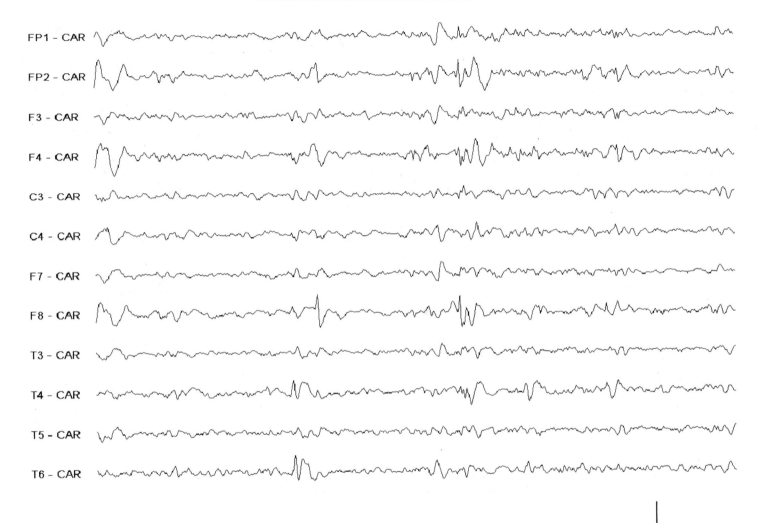

FIG. 9–20. Multifocal spikes on the common average reference (CAR). The restricted fields of these spikes do not "contaminate" the CAR and therefore their multifocality is more easily appreciated. Calibration signal 1 sec, 100μV.

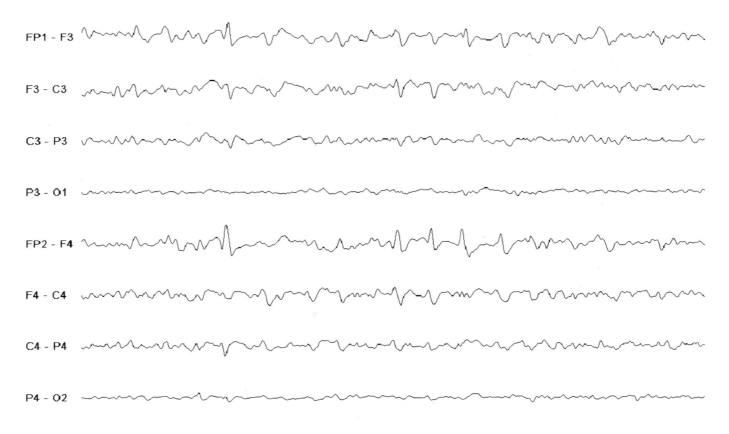

FIG. 9–21. Triphasic waves on longitudinal bipolar montage. In this instance, triphasic waves and delta are only rudimentarily expressed in this bipolar montage. Calibration signal 1 sec, 100μV.

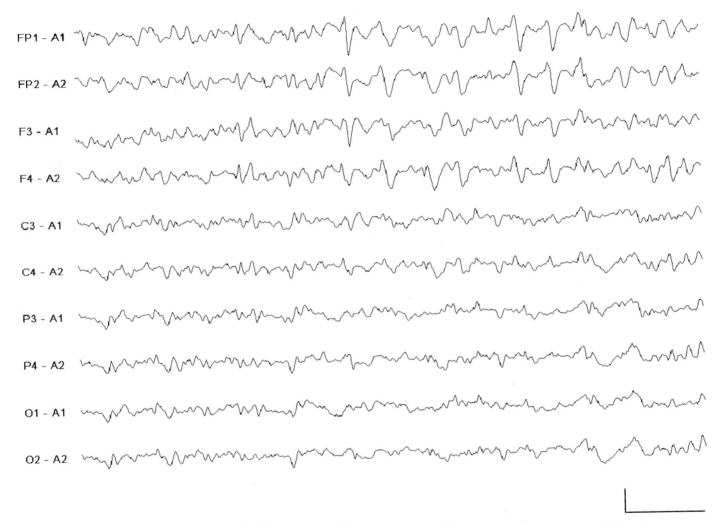

FIG. 9–22. Triphasic waves and delta on ear reference montage. These same phenomena are better depicted on an ear reference montage in this instance, as there are less cancellation effects within the principally involved (anterior) derivations. No frequency filter alteration (LLF = 0.3 Hz). Calibration signal 1 sec, 100μV.

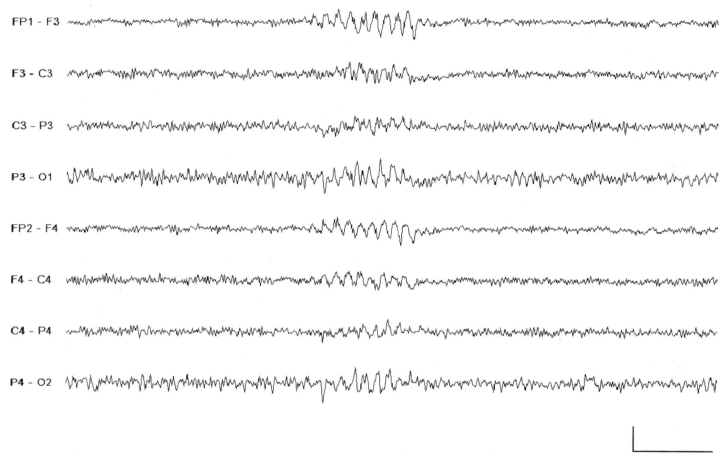

FIG. 9–23. Burst of 6 Hz theta with questionable intermingled spikes. This bipolar montage only hints at the presence of spikes intermingled within the theta burst, particularly in the F3-C3 derivation. Ongoing beta and alpha complicate the depiction of this phenomenon. Calibration signal 1 sec, 70μV.

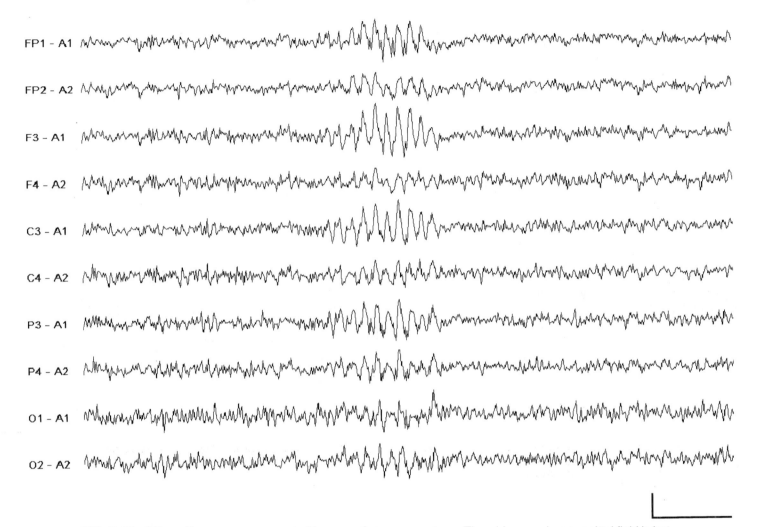

FIG. 9–24. 6 Hz spike-waves as revealed by ear reference montage. The widespread parasagittal field is better detected on this referential montage in which A1 and A2 are not involved in the spike-wave fields. Although the spikes are buried in ongoing potentials in some derivations, they are clearly seen more anteriorly, particularly in the Fp1-A1 derivation. Calibration signal 1 sec, 70μV.

P3 - A1

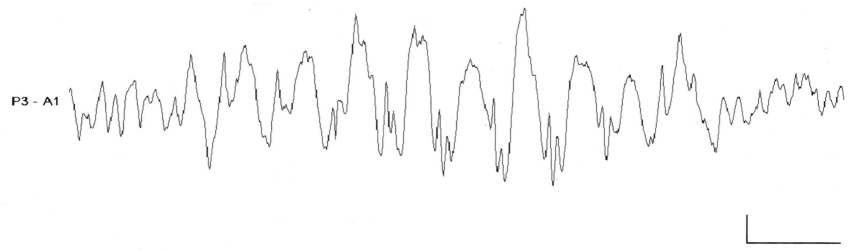

FIG. 9–25. 6 Hz spike-waves with enhanced sensitivity and faster sweep speed. These two modifications allow a more definitive display of this 6 Hz spike-wave phenomenon. Compare with the previous two tracings. Calibration signal 0.25 sec, 20μV.

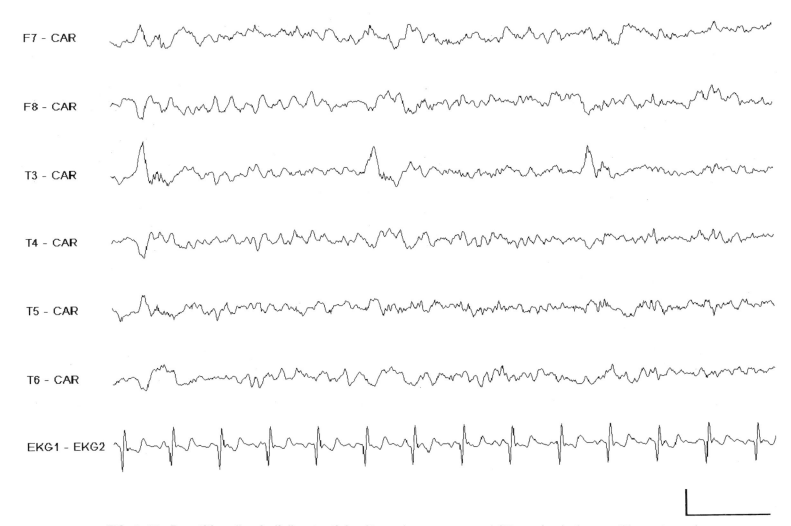

FIG. 9–26. Repetitive, "periodic" potentials. At regular sweep speed (30 mm/sec), the repetitive nature of these T3 broad spikes can be discerned, somewhat. Compare with the following tracing in Fig. 9–27. Calibration signal 1 sec, 50μV.

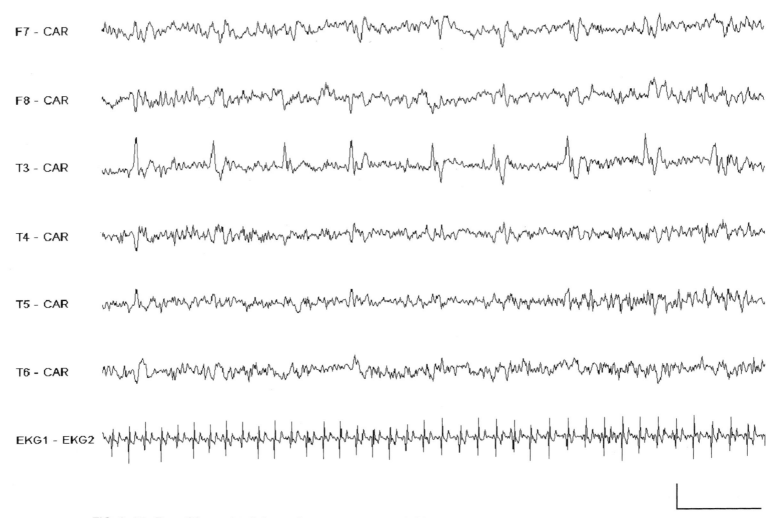

FIG. 9–27. Repetitive potentials at slower sweep speed. Displaying the same epoch at 10 mm/sec better il-lustrates the consistency of the repetitive discharges. Moreover, involvement of other regions, particularly F7, can be more clearly discerned. Calibration signal 3 sec, 50μV.

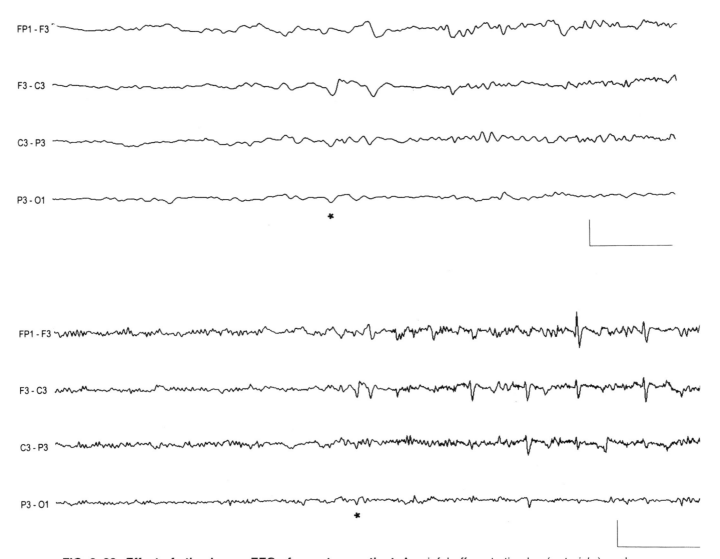

FIG. 9–28. Effect of stimulus on EEG of comatose patient. A painful afferent stimulus (*asterisks*) evokes a distinct electrographic change at slow sweep speed (*lower trace*). This is seen adequately in the upper trace at usual sweep speed but somewhat less distinctly. Calibration signal 1 sec, 100μV (*upper trace*), calibration signal 3 sec, 100μV (*lower trace*).

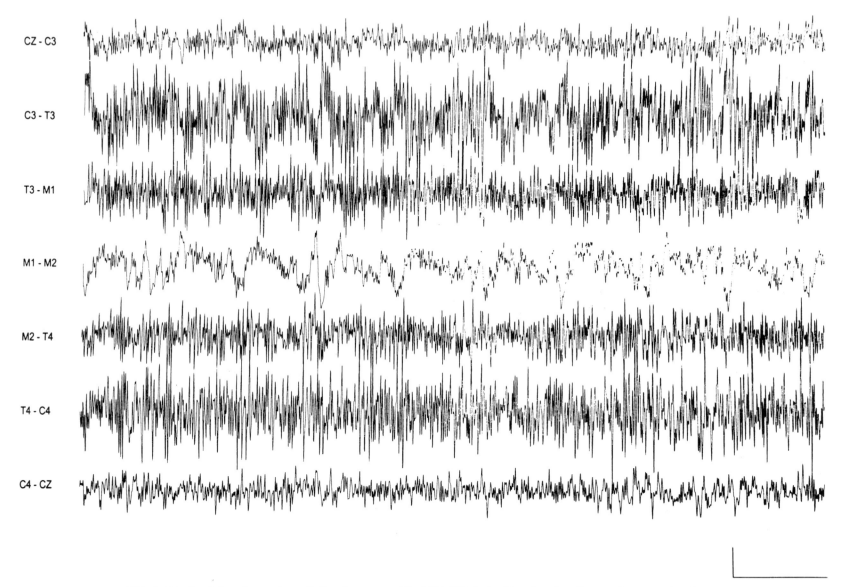

FIG. 9–29. Sustained muscle activity obscures all but M1-M2 derivation, leaving the reader guessing from which side the spikes originate. High linear filter (HLF) 70 Hz. Calibration signal 1 sec, 50μV.

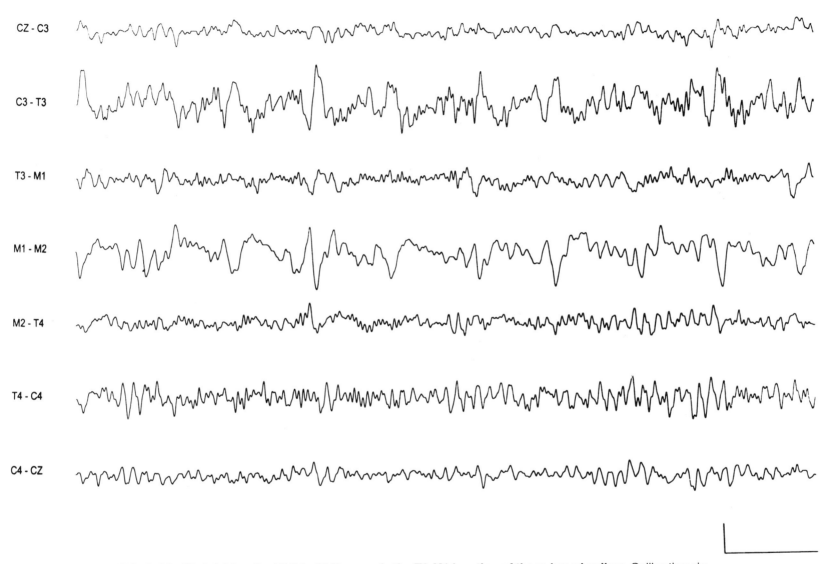

FIG. 9–30. Diminishing the HLF to 15 Hz reveals the T3-M1 location of these broad spikes. Calibration signal 1 sec, 50μV.

References

1. Jasper HH. The ten-twenty electrode system of the International Federation. *Electroencephalogr Clin Neurophysiol* 1958;10:371–373.
2. Sadler RM, Goodwin J. Multiple electrodes for detecting spikes in partial complex seizures. *Can J Neurol Sci* 1989;16:326–329.
3. Brittenham DM. Artifacts. Activities not arising from the brain. In: Daly DD, Pedley TA, eds. *Current practice of clinical electroencephalography.* New York: Raven Press, 1990:85–106.
4. Fisch BJ. *Fisch and Spehlmann's EEG primer. Basic principles of digital and analog EEG,* 3rd edition. Amsterdam: Elsevier Science, 1999.
5. Blume WT, Kaibara M. *Atlas of pediatric electroencephalography,* 2nd edition. Philadelphia: Lippincott-Raven Publishers, 1999.
6. Wolf P, Gooses R. Relation of photosensitivity to epileptic syndromes. *J Neurol Neurosurg Psychiatry* 1986;49:1386–1391.
7. Walter VJ, Walter WG. The central effects of rhythmic sensory stimulation. *Electroencephalogr Clin Neurophysiol* 1949;1:57–86.
8. Epstein CM. Visual evoked potentials. In: Daly DD, Pedley TA, eds. *Current practice of clinical electroencephalography.* New York: Raven Press, 1990:593–624.
9. Perez-Borja C, Chatrian GE, Tyce FA, et al. Electrographic patterns of the occipital lobe in man: A topographic study based on use of implanted electrodes. *Electroencephalogr Clin Neurophysiol* 1962;14:171–182.
10. Reiher J, Lebel M. Wicket spikes: Clinical correlates of a previously undescribed EEG pattern. *Can J Neurol Sci* 1977;4:39–47.
11. Kellaway P, Fox BJ. Electroencephalographic diagnosis of cerebral pathology in infants during sleep. *J Pediatr* 1952;41:262–287.
12. Kellaway P. An orderly approach to visual analysis: Characteristics of the normal EEG of adults and children. In: Daly DD, Pedley TA, eds. *Current practice of clinical electroencephalography* New York: Raven Press, 1990:139–199.
13. Gibbs FA, Gibbs EL. *Atlas of Electroencephalography.* Cambridge, MA: Addison Wesley, 1950.
14. Erwin CW, Summerville ER, Radtke RA. A review of electroencephalographic features of normal sleep. *J Clin Neurophysiol* 1984;1(3)253–274.
15. Sharbrough FW. Nonspecific abnormal EEG patterns. In: Niedermeyer E, Lopes da Silva F, eds. *Electroencephalography: Basic principles, clinical applications, and related fields.* Baltimore: Williams & Wilkins, 1993:197–215.
16. Santamaria J, Chiappa KH. *The EEG of drowsiness.* New York: Demos Publications, 1987.
17. Silverman D. Phantom spike-waves and the fourteen and six per second positive spike pattern: A consideration of their relationship. *Electroencephalogr Clin Neurophysiol* 1967;23:207–213.
18. Ebersole JS, Wade PB. Spike voltage topography identifies two types of frontotemporal epileptic foci. *Neurology* 1991;41:1425–1433.
19. Reiher J, Carmant L. Clinical correlates and electroencephalographic characteristics of two additional patterns related to 14 and 6 per second positive spikes. *Can J Neurol Sci* 1991;18:488–491.
20. Goodin DS, Aminoff MJ, Laxer KD. Detection of epileptiform activity by different non-invasive EEG methods in complex partial epilepsy. *Ann Neurol* 1990;27:330–334.
21. McLachlan RS, Blume WT. Isolated fear in complex partial status epilepticus. *Ann Neurol* 1980;8:640–641.
22. Daly DD. Epilepsy and syncope. In: Daly DD, Pedley TA, eds. *Current practice of clinical electroencephalography.* New York: Raven Press, 1990:269–334.
23. Noriega-Sanchez A, Markand ON. Clinical and electroencephalographic correlation of independent multifocal spike discharges. *Neurology* 1976;26:667–672.
24. Bauer G, Aichner F, Saltuari L. Epilepsies with diffuse slow spikes and waves of late onset. *Eur Neurol* 1983;22:344–350.
25. Weir B. The morphology of the spike-wave complex. *Electroencephalogr Clin Neurophysiol* 1965;19:284–290.
26. Lemieux JF, Blume WT. Topographical evolution of spike-wave complexes. *Brain Res* 1986;373:275–287.
27. Westmoreland BF. Benign EEG variants and patterns of uncertain clinical significance. In: Daly DD, Pedley TA, eds. *Current practice of clinical electroencephalography.* New York: Raven Press, 1990:243–252.

28. Hughes JR. Two forms of the 6/sec spike and wave complex. *Electroencephalogr Clin Neurophysiol* 1980;48:535–550.

29. Niedermeyer E. Sleep and EEG. In: Niedermeyer E, Lopes da Silva F, eds. *Electroencephalography: Basic principles, clinical applications, and related fields.* Baltimore: Williams & Wilkins, 1993:153–166.

30. Gastaut H, Roger J, Soulayrol R, et al. Childhood epileptic encephalopathy with diffuse slow spike-waves (otherwise known as "petit mal variant") or Lennox Syndrome. *Epilepsia* 1966;7:139–179.

31. Brenner RP, Atkinson R. Generalised paroxysmal fast activity: Electroencephalographic and clinical features. *Ann Neurol* 1982;11:386–390.

32. Engel J, Jr. A practical guide for routine EEG studies in epilepsy. *J Clin Neurophysiol* 1984;1(2):109–142.

33. Gastaut H, Broughton R. *Epileptic seizures. Clinical and electrographic features, diagnosis and treatment.* Springfield, IL: Charles C. Thomas; 1972.

34. Klass DW, Fischer-Williams M. Sensory stimulation, sleep and sleep deprivation. In: Remond A, ed. *Handbook of electroencephalography and clinical neurophysiology;* Vol 3D. Amsterdam: Elsevier Science, 1976:5–73.

35. Takahashi T. Activation methods. In: Niedermeyer E, Lopes da Silva F, eds. *Electroencephalography: Basic principles, clinical applications, and related fields.* Baltimore: Williams & Wilkins, 1993:241–262.

36. Harden A, Pampiglione G, Picton-Robinson N. Electroretinogram and visual evoked response in a form of "neuronal lipidosis" with diagnostic EEG features. *J Neurol Neurosurg Psychiatry* 1973;36:61–67.

37. Kaibara M, Blume WT. The postictal electroencephalogram. *Electroencephalogr Clin Neurophysiol* 1988;70:99–104.

38. Blume WT, Borghesi JL, Lemieux JF. Interictal indices of temporal seizure origin. *Ann Neurol* 1993;34:703–709.

39. Blume WT, Young GB, Lemieux JF. EEG morphology of partial epileptic seizures. *Electroencephalogr Clin Neurophysiol* 1984;57:295–302.

40. Blume WT, Kaibara M. The start-stop-start phenomenon of subdurally recorded seizures. *Electroencephalogr Clin Neurophysiol* 1993;86:94–99.

41. Lombroso CT. Neonatal EEG polygraphy in normal and abnormal newborns. In: Niedermeyer E, Lopes da Silva F, eds. *Electroencephalography: basic principles, clinical applications, and related fields.* Baltimore: Williams & Wilkins, 1993:803–875.

42. Rae-Grant AD, Strapple C, Barbour PJ. Episodic low-amplitude events: An under-recognized phenomenon in clinical electroencephalography. *J Clin Neurophysiol* 1991;8(2):203–11.

43. Niedermeyer E. Abnormal EEG patterns: epileptic and paroxysmal. In: Niedermeyer E, Lopes da Silva F, eds. *Electroencephalography: Basic principles, clinical applications, and related fields.* Baltimore: Williams & Wilkins, 1993:217–240.

44. Howell DA. Unusual centrencephalic seizure patterns. *Brain* 1955;78:199–208.

45. Reiher J, Grand'Maison F, Leduc CP. Partial status epilepticus: Short-term prediction of seizure outcome from on-line EEG analysis. *Electroencephalogr Clin Neurophysiol* 1992;82:17–22.

46. de la Paz D, Brenner RP. Bilateral independent periodic lateralized epileptiform discharges. Clinical significance. *Arch Neurol* 1981;38:713–715.

47. Walsh JM, Brenner RP. Periodic lateralized epileptiform discharges—long-term outcome in adults. *Epilepsia* 1987;28:533–536.

48. Zifkin BG, Cracco RQ. An orderly approach to the abnormal EEG. In: Daly DD, Pedley TA, eds. *Current practice of clinical electroencephalography.* New York: Raven Press, 1990:253–267.

49. Schwartz MS, Scott DF. Pathological stimulus-related slow wave arousal responses in the EEG. *Acta Neurol Scand* 1978;57:300–304.

50. Cobb WA, Guiloff RJ, Cast J. Breach rhythm. The EEG related to skull defects. *Electroencephalogr Clin Neurophysiol* 1979;47:251–271.

51. Arenas AM, Brenner RP, Reynolds CF III. Temporal slowing in the elderly revisited. *Am J EEG Technol* 1986;26:105–114.

52. Blume WT, Whiting SE, Girvin JP. Epilepsy surgery in the posterior cortex. *Ann Neurol* 1991;29:638–645.

53. Katz RI, Horowitz GR. Electroencephalogram in the septuagenarian: Studies in a normal geriatric population. *J Am Geriatr Soc* 1982;30:273–275.

54. Burger LJ, Rowan AJ, Goldensohn ES. Creutzfeldt-Jakob disease. An electroencephalographic study. *Arch Neurol* 1972;26:428–433.

55. Markand ON. Organic brain syndromes and dementias. In: Daly DD, Pedley TA, eds. *Current practice of clinical electroencephalography.* New York: Raven Press, 1990:401–423.

56. Dreyfus-Brisac C. The electroencephalogram of the premature infant and full-term newborn: Normal and abnormal development of waking and sleeping patterns. In: Kellaway P, Petersen I, eds. *Neurological and electroencephalographic correlative studies in infancy.* New York: Grune & Stratton, 1964:186–206.

57. Young GB. The EEG in coma. *J Clin Neurophysiol* 2000;17:473–85.

58. Young GB, Kreeft JH, McLachlan RS, et al. EEG and clinical associations with mortality in comatose patients in a general intensive care unit. *J Clin Neurophysiol* 1999;16:354–60.

59. Young GB, McLachlan RS, Kreeft JH, et al. An electroencephalographic classification for coma. *Can J Neurol Sci* 1997;24:320–325.

60. Young GB, Blume WT, Campbell V, et al. Alpha, theta and alpha-theta coma: a clinical outcome study utilizing serial recordings. *Electroencephalogr Clin Neurophysiol* 1994;91:93–99.

61. Young GB, Campbell VC. EEG monitoring in the intensive care unit: pitfalls and caveats. *J Clin Neurophysiol* 1999;16:40–45.

Subject Index

A

Absence status epilepticus, with electrodecremental events, 329
"Activation," of delta, in light sleep, 396
Adjacent artifacts, 9
Alerting, normal drowsiness and, 154
Alpha
  abundant, on referential montage, 51
  and beta, 59
  central, 50
  and common average reference, 55
  left hemisphere, abnormal lower, 360
  low-voltage, 73, 74
  mu rhythm and, with skull defect, on coronal montage, 385
  normal
    and beta activity, 75
    and slow alpha variant, 71
  sharply contoured, from mixture of wave forms, 60
  and theta, 52
Alpha activity
  enhancement by left central-parietal skull defect, 383
  enhancement with posterior skull defect, 388
  eye opening effects on, 63
  normal, 41–48
  in right hemisphere, reduction of, 357, 358
Alpha asymmetry, 57
  with coronal montage, 362
Alpha attenuation
  with eye opening, 61
  transient and incomplete, 62
Alpha field
  asymmetry of, referential recordings depiction of, 361

symmetry of, common average reference depiction of, 356
Alpha symmetry
  normal, 53
  shifting of, 56
  transient, 54
Alpha variant
  fast, 67
    on eye closure, 68
  slow, 69, 70
    normal alpha and, 71
    on referential montage, 72
Alpha-theta coma, 485
Alphoid rhythm
  left temporal polyspikes and, 188
  temporal, 190
    apiculate, 189
Amorphous, then normal EEG, 66
Amorphous drowsy pattern, 114
Ampiculate waves, polyspikes among, 254
Amplitude asymmetry, spurious, from interchange of electrode positions, 14
Amplitude reduction, left temporal excessive theta and, 442
Anterior coronal bipolar, 506
Anterior coronal montage, frontal polar spikes on, 225
Anterior head, periodic complexes in, 493
Anterior-posterior bipolar, 502
Anterior-posterior bipolar montage
  and coronal montage
    left temporal polyspikes on, 186
    of temporal spikes, 174
  light sleep potentials on, 131

small sharp spikes on, 167
V-waves and spindles in light non-REM sleep on, 145, 146
Arousal
  abnormal, 162, 163
    right hemisphere attenuation and, 379
  from drowsiness
    brief arousal, 155
    instantaneous arousal, 157
  focal abnormality revealed on, 402
  from light sleep, 159
    on referential montage, 158
  from moderate sleep, 160
  spindle asymmetry and, on ear reference montage, 377
  V-waves in, 153
  wave forms during, 156
Arrhythmic delta, low-voltage, 477
Artifact(s), 7–40
  adjacent, 9
  delta activity from multiple high-impedance electrodes, 11
  ECG
    and bipolar montage, 34
    V-waves, spindles and, 139
  electrode, 8
  eye movement, right temporal delta and theta and, 394
  from faulty ground electrode, 16
  glossokinetic, 27, 28
    lateral, on coronal montage, 29
    on referential montage, 30
  head movement, during hyperventilation, 10

Artifact(s) (*contd.*)
  instrumental, 17
  "jiggle," 499
  metals, 37
  muscle, 25
    beta activity and, 81
    bitemporal, left temporal delta and theta with, 401
    focal delta activity within eye blink and, 428
    left temporal delta activity within, 398
    periocular, 26
    right temporal delta and theta and, 394
  pulse
    and delta activity, 397
    PLEDS-like, 36
    smooth type, 35
  on referential recordings, 12
  rhythmic, of physiotherapy, 498
  right temporal spikes, delta and, as part of larger
      field, 207
Asymmetry
  alpha, 57
    with coronal montage, 362
  spindle, and arousal, on ear reference montage, 377
Attenuation
  with afferent stimuli, 467
  alpha
    with eye opening, 61
    transient and incomplete, 62
  of background rhythms, left central-parietal-temporal
      delta and, 417, 418
  on coronal montage, 370
  left hemisphere, 367
    and delta, 373
    in sleep, 376
  posterior, 380
  on referential montage, 371
  regional, from subgaleal edema, 40
  right hemisphere
    and abnormal arousal, 379
    IRDA, 382

from subgaleal fluid, 38
subtle onset of temporal lobe seizure as, 296–297
unilateral
  and delta, 374
  and diffuse abnormalities, 368
  effect of hyperventilation on, 369
Average reference, 6, 510

B

Background potentials, asymmetry of
  abnormal, 353–354
  in Jakob-Creutzfeldt disease, 465
Background rhythms
  attenuation of, left central-parietal-temporal delta
      and, 417, 418
  minimal disruption of, left central-parietal-temporal
      delta with, 419
  slow, 452
Benzodiazepine(s), overdose of, and skull defect, 476
Beta
  and alpha, 59
  beating of, 80
  bursting, drowsiness and, 122
  central, 76
  drowsiness with, 124
  left temporal delta activity within, 398
  and muscle artifact, 81
  normal alpha and, 75
  normal bursts of, 79
  and V-waves, 129, 130
  spindles and, 138
Beta asymmetry, 366
  increasing sensitivity and, 359
Bifrontal polar electropositive spikes, 217
Bifrontal spikes, maximum right, with triphasic
    morphology, 221
Bilateral delta, normal, 458, 459
Bilaterally synchronous periodic spikes, 492
Bioccipital delta, 406

Bioccipital spikes, in wakefulness, 268
BIPLEDs, 351
Bipolar anterior-posterior montage, PLEDs on, 346
Bipolar montage
  anterior-posterior
    and coronal montage
      left temporal polyspikes on, 186
      of temporal spikes, 174
    light sleep potentials on, 131
    small sharp spikes on, 167
    V-waves and spindles in light non-REM sleep on,
        145, 146
  bisynchronous spikes and polyspikes on, 262
  classical spike-wave on, 239
  coronal, with sagittal leads, 503, 504
  ECG artifact and, 34
  lateral eye movements on, 21
  POSTS on, 100
  3-Hz spike-waves on, 238
Bisynchronous spikes
  low flash rates and, 278
  posterior, 513
    with common average reference, 514
    on coronal montage, 515
    on ear reference montage, 516, 517
Bitemporal muscle artifact, left temporal delta and theta
    with, 401
Bitemporal persistent delta, and IRDA, 433
Blunt V-waves, on referential montage, 136
Breach rhythm
  and delta activity, 386
  focal delta, and spikes, 390
Burst(s)
  delta, in drowsiness, of adults over 60 years, 135
  nonspecific
    and spike-waves, 235
    spike-waves heralded by, 241
Burst-suppression
  with epileptiform discharges, 487–489
  without epileptiform discharges, 486

C

Central alpha, 50
Central beta, 76
Central sagittal reference, 511
    longitudinal temporal bipolar and, 512
Central-parietal delta, right, 414, 447
    and theta, 446
Central-parietal-temporal delta, left
    and attenuation of background rhythms, 417, 418
    with minimal disruption of background, 419
Coma
    alpha-theta, 485
    theta pattern, 484
Comatose patients
    effect of stimulus on EEG of, 529
    subtle regional seizures in, 322–325
Common average reference
    abnormal mu rhythm and, 365
    alpha and, 55
    bisynchronous posterior spikes with, 514
    and delta activity, 413
    frontal spikes with, 214
    multifocal spikes on, 521
    posterior delta activity and, 409
    right anterior temporal spikes on, 175
    right frontal temporal delta and right hemisphere
        abnormalities on, 423
    right parietal-central-temporal delta and, 415
    small sharp spikes and, 168, 185
    wicket spikes and temporal theta on, 108
Coronal montage
    abnormal mu rhythm on, 364
    alpha asymmetry with, 362
    anterior, frontal polar spikes on, 225
    and anterior-posterior bipolar montage
        left temporal polyspikes on, 186
        of temporal spikes, 174
    attenuation on, 370
    bipolar
        anterior, 6

    with sagittal leads, 5, 503, 504
    without sagittal leads, 5
    focal delta activity on, 405
    focal theta activity on, 449
    lateral glossokinetic artifact on, 29
    left anterior temporal spikes on, 182
    left frontal-central-temporal delta on, 427
    left temporal spikes on, 181
    mu rhythm and alpha with skull defect on, 385
    periodic complexes in herpes simplex encephalitis on,
        350
    posterior, occipital spikes with, 202
    posterior bisynchronous spikes on, 515
    right hemisphere spikes on, 210
    right temporal spikes on, 195
    6-Hz spike and wave complexes on, 250
    slow lateral eye movements on, 23
    small sharp spikes on, 165
        and interhemispheric derivations, 166
    spindle asymmetry on, 378
    subgaleal fluid and, 39
    V-waves on, 125
    wicket spikes on, 107
Coronal-bitemporal bipolar, 6, 505

D

Delta, 375
    "activation" of, in light sleep, 396
    arrhythmic, low-voltage, 477
    bilateral, normal, 458, 459
    bioccipital, 406
    bitemporal persistent, and IRDA, 433
    diffuse, 410, 456
        with dementia, 468
        periodic spikes and, 463
        triphasic waves and, 460
    focal, 410
        breach rhythm, and spikes, 390
        IRDA and, 432, 438

    focal persistent, and IRDA, 435
    frontal-central-temporal, left, on coronal montage,
        427
    generalized, high-voltage, persistent, 475
    lateralized, burst of, small sharp spikes while awake
        with, 180
    left central-parietal-temporal
        and attenuation of background rhythms,
            417, 418
        with minimal disruption of background, 419
    left frontal, with eye opening, 421
    left frontal-central theta and, 426
    left hemisphere, and eye movements, 425
    left hemisphere attenuation and, 373
    left temporal
        accentuation of, with hyperventilation, 399
        with bitemporal muscle artifact, 401
        state-dependent, 404
    in left temporal region, 383
    persistent, right frontal IRDA and, 439
    prominent right frontal spikes and, 212
    right central parietal, 208, 414
    right central-parietal theta and, 447
    right frontal temporal, and right hemisphere
        abnormalities, on common average reference,
        423
    right frontal theta and, 448
    right hemisphere
        principally right frontal, 422
        right frontal spikes and, 220
    right hemisphere electronegative and electropositive,
        209
    right parietal-central-temporal, and common average
        reference, 415
    right parietal-occipital, background activity disrupted
        by, 407
    right temporal
        and artifact, as part of larger field, 207
        and theta, and muscle and eye movement artifact,
        394

Delta (*contd.*)
  transient left anterior-midtemporal, 392
  triphasic waves and, on ear reference montage, 523
  unilateral attenuation and, 374
Delta activity
  breach rhythm and, 386
  common average reference and, 413
  diffuse, 457
    right frontal polyspikes and, 230
  diffuse periodic spike-waves and, 466
  focal
    on coronal montage, 405
    within eye blink, and muscle artifact, 428
  intermittent rhythmic. *See* Intermittent rhythmic delta
      activity (IRDA)
  left frontal, 420
    on ear reference montage, 424
  left hemisphere, 420
    then IRDA, 437
  left temporal, 403
    after eye closure, 434
    within muscle artifact, beta, and eye movements,
      398
  low-frequency filters effect on, 429, 430
  posterior, and common average reference, 409
  pulse artifact and, 397
  regional, rhythmic, 411
  rhythmic, on ear reference montage, 412
  right parietal-occipital, eye opening effects on, 408
  right temporal, 391
  temporal, intermittent, 400
Delta bursts, in drowsiness, of adults over 60 years, 135
Dementia
  dialysis, subtle spike waves mimicking triphasic
      waves in, 481
  diffuse delta with, 468
Dialysis dementia, subtle spike waves mimicking
    triphasic waves in, 481
Dialytic encephalopathy, subtle spike waves mimicking
    triphasic waves in, 481

Diffuse delta, 410, 456
  with dementia, 468
  periodic spikes and, 463
  triphasic waves and, 460
Diffuse delta activity, 457
Diffuse delta with herpes simplex encephalitis, periodic
      left temporal sharp waves and, 348
Diffuse discharges
  Jakob-Creutzfeldt disease with, 462
  Jakob-Creutzfeldt disease without, 461
Diffuse periodic spike-waves, and delta activity, 466
Diffuse theta, 444
  excess, 450, 471
Digital EEG, 501–531
Drowsiness, 123
  amorphous patterns with, 114
  arousal from
    brief, 155
    instantaneous, 157
  with beta, 124
  with blunt V-waves, 132, 133
  and bursting beta, 122
  delta bursts in, of adults over 60 years, 135
  and ear reference montage, 121
  with moderately bursting theta, 119
  normal, and alerting, 154
  with theta, 115, 117, 124
    symmetrical and asymmetrical, 120
    in temporal montage, 118
  V-waves in, 129, 153
Drowsiness-arousal, rhythmic waves in, in adult, 161

E

Ear reference montage, 6, 121
  bisynchronous posterior spikes on, 516, 517
  bisynchronous spikes and polyspikes on, 262
  14-Hz and 6-Hz positive spikes on, 170
  left frontal delta activity on, 424
  polyspikes on, 263

rhythmic delta activity on, 412
right frontal polar spikes on, 227
6-Hz spike-waves revealed by, 525
spike-waves on, 263
  3-Hz, 238
spindle asymmetry and arousal on, 377
triphasic waves and delta on, 523
Ear reference recording
  right hemisphere spikes on, 215
  spindles and V-waves, 137
ECG. *See* Electrocardiogram (ECG)
Edema, subgaleal, regional attenuation from, 40
EEG. *See* Electroencephalography (EEG)
Elderly, blunt V-waves of, 134
Electrocardiogram (ECG), and referential montage, 33
Electrocardiogram (ECG) artifact
  and bipolar montage, 34
  V-waves, spindles and, 139
Electrode(s)
  ground, faulty, artifacts from, 16
  high-impedance, artifactual delta activity from, 11
  interchange of
    effect on background activity, 13
    effect on frontal activity, 15
  international 10–20 placement system for, 1
  mandibular notch, right anterior temporal spikes and,
      193
  position of, interchange of, spurious amplitude
      asymmetry from, 14
Electrode artifacts, 8
Electroencephalography (EEG)
  amorphous and, 66
  amorphous normal, 82
  digital, 501–531
  in ICU, 469–499
Encephalitis, herpes simplex
  on coronal montage, periodic complexes in, 350
  diffuse delta with, periodic left temporal sharp waves
      and, 348
  repetitive temporal complexes in, 349

Encephalopathy
  with abnormal reactivity, 474
  dialytic, subtle spike waves mimicking triphasic
    waves in, 481
  epileptiform activity and, 494
  metabolic, triphasic waves in, 480
Epileptiform abnormalities, 283–351. *See also*
    Seizure(s)
Epileptiform activity, and encephalopathic features, 494
Epileptiform discharges
  burst-suppression with, 487–489
  burst-suppression without, 486
Epileptogenesis, left temporal, interictal recording of,
    289
Excess diffuse theta, 450, 471
  mild, 451
Eye blink, focal delta activity within, and muscle
    artifact, 428
Eye blinks, 20
Eye closure
  fast alpha variant on, 68
  left temporal delta activity after, 434
  photoparoxysmal response with, 272
  polyspikes on, 274
    minimal expression of, 275
  polyspikes with, 265
  spikes elicited by, 276
Eye flutter, with photic stimulation, 19
Eye movement(s)
  generalized suppression and, 490
  lateral
    on bipolar montage, 21
    rapid, 22
    slow
      on common average reference montage, 24
      on coronal montage, 23
  left hemisphere delta and, 425
  left temporal delta activity within, 398
  and muscle artifact, right temporal delta and theta
    and, 394

and periocular muscle potentials, 222
  right temporal theta and, 443
  vertical, and infraorbital leads, 18
Eye opening
  alpha activity abolished by, 63
  alpha attenuation with, 61
  effects on right parietal-occipital delta activity, 408
  left frontal delta with, 421
  mu revealed by, 64, 65

F
Filter(s), low-frequency, effect on delta activity, 429,
    430
Fluid, subgaleal
  attenuation from, 38
  and coronal montage, 39
Focal abnormalities, 473
Focal delta, 410
  breach rhythm, and spikes, 390
  IRDA and, 432, 438
Focal delta activity
  on coronal montage, 405
  within eye blink, and muscle artifact, 428
Focal left temporal theta activity, 441
Focal parietal-central theta, 445
Focal persistent delta, and IRDA, 435
Focal seizures, 290–293, 495–496
Focal theta, 444
  on coronal montage, 449
14-Hz positive spikes, 169
  on ear reference montage, 170
Frontal delta activity, left, on ear reference montage,
    424
Frontal IRDA, 472
Frontal seizures, right, partially obscured by spindles,
    326–327
Frontal spikes. *See* Spike(s), frontal
Frontal temporal delta, right, and right hemisphere
    abnormalities, on common average reference,
    423

Frontal theta, right, and delta, 448
Frontal-central seizures, left, gradual onset of, 315–321
Frontal-central-temporal delta, left, on coronal montage,
    427

G
Generalized, high-voltage, persistent delta, 475
Generalized abnormalities, 473
Generalized seizures
  as polyspikes, 333
  with possible regional onset, 338–339
Generalized status epilepticus, 337
Generalized suppression, 491
  and eye movements, 490
Generalized tonic-clonic seizure, with diffuse
    polyspikes, 340
Glossokinetic artifact, 27, 28
  lateral, on coronal montage, 29
  on referential montage, 30

H
Head
  anterior, periodic complexes in, 493
  posterior, suppression in, 478, 479
Head movement artifacts, during hyperventilation, 10
Herpes simplex encephalitis
  on coronal montage, periodic complexes in, 350
  diffuse delta with, periodic left temporal sharp waves
    and, 348
  repetitive temporal complexes in, 349
Hyperventilation
  before, 85
  accentuation of left temporal delta with, 399
  early, 85
  effect on unilateral attenuation, 369
  head movement artifacts during, 10
  late, 85
  light sleep after, 87

Hyperventilation response
    early, 83
    normal sharply contoured, 86

I

ICU. *See* Intensive care unit (ICU)
Infraorbital leads, vertical eye movements and, 18
Infraorbital region, sequential right frontal spikes
        extending to, 228
Instrumental artifact, 17
Intensive care unit (ICU), EEG in, 469–499
Intermittent rhythmic delta activity (IRDA), 431
    bitemporal persistent delta and, 433
    and focal delta, 432, 438
    focal persistent delta and, 435
    frontal, 472
    left hemisphere delta activity and, 437
    right frontal, and more persistent delta, 439
    in temporal regions, 436
International 10–20 electrode placement system for, 1
Ipsilateral skull defect, left central-parietal theta and,
        387
IRDA. *See* Intermittent rhythmic delta activity (IRDA)

J

Jakob-Creutzfeldt disease, 463, 466, 467
    asymmetry of background potentials in, 465
    with diffuse discharges, 462
    periodic spikes in, 464
    without diffuse discharges, 461
"Jiggle" artifact, 499

L

Lambda waves, 88
    continuous, 89
    normal, 90
    photic driving response, 94
    photic following response, 92

photic response in elderly, 93, 98
    prominent photic responses at low flash rates, 91
Left anterior-midtemporal delta, transient, 392
Left central-parietal skull defect, alpha activity
        enhancement by, 383
Left central-parietal theta, and ipsilateral skull defect,
        387
Left central-parietal-temporal delta
    and attenuation of background rhythms, 417, 418
    with minimal disruption of background, 419
Left frontal delta, with eye opening, 421
Left frontal delta activity, 420
    on ear reference montage, 424
Left frontal-central theta, and delta, 426
Left frontal-central-temporal delta, on coronal montage,
        427
Left hemisphere attenuation, 367
    and delta, 373
    in sleep, 376
Left hemisphere delta, and eye movements, 425
Left hemisphere delta activity, 420
    then IRDA, 437
Left mandibular notch reference, 509
Left temporal delta
    accentuation of, with hyperventilation, 399
    state-dependent, 404
    and theta, with bitemporal muscle artifact, 401
Left temporal delta activity, 403
    after eye closure, 434
    within muscle artifact, beta, and eye movements, 398
Left temporal epileptogenesis, interictal recording of,
        289
Left temporal excess theta, and amplitude reduction,
        442
Left temporal region, theta and delta in, 383
Left temporal seizure
    continuation of, 286
    onset of, 285
    postictal phase of, 288

Left temporal theta, 395, 440
    and delta, with bitemporal muscle artifact, 401
Left temporal theta activity, focal, 441
Longitudinal bipolar and posterior coronal montage,
        posterior synchronous discharges with, 518
Longitudinal bipolar montage, triphasic waves on, 522
Longitudinal temporal bipolar, and central sagittal
        reference, 512
Low-frequency filters, effect on delta activity, 429, 430
Low-voltage alpha, 73, 74
Low-voltage arrhythmic delta, 477

M

Mandibular notch electrode, right anterior temporal
        spikes and, 193
Mandibular notch reference, 507
    left, 509
    right, 508
Medication effect, 453, 454
    change in appearance of, with sensitivity reduction,
        455
Metabolic encephalopathy, triphasic waves in, 480
Metals artifact, 37
Mild excess theta diffusely, 451
Mild focal abnormality, 372
Mitten pattern, 140
    and spindles, of deep non-REM sleep, 143
Montage
    advantages and disadvantages of, 5–6
    bipolar
        anterior-posterior
            and coronal montage
                left temporal polyspikes on, 186
                of temporal spikes, 174
            light sleep potentials on, 131
            PLEDs on, 346
            small sharp spikes on, 167
            V-waves and spindles in light non-REM sleep
                on, 145, 146
        bisynchronous spikes and polyspikes on, 262

classical spike-wave on, 239
coronal, with sagittal leads, 503, 504
ECG artifact and, 34
lateral eye movements on, 21
longitudinal, triphasic waves on, 522
POSTS on, 100
3-Hz spike-waves on, 238
common average reference, right anterior temporal
    spikes on, 175
coronal
    abnormal mu rhythm on, 364
    alpha asymmetry with, 362
    anterior, frontal polar spikes on, 225
    and anterior-posterior bipolar montage
        left temporal polyspikes on, 186
        of temporal spikes, 174
    attenuation on, 370
    focal delta activity on, 405
    focal theta activity on, 449
    lateral glossokinetic artifact on, 29
    left anterior temporal spikes on, 182
    left frontal-central-temporal delta on, 427
    left temporal spikes on, 181
    mu rhythm and alpha with skull defect on, 385
    periodic complexes in herpes simplex encephalitis
        on, 350
    posterior, occipital spikes with, 202
    posterior bisynchronous spikes on, 515
    right hemisphere spikes on, 210
    right temporal spikes on, 195
    6-Hz spike and wave complexes on, 250
    slow lateral eye movements on, 23
    small sharp spikes on, 165
        and interhemispheric derivations, 166
    spindle asymmetry on, 378
    subgaleal fluid and, 39
    "V-waves" on, 125
    wicket spikes on, 107
ear reference, 121
    bisynchronous posterior spikes on, 516, 517
    bisynchronous spikes and polyspikes on, 262

14-Hz and 6-Hz positive spikes on, 170
polyspikes on, 263
rhythmic delta activity on, 412
right frontal polar spikes on, 227
6-Hz spike-waves revealed by, 525
spike-waves on, 263
    3-Hz, 238
triphasic waves and delta on, 523
reference
    ear, spindle asymmetry and arousal on, 377
    slow lateral eye movements on, 24
referential
    abundant alpha on, 51
    activity revealed by, 381
    arousal from light sleep on, 158
    attenuation on, 371
    ECG and, 33
    glossokinetic artifact on, 30
    occipital spikes with, 202
    PLEDs on, 343
    right occipital spikes on, 204
    6-Hz spike and wave on, 249
    slow alpha variant on, 72
    temporal, drowsiness with theta in, 118
Mu, eye opening and, 64, 65
Mu rhythm
    abnormal
        and common average reference, 365
        on coronal montage, 364
    and alpha, with skull defect, on coronal montage, 385
    asymmetrical, 363
    prominent, with skull defect, 384
Multifocal spikes
    on common average reference, 521
    display with montage and time constant
        modifications, 519
    with shorter time constant, 520
Muscle and eye movement artifact, right temporal delta
    and theta and, 394
Muscle artifact, 25
    beta activity and, 81

bitemporal, left temporal delta and theta with, 401
focal delta activity within eye blink and, 428
left temporal delta activity within, 398
periocular, 26
Myoclonus, palatal, 32

N
Nonepileptiform abnormalities, 353–468
Non-REM sleep
    deep, Mitten pattern and spindles of, 143
    frontal polar spikes in, 218
    light
        spindles and V-waves in, on anterior-posterior
            bipolar montage, 145, 146
        V-waves and spindles in, 141, 142
Normal bilateral delta, 458, 459

O
Occipital polyspikes
    and occipital spikes, in sleep, 205
    right parietal, 206
Occipital spikes, 200
    and polyspikes, in sleep, 205
    with posterior coronal and referential montages, 202
    right, 198, 201, 203
        on referential montage, 204
        and right hemisphere spindle reduction, 199

P
Palatal myoclonus, 32
Parietal-central theta, focal, 445
Parietal-central-temporal delta, right, and common
    average reference, 415
"Paroxysmal fast activity," symmetrical, and
    asymmetrical tonic seizures, 330–332
Periocular muscle artifact, 26

Periocular muscle potentials, eye movements and, 222
Periodic complexes
  in anterior head, 493
  in herpes simplex encephalitis on coronal montage, 350
Periodic lateralized epileptiform discharges (PLEDs)
  on bipolar anterior-posterior montage, 346
  evolving into seizure, 497
  left hemisphere, 342
  on referential montage, 343
  right parietal, 344
  right temporal, 345
Periodic lateralized epileptiform discharges (PLEDs) plus, 347
Periodic left temporal sharp waves, and diffuse delta with herpes simplex encephalitis, 348
"Periodic" potentials, repetitive, 527
Periodic spikes
  bilaterally synchronous, 492
  and diffuse delta, 463
  in Jakob-Creutzfeldt disease, 464
Periodic spike-waves, diffuse, and delta activity, 466
Photic response
  driving, 94, 95
  in elderly, 98
  at higher flash rates, 99
  preservation of, 416
  widespread field of, 96, 97
Photic stimulation
  eye flutter with, 19
  with eyes closed, 276
Photomyoclonic response, to low-frequency flash with eyes closed, 279
Photomyogenic response, 271, 280
Photoparoxysmal response, 269, 270, 271
  with eye closure, 272
  prominence of, variations in, with frequency, 277
  subtle, 273

Physiotherapy, rhythmic artifact of, 498
PLEDs. *See* Periodic lateralized epileptiform discharges (PLEDs)
PLEDs-like pulse artifact, 36
Polyspike(s)
  among apiculate waves, 254
  bisynchronous, on bipolar and ear reference montages, 262
  burst of, in wakefulness, 264
  diffuse, 255
    bursts of, 266
  on ear reference montage, 263
  on eye closure, 274
    minimal expression of, 275
  with eye closure, 265
  frontal, right, and diffuse delta activity, 230
  generalized, and asymmetrical background, 259
  generalized seizures as, 333
  generalized tonic-clonic seizure with, 340
  minimal expression of, 260
  occipital
    and occipital spikes, in sleep, 205
    right parietal, 206
  regionally accentuated, 229
  runs of, 253
    in wakefulness, 256
  temporal, left, 187
    and alphoid rhythm, 188
    on combined coronal and anterior-posterior bipolar montage, 186
  tonic seizure with, 336
Polyspike-waves
  in apiculate background, 257
  unilateral, 267
Positive occipital sharp transients of sleep (POSTS)
  on bipolar montage, 100
  high-frequency, 102
  prominent, 101
Posterior attenuation, 380

Posterior bisynchronous spikes, on coronal montage, 515
Posterior coronal and longitudinal bipolar montage, posterior synchronous discharges with, 518
Posterior coronal montage, occipital spikes with, 202
Posterior delta activity, and common average reference, 409
Posterior head, suppression in, 478, 479
Posterior skull defect, alpha activity enhancement with, 388
Posterior slow waves of youth, 58
Posterior spikes, bisynchronous, on ear reference montage, 516, 517
Posterior synchronous discharges, with posterior coronal and longitudinal bipolar montage, 518
POSTS. *See* Positive occipital sharp transients of sleep (POSTS)
Potential(s), repetitive, 527, 528
Psychomotor variant, 109
  rhythmic, 110
  vs. wicket spikes, 111
Pulse artifact
  and delta activity, 397
  PLEDS-like, 36
  smooth type, 35

R

Rapid eye movement (REM) sleep, 151, 152
Reference montage
  abundant alpha on, 51
  activity revealed by, 381
  arousal from light sleep on, 158
  attenuation on, 371
  blunt V-waves on, 136
  ear, spindle asymmetry and arousal on, 377
  ECG and, 33
  glossokinetic artifact on, 30
  occipital spikes with, 202
  PLEDs on, 343

right occipital spikes on, 204
6-Hz spike and wave on, 249
slow alpha variant on, 72
slow lateral eye movements on, 24
Regional delta activity, rhythmic, 411
REM sleep. *See* Rapid eye movement (REM) sleep
Repetitive, "periodic" potentials, 527
Repetitive potentials, 528
Rhythmic artifact of physiotherapy (RAP), 498
Rhythmic delta activity, on ear reference montage, 412
Rhythmic regional delta activity, 411
Rhythmic waves
  fast, minimal expression of, 260
  temporal, right, and intermingled spikes, 196
Right central-parietal delta, 414
Right central-parietal theta, 446
  and delta, 447
Right frontal IRDA, and more persistent delta, 439
Right frontal temporal delta, and right hemisphere
    abnormalities, on common average reference,
    423
Right frontal theta, and delta, 448
Right hemisphere, abnormalities of, right frontal
    temporal delta and, on common average
    reference, 423
Right hemisphere attenuation
  and abnormal arousal, 379
  IRDA, 382
Right hemisphere delta, principally right frontal, 422
Right hemisphere spindle reduction, right occipital
    spikes and, 199
Right mandibular notch reference, 507
Right parietal-central-temporal delta, and common
    average reference, 415
Right parietal-occipital delta, background activity
    disrupted by, 407
Right parietal-occipital delta activity, eye opening
    effects on, 408
Right temporal delta, and theta, and muscle and eye
    movement artifact, 394

Right temporal delta activity, 391
Right temporal theta
  and delta, and muscle and eye movement artifact, 394
  and eye movements, 443

S
Secondary bilateral synchrony, 245
  on compressed display, 246
Seizure(s), 283–351
  focal, 290–293, 495–496
  generalized
    as polyspikes, 333
    with possible regional onset, 338–339
    secondarily, 312–314
  as generalized paroxysmal fast activity, and theta,
    334–335
  gradual onset of, 306–309
  left frontal-central, gradual onset of, 315–321
  left hemisphere, of multiple morphologies, 341
  left occipital, 312–314
  left temporal
    continuation of, 286
    onset of, 285
    postictal phase of, 288
  partial, gradual onset of, 300–303
  PLEDs evolving into, 497
  right frontal, partially obscured by spindles, 326–327
  subtle onset of, 306–309
  subtle regional, in comatose patient, 322–325
  termination of, 287, 295, 298–299, 304–305
  tonic
    asymmetrical, symmetrical "paroxysmal fast
     activity" and, 330–332
    with generalized spike-waves and polyspikes, 336
  tonic-clonic, generalized, with diffuse polyspikes,
    340
Sensitivity reduction, change in appearance of
    medication effect with, 455
Sequential vertex waves ("V-waves"), on coronal
    montage, 125

7-Hz rhythmic waves, sequential spikes with burst of,
    258
Sharp waves, 219
Sine waves, superimposed, morphologies of, 4
6-Hz positive spikes, 169, 171
  on ear reference montage, 170
6-Hz spike and wave, 171
  on referential montage, 249
6-Hz spike and wave complexes, on coronal montage,
    250
6-Hz spike-wave/positive spikes, incomplete expression
    of, 172
6-Hz spike-waves, 248
  by ear reference montage, 525
  with enhanced sensitivity and faster sweep speed, 526
6-Hz theta, burst of, with questionable intermingled
    spikes, 524
Skull defect
  benzodiazepine overdose and, 476
  bursts of spike-like waves with, 389
  ipsilateral, left central-parietal theta and, 387
  left central-parietal, alpha activity enhancement by,
    383
  mu rhythm and alpha, on coronal montage, 385
  posterior, alpha activity enhancement with, 388
  prominent mu rhythm with, 384
  theta with, left temporal spikes and, 179
Sleep
  asynchronous normal, spindles of, 147
  deep stage 3, 148, 149
  left hemisphere attenuation in, 376
  light
    "activation" of delta in, 396
    after hyperventilation, 87
    arousal from, 159
    on referential montage, 158
  moderate, arousal from, 160
  non-REM
    deep, Mitten pattern and spindles of, 143

Sleep (*contd.*)
    frontal polar spikes in, 218
    light
        spindles and V-waves in, on anterior-posterior
            bipolar montage, 145, 146
        V-waves and spindles in, 141, 142
    occipital spikes and polyspikes in, 205
    phenomena of, multiple, 150
    REM, 151, 152
Sleep potentials, light, on anterior-posterior bipolar
    montage, 131
Slow background rhythm, 452
Small sharp spikes (SSSs), 164, 185
    on anterior-posterior bipolar montage, 167
    and common average reference, 168, 185
    on coronal montage, 165
        and interhemispheric derivations, 166
    of unusual morphology, 184
    while awake, with burst of lateralized delta, 180
Spike(s)
    bifrontal, maximum right, with triphasic morphology,
        221
    bifrontal polar electropositive, 217
    bisynchronous, 251
        on bipolar and ear reference montages, 262
        low flash rates and, 278
        posterior, on coronal montage, 515
    bisynchronous posterior, 513
        with common average reference, 514
    breach rhythm, and focal delta, 390
    electropositive right central parietal, in wakefulness,
        211
    foci of, multiple independent, 231
    14-Hz and 6-Hz positive, 169
        on ear reference montage, 170
    frontal
        with common average reference, 214
        right, 213
            prominent, and delta, 212

and right hemisphere delta, 220
    sequential, 216
        extending to infraorbital region, 228
    right frontal polar-inferior, 226
frontal polar, in non-REM sleep, 218
    on anterior coronal montage, 225
    right, 224
        on ear reference montage, 227
        low-voltage, 223
intermingled, burst of 6-Hz theta with, 524
intermingled with right temporal rhythmic waves,
    196
lack of, 78, 243
    sharply contoured waves and, 261
multifocal
    on common average reference, 521
    display with montage and time constant
        modifications, 519
    with shorter time constant, 520
occipital, 200
    and occipital polyspikes, in sleep, 205
    with posterior coronal and referential montages,
        202
    right, 198, 201, 203
        on referential montage, 204
        and right hemisphere spindle reduction, 199
periodic
    bilaterally synchronous, 492
    and diffuse delta, 463
    in Jakob-Creutzfeldt disease, 464
posterior, bisynchronous, on ear reference montage,
    516, 517
right hemisphere
    on coronal montage, 210
    on ear reference recording, 215
right hemisphere electronegative and electropositive,
    209
sequential, within burst of 7-Hz rhythmic waves, 258

sequential right frontal broad, 219
6-Hz positive, 169, 171
    on ear reference montage, 170
6-Hz spike-wave positive, incomplete expression of,
    172
small sharp. *See* Small sharp spikes (SSSs)
temporal
    with abnormal background, 177
    coronal and anterior-posterior bipolar montage of,
        174
    delta, and artifact, as part of larger field, 207
    left, 178
        on coronal montage, 181
        and theta with skull defect, 179
    left anterior, on coronal montage, 182
    right
        on coronal montage, 195
        frequent, with stereotyped field and morphology,
            104
        and sharply contoured temporal theta, 197
    right anterior
        on common average reference montage, 175
        and mandibular notch electrode, 193
    sequential left, 176
wicket, 103–105. *See* Wicket spikes
    on coronal montage, 107
    temporal, left, 191
    and temporal theta, on common average reference,
        108
    and theta, 106
    vs. psychomotor variant, 111
Spike-like waves, bursts of, with skull defect, 389
Spike-waves
    bisynchronous, posterior, 252
    classical, on bipolar montage, 239
    on ear reference montage, 263
    generalized
        distorted, 244
        tonic seizure with, 336

"generalized," prolonged burst of, 328
left hemispheric and bilaterally synchronous, 242
lingering, 237
nonspecific burst and, 235
nonspecific bursts heralding, 241
6-Hz, 248
    by ear reference montage, 249, 525
    with enhanced sensitivity and faster sweep speed,
        526
slow
    on bipolar and ear reference montages, 238
    right hemisphere, 247
subtle, mimicking triphasic waves, in dialytic
        encephalopathy, 481
3-Hz, 234, 240
    and slow spike-waves, on bipolar and ear reference
        montages, 238
varying field of, 236
Spindle(s)
asynchronous normal sleep, 147
of deep non-REM sleep, 143
and V-waves
    abundant, 144
    ear reference recording, 137
    in light non-REM sleep, on anterior-posterior
        bipolar montage, 145, 146
V-waves
    and beta activity, 138
    in light non-REM sleep, 141, 142
Spindle asymmetry
    and arousal, on ear reference montage, 377
    on coronal montage, 378
"Spindle coma pattern," 482
"Spindle-like bursts," 483
SREDA. See Subclinical rhythmic EEG discharge of
        adults (SREDA)
"Start-stop-start" phenomenon, 326–327
State-dependent left temporal delta, 404

Status epilepticus
    absence, with electrodecremental events, 329
    generalized, 337
Subclinical attack at delta focus, 310–311
Subclinical rhythmic EEG discharge of adults
        (SREDA), 112
    at slow sweep speed, 113
Subgaleal edema, regional attenuation from, 40
Subgaleal fluid
    attenuation from, 38
    and coronal montage, 39
Subtle regional seizures, in comatose patients, 322–325
Suppression
    generalized, 491
        and eye movements, 490
    in posterior head, 478, 479
Symmetrical "paroxysmal fast activity," and
        asymmetrical tonic seizures, 330–332

T

Temporal activity, normal, for age, 49
Temporal alphoid rhythm, 190
    apiculate, 189
Temporal delta activity, intermittent, 400
Temporal lobe seizure, subtle onset of, as attenuation,
        296
Temporal montage, drowsiness with theta in, 118
Temporal polyspikes, left, 187
    and alphoid rhythm, 188
    on combined coronal and anterior-posterior bipolar
        montage, 186
Temporal regions, IRDA in, 436
Temporal rhythmic waves, right, and intermingled
        spikes, 196
Temporal spikes
    with abnormal background, 177
    coronal and anterior-posterior bipolar montage of,
        174

left, 178
    on coronal montage, 181
    and theta with skull defect, 179
left anterior, on coronal montage, 182
right
    on coronal montage, 195
    delta, and artifact, as part of larger field, 207
    frequent, with stereotyped field and morphology,
        194
    and sharply contoured temporal theta, 197
right anterior
    on common average reference montage, 175
    and mandibular notch electrode, 193
sequential left, 176
Temporal theta
    right, and eye movements, 443
    wicket spikes and, on common average reference,
        108
Temporal wicket spikes, left, 191
Theta
    and alpha, 52
    diffuse, 444
        excessive, 471
    drowsiness with, 115, 117, 124
        in temporal montage, 118
    excess diffuse, 450
        mild, 451
    focal, 444
        on coronal montage, 449
    focal parietal-central, 445
    left central-parietal, and ipsilateral skull defect, 387
    left frontal-central, and delta, 426
    left temporal, 395, 440
        with bitemporal muscle artifact, 401
    left temporal excess, and amplitude reduction, 442
    in left temporal region, 383
    minimal evidence of, 116
    moderately bursting, drowsiness with, 119
    right central-parietal, 208, 446
        and delta, 447

Theta (*contd.*)
  right frontal, and delta, 448
  right temporal
    and delta, and muscle and eye movement artifact, 394
    and eye movements, 443
  seizures as generalized paroxysmal fast activity, 334–335
  6 Hz, burst of, with questionable intermingled spikes, 524
  with skull defect, left temporal spikes and, 179
  symmetrical and asymmetrical, in drowsiness, 120
  temporal
    sharply contoured, and right temporal spikes, 197
    wicket spikes and, on common average reference, 108
  wicket spikes and, 106
Theta activity, focal left temporal, 441
Theta pattern coma, 484
3-Hz spike-waves, 234, 240
  and slow spike-waves on bipolar and ear reference montages, 238
Tonic seizures
  asymmetrical, symmetrical "paroxysmal fast activity" and, 330–332
  with generalized spike-waves and polyspikes, 336
Tonic-clonic seizures, generalized, with diffuse polyspikes, 340
Toranomaki, 281
Transient left anterior-midtemporal delta, 392
Tremor(s), 31

Triphasic waves
  and delta, on ear reference montage, 523
  and diffuse delta, 460
  on longitudinal bipolar montage, 522
  in metabolic encephalopathy, 480
  subtle spike waves mimicking, in dialytic encephalopathy, 481

U
Unilateral attenuation
  and delta, 374
  and diffuse abnormalities, 368
  effect of hyperventilation on, 369

V
Variant(s), psychomotor, 109
  rhythmic, 110
  vs. wicket spikes, 111
V-waves
  in arousal and drowsiness, 153
  and beta, 129, 130
  blunt
    drowsiness with, 132, 133
    of elderly, 134
    on referential montage, 136
  on coronal montage, 125
  drowsiness and, 129
  sequential, in youth, 126

spindles and
  abundant, 144
  and beta activity, 138
  ear reference recording, 137
  and ECG artifact, 139
  in light non-REM sleep, 141, 142
  on anterior-posterior bipolar montage, 145, 146
varieties of, 127

W
Wakefulness
  bioccipital spikes in, 268
  electropositive right central parietal spikes in, 211
  polyspike bursts in, 264
  polyspikes in, 256
Wave(s)
  sharp, 219
  sharply contoured, without spikes, 261
Wave forms
  "classical" appearance of, 2–3
  mixture of, sharply contoured alpha from, 60
  normal sharply contoured, 77
Wicket spikes, 103–105
  abrupt, 192
  on coronal montage, 107
  temporal, left, 191
  and temporal theta, on common average reference, 108
  and theta, 106
  vs. psychomotor variant, 111